Heinerman's Encyclopedia of

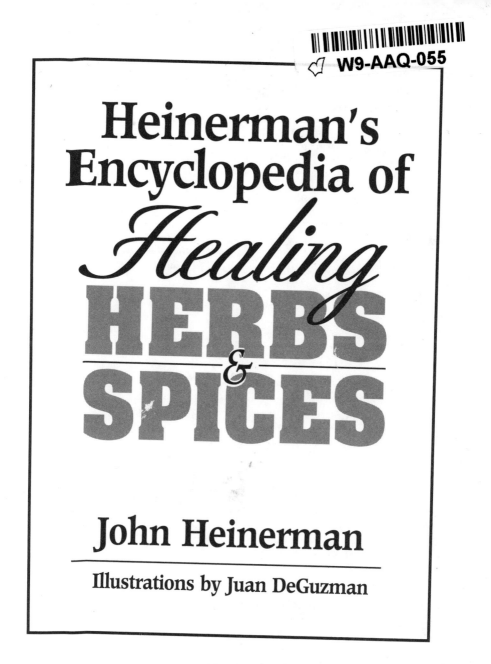

Healing

HERBS

&

SPICES

John Heinerman

Illustrations by Juan DeGuzman

PRENTICE HALL
Englewood Cliffs, New Jersey 07632

Library of Congress Cataloging-in-Publication Data

Heinerman, John.
    [Encyclopedia of healing herbs and spices]
    Heinerman's Encyclopodia of healing herbs and spices / by John Heinerman.
        p. cm.
    Includes bibliographical references and index.
    ISBN 0-13-310202-5—ISBN 0-13-310210-6 (pbk.)
        1. Herbs—Therapeutic use—Encyclopedias. I. Title.
    RM666.H33h4415   1995
    615′.321′03—dc20

                                                        95-34371
                                                        CIP

Printed in the United States of America

10 9 8 7 6

ISBN 0-13-310202-5   ISBN 0-13-310210-6(PBK)

ATTENTION: CORPORATIONS AND SCHOOLS

Parker Publishing Company books are available at quantity discounts with bulk
purchase for educational, business, or sales promotional use. For information, please
write to: Prentice Hall Career & Personal Development Special Sales, 113 Sylvan Avenue,
Englewood Cliffs, NJ 07632. Please supply: title of book, ISBN number, quantity, how
the book will be used, date needed.

PARKER PUBLISHING COMPANY
West Nyack, NY 10994

A Simon & Schuster Company

On the World Wide Web at http://www.phdirect.com

Prentice-Hall International (UK) Limited, *London*
Prentice-Hall of Australia Pty. Limited, *Sydney*
Prentice-Hall Canada Inc., *Toronto*
Prentice-Hall Hispanoamericana, S.A., *Mexico*
Prentice-Hall of India Private Limited, *New Delhi*
Prentice-Hall of Japan, Inc., *Tokyo*
Simon & Schuster Asia Pte. Ltd., *Singapore*
Editora Prentice-Hall do Brasil, Ltda., *Rio de Janeiro*

To Heber C. Kimball,
a devoted friend to the Mormon prophet Joseph Smith, a stalwart counselor to Brigham Young, and an energetic champion of truth and liberty!

OTHER BOOKS BY THE SAME AUTHOR

DOUBLE THE POWER OF YOUR IMMUNE SYSTEM

HEINERMAN'S NEW ENCYCLOPEDIA OF FRUITS AND VEGETABLES

HEINERMAN'S ENCYCLOPEDIA OF HEALING JUICES

HEINERMAN'S ENCYCLOPEDIA OF NUTS, BERRIES AND SEEDS

INTRODUCTION
THE TEN CARDINAL RULES OF HERB USAGE

Rule I. Never take herbs in *any* form at the same time you take prescription or over-the-counter medications. The two will always be *incompatible* with each other. Keep them separate and take apart from each other by at least 4-5 hours.

Rule II. If any herb is causing an unpleasant side effect of extreme proportions, *discontinue immediately* until the problem can be explained or rectified somehow. Remember that what may pass for a so-called "healing" or "cleansing crisis" could, in fact, be life threatening. "When in doubt, *do without.*"

Rule III. Learn to educate yourself on herbs before using them. A medical doctor isn't always the best person to consult for information about herbs, nor is a pharmacist. Neither of them has had any specific training in that area. You need to consult with a professional herbalist, homeopathic or naturopathic doctor, folk healer, or any similar person skilled in the *medicinal* application of herbs. Or refer to books on medicinal plants that are reliable and trustworthy. Besides this book, I would also recommend the following titles:

> *The Way of Herbs* by Michael Tierra, N.D. (Santa Cruz, CA: Unity Press, 1980).
>
> *Medicinal Plants of the Mountain West* (1979) and *Medicinal Plants of the Desert and Canyon West* (1989), both by Michael Moore (Santa Fe, NM: University of New Mexico Press).
>
> *A Modern Herbal* (2 volumes) by Maude Grieve (New York: Dover Publications, 1971).
>
> *Herbs That Heal* by Michael A. Weiner, Ph.D. and Janet A. Weiner (Mill Valley, CA: Quantum Books, 1994).
>
> *Lehrbuch der Phytotherapie* (6th Edition) by Rudolf Fritz Weiss, M.D. (Stuttgart, Germany: Hippokrates Verlag GmbH, 1985). For those who can read and understand German, I highly recommend it.
>
> *Herbes Medicinales* by Hans Fluck, Ph.D. (2nd French edition) (Neuchatel, Switzerland: Delachaux & Niestle S.A., 1973). Very good reference for those who can read and translate it.

Rule IV. When attempting self-treatment for any *serious* health problem, several very important determinations must be made by the individual.

(A) Is the problem treatable using alternative medicines instead of conventional therapies? In some cases they are, but in others they aren't. Arthritis and fever certainly can be treated with herbs alone. But a third-degree burn or lacerated artery requires emergency medical attention *immediately!* Still other problems fall somewhere in between either of these extremes. Cancer is one of these. Some types (leukemia or colorectal tumors) may be successfully treated using *only* natural remedies, provided they are detected *early enough.* However, other kinds of malignant growths (brain or bone marrow cancers) do not easily respond to herbs alone, and usually require some elective surgery, cobalt radiation or chemotherapy to bring under control.

(B) Do you thoroughly understand the nature of the problem at hand? Don't leave anything to guesswork as to the type of problem you have or the extent of its seriousness. *Get four separate opinions.* The first diagnosis should always be from a competent medical doctor; the second evaluation needs to come from a doctor of homeopathy, naturopathy, osteopathy, or chiropractic. All of these specialists have received extensive training in human anatomy with some dissection work on cadavers; therefore, their understanding of the body and its many biological functions is more complete and thorough than it will be for other professions listed hereafter. The third opinion *must* come from someone steeped in traditional folk medicine; this can be an herbalist, a Native American shaman or medicine man, an Oriental practitioner or acupuncturist, a foot reflexologist, a massage therapist, an iridologist, or an unlicensed nutritionist. And since a definite connection has already been established between the mind and body in causes of illness, it is imperative that someone like a priest, rabbi, minister, psychologist, psychiatrist, social worker, or metaphysical counselor be consulted. Such indivduals can more easily discern the mental, emotional or spiritual frustrations that are greatly aggravating the biological problems.

(C) For how long should treatment with herbs continue? This is a determination that can only be made between yourself and your several therapists. Some conditions (cancer) may require that an herb (red clover or chaparral) be used all the time; but other problems (headache, fever) may only need certain herbs (wood betony, catnip) for a short duration.

(D) If confusion and uncertainty still exist, even after following these few simple guidelines, then get more information through yet another opinion or by reading an herb book. But above all, do not neglect prayer. Imploring the Creator, who made us and plants, for further inspired guidance isn't a shameful thing at all, but rather is the mark of a true believer in Divine Providence!

Rule V. Generally speaking, herbal medicines are just that, *medicine!* As such, most herbs should only be used when body health is placed in some kind of jeopardy. Otherwise, most *medicinal herbs* should be left alone. There are, however, some very qualified exceptions to this fundamental rule.

EXCEPTION ONE: Plants of definite nutritive value may be used on a fairly consistent basis, because their rich blend of vitamins, minerals, trace elements, amino acids, enzymes, and hormones afford the body *solid* protection against potential illnesses. Such herbs might include: alfalfa, beet root, chamomile, dandelion, evening primrose, flaxseed, ginger, hops, kelp, marshmallow, nettle, onion, parsley, radish, stinging nettle, turmeric, watercress and yarrow.

EXCEPTION TWO: A lingering or lifetime illness that demands the constant use of certain herbs. Goldenseal for diabetes and garlic for yeast infection are two that come to mind. Sometimes a chronic condition that could merit consistent use of a particular plant may also, in fact, necessitate short periods of discontinuation because the herb is liable to do some potential harm to the body. The prolonged consumption of juniper berry, for example, for congestive heart failure or elevated serum cholesterol will irritate the kidneys.

Rule VI. Some herbs are easily contraindicated in particular health situations, making them quite undesirable. Cayenne pepper, garlic, goldenseal, onion and pau d'arco are *strongly* hypoglycemic and should *never* be taken *individually* by those suffering from low blood sugar or hypoglycemia; otherwise they may well have unexplained fatigue and mood swings. (An exception to this would be taking Kyolic aged garlic extract made by Wakunauga of America. Due to the lengthy aging process involved, the specific elements responsible for these unpleasant reactions are removed; so people with hypoglycemia can safely take Kyolic garlic without worrying.) Juniper berry provokes uterine contractions, and in women who are pregnant this could cause an early abortion of the developing fetus. Therefore, a certain amount of caution needs to be exercised with regard to a small group of herbs for a *few* health problems.

Rule VII. Know *when* and *how much* to take of individual herbs or herbal formulas. Because this is such a highly technical area involving a large number of qualifying factors, I've decided to simplify everything into an abbreviated version that I feel will nicely summarize all of the important points, omitting many things that are less significant. In order to do so, I chose to create *four* distinct *categories* into which *all* herbs and herbal formulations could somewhere be placed. And based on a quarter-century of personal experience with these natural medicines, I've given an *average* recommended amount for each category. Dosages for children (ages 4-12) are usually *one-half* the amounts suggested for adults.

1. *Energy/Stamina:* Single herbs and herbal formulas especially designed for this category are best taken on an empty stomach or in between meals, usually in the morning or early afternoon. Dosages: 2-4 capsules/tablets; 10-18 drops fluid extract/ tincture beneath the tongue; or 1 cup *warm* tea.

2. *Vitality/Nutrition:* Single herbs and herbal formulas intended main-ly for nutritional support are best taken with meals any time of the day or night. Dosages: 4-6 capsules/ tablets; 10-15 drops fluid extract/tincture beneath the tongue or in a glass of water, three times daily; or 2 cups warm or cool tea.

3. *Weight Loss/Cleansing:* Single herbs and herbal formulas intended to shed unwanted pounds and detoxify the system of impurities are best taken in between meals or on an empty stomach, usually in the early morning or late afternoon. Dosages: 3-5 capsules/tablets; 12 drops fluid extract/ tincture three times daily in a glass of water; or 1 cup *lukewarm* tea morning, noon and night. CAUTION: Whenever taking any herbs for such weight loss/ cleansing purposes, always be sure to take an adequate vitamin-mineral supplement of some kind (up to 4 tablets daily) to insure replacement of nutrients lost.

4. *Relief:* Single herbs and herbal formulas designed to relieve pain are best taken in between meals, and *periodically* throughout the day (say every 4-6 hours or on an "as need" basis). Dosages: 2 capsules/tablets every 4 hours; 15 drops fluid extract/ tincture beneath the tongue or in a glass of water, every 4 hours; or 1 cup warm or cool tea (depending on the situation) every 4 hours.

Rule VIII. The effectiveness of an herb depends upon a wide variety of factors, some of which are human-related and others environmentally based. Two lists of them appear in the following table. Several of each from either group may account for why a specific plant isn't working as well for you as the way it is supposed to.

Human Factors	*Environmental Factors*
Sex (M/F)	Soil
Age	Climate
Ethnicity	Altitude
Genetics	Geography (Place of Growth)
Rate of Metabolism	Time of Harvest
Diet	Drying
Social Habits (i.e., drinking or smoking)	Milling
	Storage
State of Health	
Manufactured Products Used (i.e., capsule/tablet, tincture, tea, oil or poultice)	
Adulteration (substituting a cheaper and inferior herb for an expensive and superior one, or including non-botanical fillers)	

Rule IX. When purchasing herbs, always keep in mind that the best values are often to be found in an herb shop, health food store, or, nutrition center. There is no inflationary markup in costs as there *always* is in direct marketing companies, which have legions of sponsored distributors who must be paid monthly bonuses on what they sell. Eliminate such middlemen and your herbs immediately become more affordable!

Rule X. Fresh herbs and dried herbs have near equal advantages. The former contain essential oils which are lost in the drying process (melaleuca is a good example of this). On the other hand, were it not for the drying process, some herbs would still retain volatile components that can evoke drastic side effects. (For instance, *fresh* cascara sagrada bark produces a violent purgative or vomiting effect; whereas, when the same bark is slowly *dried* over a period of several months, it is transformed into a gentle laxative.) The nutritional content of herbs in both states varies considerably and , again, has mixed blessings. Vitamin C is really heat-sensitive, so obviously *fresh* rosehips will contain a whopping amount of this important nutrient, whereas *dried* rosehips will lose a great deal of their vitamin C content. However, mineral and trace element contents of many *dried* herbs seem to dramatically increase when they're left in the sun for a while after harvesting. The amount of calcium, magnesium, potassium and iron, for example, isalways higher in *dried* parsley and yellow dock than it is in the fresh plants. The potency of herbs can either decrease or increase in the dried state. Witness what happens when *fresh* garlic is brought into close contact with the eyes—tears immediately form; but the same effect is pretty much lost when *dried* garlic *powder* is held close to the eyes instead. By the same token, though, *fresh* peppermint leaves will never produce the same *strong* minty sensation that the *dried* leaves will, especially after they've been carefully stored in a wide-mouth gallon glass jar for *seven years*! Finally, *fresh* herbs grow moldy fast once they're picked, but *dried* herbs will keep for several years with proper storage.

> God made the herbs and plants that be
> For the likes of you and me;
> And endowed them with life therein,
> To keep us well men and women.

> May you the reader, find my book
> Worth the having and the look,
> That with this information wealth
> You'll live long and enjoy good health!

—John Heinerman
July 12, 1995
Salt Lake City, UT

SYMPTOMS CONTENTS

ABDOMINAL CRAMPS & INFLAMMATIONS (see also CRAMPS): apple bark 22, ginger 251, lilac 308, prickly ash 378, rhubarb 397, sweet cicely 440.

ABORTION (INDUCE): cotton 190.

ABORTION (PREVENT): black haw 73.

ABRASIONS (see also BRUISES): adder's tongue 3, cattail 124, shepherd's purse 425, witch hazel 475.

ABSCESSES: Chinese cucumber 152, mullein 341, peony 369.

ABSENTMINDEDNESS: (see MEMORY LOSS)

ACHES (see also PAIN): lemongrass 305, thyme 445.

ACID INDIGESTION: belladonna 58, bitters 68, caraway 116, chicory 150, cinnamon 160, lilac 308, sweet cicely 440.

ACNE: amaranth 13, asparagus 36, birch 63, burdock 103, celandine 134, pine 370, poplar 377, rhubarb 397, roses 400, thyme 445, turmeric 450, walnut 462, wheat grass 466.

ADDICTIONS: (see DRUG ADDICTIONS)

AGING (see also OLD AGE SPOTS and WRINKLES): chaparral 140, ho-shou-wu 283.

AGITATION: ashwagandha 35.

AIDS (see also CANCER): anemone 15, astragalus 38, chamomile 138, Chinese cucumber 152, echinacea 211.

AIR-SWALLOWING: tarragon 441.

ALCOHOLISM: ashwagandha 35, cloves 168.

ALLERGIC RHINITIS (see ALLERGIES)

ALLERGIES: agrimony 5, Brigham tea 93, chamomile 138, eyebright 229, osha 362, thyme 445, uva ursi 454, wood betony 475.

ALZHEIMER'S DISEASE (see also MEMORY LOSS): ginkgo 255.

AMEBIASIS: Brigham tea 93.

ANEMIA: angelica 17, prickly ash 378, suma 438.

ANGINA (see also CARDIAC DISORDERS): aconite 1, arnica 23, chrysanthemum 155, mullein 341.

ANOREXIA NERVOSA: chives 154.

ANXIETY NEUROSIS: ashwagandha 35, Japanese honeysuckle 288, kava kava 296, lavender 299, lily 309, spruce 432, tarragon 441.

APPETITE (POOR): asafoetida 30, bouquet garni 90, cinchona 158, fennel seed 230, fungus 241, ginger 251, licorice root 307, sweet cicely 440, tarragon 441, thyme 445, wild black cherry 470.

ARTERIOSCLEROSIS (see also CARDIAC DISORDERS and CHOLESTEROL, ELEVATED): arnica 23, skullcap 427.

ARTHRITIS: angelica 17, ash 34, ashwagandha 35, bay 50, bean 52, belladonna 58, cayenne pepper 127, feverfew 234, pine 370, prickly ash 378, rhubarb 397, sassafras 424, skullcap 427, turmeric 450, wormwood 477, yarrow 480, yucca 485.

ASTHMA: aconite 1, adder's tongue 3, agrimony 5, black haw 73, camphor 114, chamomile 138, Chinese cucumber 152, coffee 178, coltsfoot 181, elderberry 213, elecampane 218, eucalyptus 222, frankincense 240, ginger 251, ginkgo 255, juniper berry 291, lobelia 313, mountain mahogany 339, mullein 341, onion 357, osha 362, peony 369, thyme 445, yellow dock 482.

ATHEROSCLEROSIS (see also ARTERIOSCLEROSIS): alfalfa 7, digitalis 203, ginkgo 255, tea 443.

ATHLETE'S FOOT (see also FUNGAL INFECTIONS): calendula 111, chaparral 140, cinnamon 160, thyme 445.

ATTENTION DEFICIT DISORDER: ashwagandha 35, blue vervain 86.

BACKACHE: bay 50, bupleurum 102, camphor 114, ginger 251, lemongrass 305, mustard 344, prickly ash 378.

BAD BREATH: alfalfa 7, blackberry 70, chrysanthemum 155, cinnamon 160, coriander 184, dill 204, fennel seed 230, myrrh 346, parsley 363, rosemary 403, thyme 445, watercress 464.

BALDNESS: magnolia 318, stinging nettle 434.

BED SORES: aloe 11, anemone 17, arnica 23, arum 29, bearded darnel 53, malaleuca 328, witch hazel 475.

BED WETTING: cornsilk 186.

BIRTH CONTROL (MALE): chicory 150, cotton 190.

BIRTH CONTROL (FEMALE): juniper berry 291, kola nut 297.

BITTER TASTE: chrysanthemum 155.

BLACK EYE: bluebottle 81.

BLACKHEADS: asparagus 36, roses 400.

BLADDER PROBLEMS: buchu 100, cornsilk 186, eucalyptus 222, ginger 251, tarragon 441, wood betony 476.

BLEEDING: amaranth 13, aster 37, atractylis 40, bayberry 51, birthwort 66, bugleweed 101, cayenne pepper 127, cotton 190, horsetail 281, juniper berry 291, moss 337, plantain 373, shepherd's purse 425, smartweed 430, stinging nettle 435, turmeric 450, white oak 468.

BLISTERS: celandine 134.

BLOOD CIRCULATION (POOR): basil 49, flaxseed 237, ginkgo 255, thyme 445.

BLOOD CLOTS: cayenne pepper 127, ginger 251, goldenseal 261, motherwort 339, pine 370, red clover 390, sage 407.

BLOOD COAGULATION (ENCOURAGE): juniper berry 291.

BLOOD IMPURITIES: blackberry 70, burdock 103, chickweed 147, dandelion 200, sagebrush 416, sassafras 424, yellow dock 482.

BLOOD PRESSURE (see HYPERTENSION and LOW BLOOD PRESSURE)

BLOOD VESSEL PROBLEMS: calendula 111.

BLOODY STOOL/URINE: aster 37, bayberry 51, bugleweed 101, oak 356, shepherd's purse 426, white oak 468.

BLOTCHES (SKIN): horseradish 278.

ola 259, rhubarb 397, sagebrush 416, walnut 462, white oak 468, willow 473.

DIGESTION, POOR (see INDIGESTION)

DIGESTIVE DISORDERS (see INDIGESTION)

DIPHTHERIA: lobelia 313.

DISLOCATED JOINTS: daffodil 198, wormwood 477.

DISTENDED BOWELS: prickly ash 378.

DIZZINESS: bearded darnel 53, catnip 122, chrysanthemum 155, mistletoe 333.

DROPSY (see EDEMA)

DRUG ADDICTION (WITHDRAWAL): camphor 114, catnip 122, goldenseal 261, kola nut 297, lily 309, nutmeg 350, nux vomica 353, passion flower 366.

DRUG OVERDOSE: nux vomica 353.

DRY MOUTH: chrysanthemum 155.

DRY SCALP (see SCALP PROBLEMS)

DRY SKIN: flaxseed 37.

DUODENAL ULCER (see ULCERS)

DYSENTERY: agave 4, apple bark 22, butternut 107, gladiola 259, hops 275, lobelia 313, sassafras 424.

DYSMENORRHEA (see FEMALE COMPLAINTS)

EAR ACHE: melaleuca 328, mullein 341, turmeric 450.

ECZEMA: amaranth 13, ash 34, birch 63, burdock 103, club moss 169, evening primrose 225, poplar 377, rhubarb 397, sage 410, sagebrush 416, St. Johnswort 421, sassafras 424, slippery elm 428, turmeric 450, walnut 462, watercress 464, witch hazel 475.

EDEMA: aloe 11, asparagus 36, broom 97, citrin 163, cornsilk 186, digitalis 203, horsetail 281, parsley 363, turmeric 450, uva ursi 454, wood betony 476, yarrow 480.

EMOTIONAL TRAUMA: agrimony 5, licorice root 307, lily 309.

EMPHYSEMA: frankincense 240, juniper berry 291, mountain mahogany 339, pine 370, yellow dock 482.

ENERGY IMBALANCE: astragalus 38, atractylis 40, mistletoe 333.

EPIDEMICS: camphor 114, garlic 244, goldenseal 261, onion 357, thyme 445.

EPILEPTIC SEIZURES: cleavers 167, elephant grass 220, marjoram 324, safflower 407.

ERYSIPELAS: arrowroot 25, belladonna 58, club moss 169, elephant grass 220, lobelia 313.

EYE PROBLEMS: agrimony 5, basil 49, brooklime 96, burdock 103, catnip 122, chervil 145, chrysanthemum 155, eyebright 229, fennel seed 230, flaxseed 237, goldenseal 261, morning glory 335, mountain mahogany 339, roses 400, sagebrush 416, snapdragon 431, squawvine 433, thyme 445, turmeric 450.

FATIGUE: astragalus 38, barley grass 47, cattail 124, cayenne pepper 127, club moss 169, evening primrose 225, fungus 241, gentian 251, ginseng 257, guarana 267, kava kava 296, kola nut 297, mahuang 319, maple 320, pine 370, prickly ash 378, spruce 432, suma 438, thyme 445.

FEAR: lily 309.

GOITER: bladderwrack 76, kelp 297.

GONORRHEA (see also SEXUALLY TRANSMITTED DISEASES): blazing star 77, Brigham tea 93, garlic 244, sarsaparilla 423, squawvine 433.

GOUT: ash 34, asparagus 36, bean 52, buchu 100, lilac 308, peony 369, pine 370, rosemary 403, sassafras 424, tarragon 441, watercress 464, wood betony 476, yarrow 480.

GRANULOMA INGUINALE: Brigham tea 93.

GUM DISEASE & PROBLEMS: catnip 122, cinquefoil 162, eucalyptus 222, myrrh 346, thyme 445, watercress 464, willow 473.

GYNECOLOGICAL PROBLEMS (see also FEMALE COMPLAINTS): doong quai 208, motherwort 339.

HAIR LOSS (see BALDNESS)

HAIR PROBLEMS (see SCALP PROBLEMS)

HALITOSIS (see BAD BREATH)

HALLUCINATION: ashwagandha 35.

HANGOVER (see also ALCOHOLISM): barberry 46, nux vomica 353.

HAYFEVER: catnip 122, chamomile 138, coltsfoot 181, eyebright 229, fenugreek 232.

HEAD COLD (see CONGESTION)

HEAD INJURIES: ginkgo 255.

HEADACHE (see also MIGRAINES): asafoetida 30, basil 49, brooklime 96, bupleu- rum 102, cayenne pepper 127, chamomile 138, chrysanthemum 155, cinchona 158, coca 174, ginger 251, lavender 299, mint 331, mistletoe 333, morning glory 335, sagebrush 416, spruce 432, thyme 445, watercress 464, wintergreen 474, wood betony 476.

HEARING LOSS: bergamot 59, ginkgo 25.

HEART ARRHYTHMIA: belladonna 58, ginkgo 25.

HEART ATTACK: cayenne pepper 127, garlic 244, ginkgo 255, mistletoe 333.

HEART MUSCLE TWITCHING: kava kava 296.

HEART PROBLEMS (see CARDIAC DISORDERS)

HEARTBURN (see also INTESTINAL GAS): anise 18, annatto 20, belladonna 58, bitters 68, bouquet garni 90, caraway 116, cinnamon 160, sweet cicely 440, turmeric 450, willow 473.

HEMORRHAGING (see BLEEDING)

HEMORRHOIDS: brooklime 96, bugleweed 101, mountain mahogany 339, mullein 341, oak 356, uva ursi 454, white oak 468.

HEPATITIS (see also INFECTIONS and LIVER PROBLEMS): barberry 46, Brigham tea 93, calendula 111, chamomile 138, dandelion 200, milk thistle 330, rhubarb 397, wormwood 477.

HERNIA: comfrey 182, fenugreek 232, marshmallow 326.

HERPES: aloe 11, arnica 23, arum 29, astragalus 38, bearded darnel 53, birch 63, burdock 103, cascara sagrada 119, chickweed 147, cotton 190, garlic 244, henna 273, melaleuca 328, mint 331, morning glory 335, rhubarb 397, sassafras 424, slippery elm 428, turmeric 450, wild Oregon grape 472.

HIGH BLOOD PRESSURE (see HYPERTENSION)

INSECT (REPELLANT): eucalyptus 222, lemongrass 305, mountain mahogany 339, neem 349, pyrethrum 383, wormwood 477.

INSOMNIA: bearded darnel 53, belladonna 58, catnip 122, chrysanthemum 155, dill 204, fungus 241, hops 275, lavender 299, lily 309, passion flower 366, squawvine 433, tarragon 441.

INSULIN SHOCK: aconite 1.

INTESTINAL GAS (see also HEARTBURN): agave 4, annatto 20, bitters 68, bouquet garni 90, lemongrass 305, nutmeg 350, sweet cicely 440, tarragon 441, willow 473.

INTESTINAL INFLAMMATION: mullein 341, tea 442.

INTESTINAL PARASITES: ash 34, Brigham tea 93, bayberry 51, citrin 163, garlic 244, pumpkin 381, wood betony 476, wormwood 477.

INTOLERANCE: beech 55.

IRREGULAR HEART BEAT: bitters 68, mullein 341.

IRRITABLE BOWEL SYNDROME: marshmallow 326, psyllium 380, slippery elm 428.

IRRITABILTY: mistletoe 333.

ITCHING: bird-of-paradise 65, chickweed 147, sage 410, yellow dock 482.

ITCHY SCALP (see SCALP PROBLEMS)

JAUNDICE: agave 4, chicory 150, dandelion 200, rhubarb 397, wormwood 477.

JOINT PAIN & STIFFNESS: flaxseed 237, ginger 251, mustard 344, prickly ash 378.

KIDNEY PROBLEMS: agave 4, cornsilk 186, digitalis 203, mustard 344, nutmeg 350, parsley 363, rhododendron 396, tarragon 441, uva ursi 454, wood betony 476.

KIDNEY STONES: apple bark 22, buchu 100, burdock 103, cornsilk 186, ginger 251, parsley 363, rhododendron 396, rosemary 403, sorrel 432, uva ursi 454.

LABOR, DELAYED (see DELAYED LABOR)

LACTATION (IMPROVE): anise 18, caraway 116, dill 204, parsley 363.

LACTATION (ENDING): sage 410, sassafras 424.

LARYNGITIS: aconite 1, arnica 23, Chinese cucumber 152, clary sage 165, eucalyptus 222, hyssop 284, sage 410.

LEG CRAMPS: eucalyptus 222, melaleuca 328, peppermint 331.

LEG ULCER: alfalfa 7, aloe 11, arnica 23, brooklime 96, morning glory 335.

LEPROSY: anemone 17, castor bean 120, elephant grass 220, hops 275, turmeric 450.

LEUKEMIA (see also CANCER): parsley 363, pine 370, red clover 390, wheat grass 466.

LICE (see also SCALP PROBLEMS): azalea 42, chaparral 140.

LIGAMENTS, TORN (see TORN LIGAMENTS)

LIP SORES (see COLD SORES)

LIVER PROBLEMS: apple bark 22, artichoke 27, bitters 68, blackberry 70, blessed thistle 77, chamomile 138, chicory 150, cumin 194, dandelion 200, eucalyptus 222, milk thistle 330, roses 400, tea 443, turmeric 450, wormwood 477, zedoary 487.

MOTION SICKNESS: ginger 251, pine 370.

MOUTH DISORDERS (see ORAL PROBLEMS)

MOUTH SORES (see COLD SORES)

MUCUS ACCUMULATION: arnica 23, black alder 70, black haw 73, elderberry 213, eucalyptus 222, nasturtium 348, rhododendron 396, watercress 464.

MUMPS: Chinese cucumber 152, dandelion 200, lilac 308, marjoram 324, mullein 341, pennyroyal 368, pine 370, turmeric 450.

MUSCLE PROBLEMS: calendula 111, camphor 114, daffodil 198, ginger 251, licorice root 307, marijuana 321, marshmallow 326, prickly ash 378, roses 400, rosemary 403, thyme 445.

MUSCLE SPASMS: agave 4, lobelia 313, marijuana 321, mints 331, skullcap 427.

MUSCULAR STIFFNESS (see also CRAMPS, ARTHRITIS, LUMBAGO, RHEUMA-TISM, TENDONITIS, PULLED LIGAMENTS): chamomile 138, ginger 251, horse-radish 278, roses 400, wormwood 477.

MYOCARDIAL INFARCTION: cayenne pepper 127, ginger 251, sage 410.

NAIL PROBLEMS: horsetail 281.

NAUSEA (see also VOMITING): apple bark 22, bergamot 59, catnip 122, ginger 251, nutmeg 350.

NAVEL INJURY: turmeric 450.

NERVOUS TRAUMA (see SHOCK, HYSTERIA): St. Johnswort 421.

NERVOUSNESS: basil 49, blue vervain 86, cattail 124, celery 135, hops 275, Japanese honeysuckle 288, licorice root 307, lily 309, sage 410, skullcap 427, tarragon 441.

NEURALGIA: adder's tongue 3, cinchona 158, doong quai 208, ginger 251, moth-erwort 339.

NEURITIS: motherwort 339.

NIGHT BLINDNESS: dandelion 200, eyebright 229, passion flower 366, roses 400, yellow dock 482.

NOSEBLEED: bugleweed 101, shepherd's purse 425.

OBESITY: cayenne pepper 127, celery 135, chickweed 147, citrin 163, guar gum 269, kelp 297, mahuang 319, psyllium 380, stinging nettle 435, wild Mexican yam 470, yohimbine 484.

OLD AGE SPOTS: dandelion 200, horsetail 281.

OPHTHALMIA: turmeric 450.

ORAL PROBLEMS: echinacea 211, goldenseal 261, zedoary 487.

OSTEOARTHRITIS: feverfew 234.

PAIN: arnica 23, belladonna 58, coca 174, dong quai 208, elecampane 218, fun-gus 241, ginger 251, marijuana 321, pau d'arco 367, peony 369, prickly ash 378, wormwood 477.

PALSY (see also NERVOUSNESS): corydalis 188.

PANCREATITIS: mullein 341.

PANIC ATTACKS (see also ANXIETY NEUROSIS): ashwagandha 35, lily 309.

PARALYSIS: chamomile 138, pine 370, prickly ash 378.

PARASITES (see INTESTINAL PARASITES, SKIN PARASITES)

PARKINSON'S DISEASE: corydalis 188, pine 370.

RESPIRATORY DISORDERS: dandelion 200, elecampane 218, eucalyptus 222, frankincense 240, mahuang 319, mountain mahogany 339, purslane 382, yellow dock 482.

RESTLESSNESS (see NERVOUSNESS)

RHEUMATISM: agave 4, camphor 114, lemongrass 305, lilac 308, motherwort 339, prickly ash 378, roses 400, rosemary 403, sassafras 424, tarragon 441, wild Mexican yam 470.

RHEUMATOID ARTHRITIS (see ARTHRITIS)

RINGING IN THE EAR (see TINNITUS)

RINGWORM: arum 29, azalea 42, pau d'arco 367, sagebrush 416, turmeric 450, walnut 462.

RUNNY NOSE (see POST-NASAL DRIP)

SALIVA (DELAYED FLOW): anemone 17, prickly ash 378.

SCABIES (see also SKIN PROBLEMS): neem 349, pennyroyal 368.

SCALDS (see BURNS)

SCALP PROBLEMS: cactus 109, cattail 124, henna 273, horsetail 281, magnolia 318, rosemary 403, sage 410, sagebrush 416, stinging nettle 435.

SCARLET FEVER (see FEVER)

SCHIZOPHRENIA: ashwagandha 35, evening primrose 225, tarragon 441.

SCIATICA: adder's tongue 3, bean 52, buttercup 106, camphor 114, lemongrass 305, motherwort 339.

SCRAPES (see BRUISES)

SCURVY: blue spruce 83, cayenne pepper 127, pine 370.

SEIZURES (see EPILEPTIC SEIZURES)

SENILITY (see MEMORY LOSS)

SEXUAL DYSFUNCTION (see FRIGIDITY, IMPOTENCY)

SEXUAL FRIGIDITY (see FRIGIDITY)

SEXUAL PROBLEMS (see FRIGIDITY, IMPOTENCY)

SEXUALLY TRANSMITTED DISEASES: Brigham tea 93, garlic 244, melaleuca 328, pokeroot 375.

SHINGLES: belladonna 58, buttercup 106, cayenne pepper 127, garlic 244, pennyroyal 368, sassafras 424.

SHIGELLOSIS: Brigham tea 93, garlic 244, wormwood 477.

SHOCK: arnica 23, lily 309, St. Johnswort 421.

SHOULDER PAIN (see PAIN)

SICKLE CELL ANEMIA: prickly ash 378, red clover 390.

SINUS PROBLEMS: camphor 114, eyebright 229, goldenseal 261, horehound 277, horseradish 278, juniper berry 291, pine 370, walnut 462, watercress 464, yellow dock 482.

SINUSITIS (see SINUS PROBLEMS)

SKIN PARASITES: eucalyptus 222, garlic 244, melaleuca 328, neem 349, pau d'arco 367.

SKIN PROBLEMS: agrimony 5, birch 63, calendula 111, castor bean 120, chamomile 138, club moss 169, coffee 178, elderberry 213, garlic 244, henna

SWEATING (INDUCE): boneset 87, catnip 122, feverfew 234.

SWELLING (see INFLAMMATION)

SWOLLEN GLANDS: ginger 251, lavender 299, pokeroot 375.

SWOLLEN JOINTS (see ARTHRITIS)

SYPHILLIS (see also SEXUALLY TRANSMITTED DISEASES): Brigham tea 93, burdock 103, echinacea 211, garlic 244, morning glory 335, sarsaparilla 423, squawvine 433.

TAPEWORMS (see INTESTINAL WORMS)

TENDONITIS (see also INFLAMMATION): bay 50, lemongrass 305, plantain 373.

TENSION (see STRESS)

TESTICLE INFLAMMATION: burdock 103, chickweed 147, plantain 373.

TETANUS (see LOCKJAW)

THIRST (see DEHYDRATION)

THROAT DISORDERS (see COUGHS, LARYNGITIS, SORE THROAT, and TONSILLITIS)

THYROID PROBLEMS: bladderwrack 76, kelp 297.

TINNITUS: fenugreek 232, ginkgo 255.

TONSILLITIS: cinquefoil 162, echinacea 211, lobelia 313, mullein 341, pokeroot 375, sage 410, sorrel 432, walnut 462, willow 473, yellow dock 482.

TOOTH DECAY: camphor 114, prickly ash 378, rhubarb 397, sorrel 432, tea 443, thyme 445, watercress 464.

TOOTHACHE: allspice 10, apple bark 22, black pepper 74, catnip 122, cattail 124, cloves 168, coriander 184, garlic 244, ginger 251, melaleuca 328, plantain 373, prickly ash 378, ramps 387.

TORN LIGAMENTS: horsetail 281, marshmallow 326, slippery elm 428.

TRANSPLANT REJECTION: garlic 244, ginkgo 255, kava kava 296.

TREMBLING (see also NERVOUSNESS): catnip 122, corydalis 188.

TUBERCULOSIS: castor bean 120, echinacea 211, elecampane 218, hops 275, mountain mahogany 339, thyme 445.

TUMORS (see CANCER)

TWITCHES (see NERVOUSNESS and MUSCLE SPASMS)

TYPHOID (see FEVER and INFECTION)

TYPHUS (see FEVER and INFECTION)

ULCERS: aloe 11, bilberry 61, calendula 111, cayenne pepper 127, comfrey 182, licorice root 307, plantain 373, roses 400, wheat grass 466.

URIC ACID ACCUMULATION (see CALCIUM DEPOSITS and GOUT)

URINARY PROBLEMS: asparagus 36, buchu 100, horsetail 281, parsley 363.

URINARY TRACT INFECTION: agave 4, garlic 244, marshmallow 326, mullein 341, purslane 382, uva ursi 454.

URINATION (POOR): agave 4, buchu 100, Chinese cucumber 152, parsley 363, rosemary 403, tarragon 441.

UTERINE CRAMPS (see CHILDBIRTH, DIFFICULT)

UTERINE HEMORRHAGING (see BLEEDING)

VAGINITIS: amaranth 13, bayberry 51, blazing star 77, witch hazel 475.

VARICOSE VEINS: bay 50, bayberry 51, calendula 111, gotu kola 266, oak 356, pine 370, zedoary 487.

VENEREAL DISEASE (see also SEXUALLY TRANSMITTED DISEASES): blazing star 77, chickweed 147, sarsaparilla 423, sassafras 424, slippery elm 428, sumac 439.

VERTIGO: catnip 122, ginkgo 255, mints 331.

VITAMIN/MINERAL DEFICIENCY: alfalfa 7, parsley 363, purslane 382, watercress 464.

VOMITING: apple bark 22, bergamot 59, ginger 351, lemongrass 305, nutmeg 350.

VOMITING (INDUCE): ipecac 285.

WARTS: aloe 11, celandine 134, dandelion 200.

WEAKNESS (see FATIGUE)

WHITLOWS (see BOILS and CARBUNCLES)

WHOOPING COUGH (see also COUGHS): bryony 99, lobelia 313, red clover 390.

WORMS (see INTESTINAL PARASITES)

WOUNDS: adder's tongue 3, agave 4, arnica 23, bilberry 61, birch 63, brier rose 92, cactus 109, calendula 111, comfrey 182, elephant grass 220, eucalyptus 222, lily 309, marshmallow 326, melaleuca 328, morning glory 335, mullein 341, poplar 377, sagebrush 416, St. Johnswort 421, shepherd's purse 426, slippery elm 428, smartweed 430, thyme 445, turmeric 450, wheat grass 466, wild Oregon grape 472, willow 473, yarrow 480.

WRINKLES: cleavers 167, horsetail 281, roses 400, wild Mexican yam 470.

YEAST INFECTIONS (see also CANDIDIASIS and FUNGAL INFECTION): castor bean 120, squawvine 433, thyme 445.

HERBS & SPICES CONTENTS

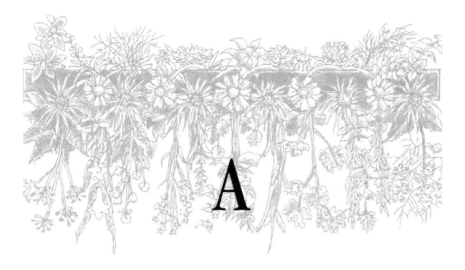

ACONITE
(ACONITE NAPELLUS)

Brief Description

This hardy plant, also called monkshood and wolfsbane, is an herbaceous perennial with a tuberous root that in shape and color somewhat resembles a small turnip. In fact, part of its generic name means that very thing—the Greek *akontion* means a dart (probably due to the herb's toxic compounds) and *napellus* means "little turnip."

The stem can reach about 3 feet. It is covered with dark green, divided glossy leaves. The flowers are usually dark blue and grow in erect clusters. Their shape is intended by nature to attract bees for pollination. The sepals are purple—this color being particularly tempting to bees—and are shaped in a fancy way, with one of them being in the form of a hood (hence, one of its common names, monkshood).

German Naturopathic Remedy for Neuralgia

Facial neuralgia can be a common problem with many adults who suffer from stress, nervousness, and other neurological disorders. Various naturopathic doctors throughout Germany have come to rely upon tincture of aconite root for resolving this problem in most of their patients suffering from genuine trigeminal neuralgia.

The usual dose prescribed ranges any where from 5 to 10 drops or more, twice or thrice daily. The standard practice is to start the patient out on a smaller dose and then gradually increase it very slowly and then decrease it again after several weeks time. One of the more popular German products widely employed for this is called Aconitystat and contains 70 grams of extracted juice from every 100 grams of plant roots. Pure aconite is also relied upon, but administered in pills, containing 0.05 to 0.2 mg.

Arthritic and Gouty Pains Disappear

It is rather remarkable that one of nature's more toxic herbs, aconite, just happens to be one of the more effective remedies in successfully clearing up the excruciating pains accompanying rheumatoid arthritis and gout. Problem is though, you can't buy aconite in most health food stores or herb shops in the U.S., simply because the proprietors either don't know enough about it or else fear it may cause undue harm to some of their customers.

But in much of Europe, where herbal medicine is more popular and widely accepted by members of the orthodox medical establishment, it isn't uncommon at all to find aconite tincture. I like to combine it with some valerian tincture for such problems. My standard recommendation has always been 10 drops of each tincture in one-half cup distilled water three times daily on an empty stomach. It has never failed to work that I know of, for arthritis or gout.

To make your own tincture, combine about 4 ounces each of coarsely cut, dried aconite and valerian roots in 1-1/2 pints of vodka, rum, gin, or brandy. Shake every day, permitting both roots to extract for about 15 days. Strain the liquid through fine wire mesh lined with cheesecloth, bottle in dark-colored glass and store in a cool, dry place.

Quick-Acting Homeopathic Drug

Author Michael Wiener has described aconite as a very "fast-acting medicine," in *The Complete Book of Homeopathy* (Garden City, NY: Avery Publishing, 1989). But, because of its short-term effects, he adds, it necessitates "repeated [dosages] frequently in acute conditions." He suggests it for "use in complaints that come on suddenly and with great intensity." Some health conditions that might qualify for this include cardiac arrest, insulin shock, paralysis due to stroke, and momentary suffocation due to an asthmatic or bronchial attack.

Warning: In such extreme cases, however, it is important to remember that the *homeopathic* preparation of aconite *must* be administered under the supervision of a skilled homeopathic or naturopathic practitioner. This is *not* an herb for every body or for casual use by lay people by any means! You have to know what you're doing when using aconite or else you could wind up in the intensive care unit of your local hospital, if you're not careful with it!

ADDER'S TONGUE
(ERYTHRONIUM AMERICANUM)

Brief Description

This fernlike herb is a perennial and grows from six to nine feet in height. It has two slender, pale green leaves of equal length (about 5 feet), with one twice as wide as the other and brown-spotted. The flowers are yellow and between 1 and 2 feet long. The root is solid, brown on the outside, white on the inside and somewhat round-shaped like an onion bulb. Both the root and herb were once listed in the *United States Pharmacopeia* from 1820 to 1850.

Good Wound Healer

A popular remedy among the despised gypsies of the French countryside is to make an ointment from the leaves and flowers of adder's tongue. One pint of extra virgin olive oil is gently warmed over a low heat. Then as much finely cut adder's tongue leaf and flower are added as the oil can absorb. They are permitted to gently brew but not boil, being stirred every so often with a wooden spoon. Then 1 cup of melted beeswax is added and the mixture cooked for another 5-7 minutes. The contents are then poured into empty baby food jars and kept uncovered until well set.

I've seen it used for all manner of wounds in man and beast alike, including sores, bruises, skin ulcers, scrapes, insect bites/stings, abrasions, minor cuts, and burns. It makes a wonderful healing balm.

Fine Relief from Sciatica and Neuralgia

In some of the provinces of France, country folks will occasionally turn to adder's tongue to help relieve their pains from sciatica and neuralgia. A hot infusion is made using one cup of water with 1/2 teaspoon of the chopped bulb, which is simmered on low heat for about 15 minutes. A clean cloth is soaked in the hot tea, the excess liquid wrung out and the pack then laid over the site of pain, with a second, folded dry cloth overlaid to help retain the heat longer. Relief from excruciating pain is reported within ten minutes or less.

Help for the Respiratory System

Small amounts (1/2 cup) of tea made from the bulb, when taken warm in *slow* sips, will help to relieve chest tightness and act as a potent decongestant in clearing out mucus accumulations in cases of asthma and bronchitis.

AGAVE
(AGAVE AMERICANA)

Brief Description

Those who've seen agave will swear it looks a lot like the yucca plant for which it has sometimes been mistaken. However, agave is much more robust and has thicker, spiney-edged leaves and a flowering stalk that, unlike the other desert plant, forms distinct armlike branches. Agave prefers the soil and climates of the many deserts found throughout the great American West and Southwest.

Guatemalan Healing Miracles

Some years ago I spent some time with various Indian folk healers called *curanderos* (if they were male) or *curanderas* (if they were female) in the Guatemalan highlands. Agave was one of the more important plants they utilized quite often for spasms, coughs, poor urination, accumulated phlegm, fevers, kidney inflammation and pain, rheumatism, skin sores, urinary tract infection and wounds.

In one instance, I saw a child bitten by a rabid dog (which was soon shot) treated by a local village healer. The woman squeezed some juice out of a fresh cut agave leaf, then heated it in a large metal spoon over a fire, before rubbing it into the bite. The child experienced no serious problems thereafter, and this procedure was repeated several more times the day I witnessed this.

The stiff rosette located in the center of the tough green leaves is sometimes boiled in a little water with salt and ingested warm for treating jaundice of the liver. It is said to be quite effective within 24 hours.

The Maya in this region of Central America will take the leaf juice internally for its soothing and demulcent properties. The agave juice forms a protective coating over inflamed tissues of the stomach and intestinal tract. This results, I was told, in a quieting effect on the stomach and reduces irritation in the intestines that might be caused by diarrhea or dysentery.

A good leaf tincture can also be made for treating indigestion, gassy fermentation, and chronic constipation. The Maya healer takes about 1/2 pound of fresh agave leaf, rinses it under running water, and chops it up into very small pieces. These are then placed in a clean glass jar with a good lid. The chopped herb material is then covered over the top with sufficient grain alcohol (similar to Everclear). Pure grain alcohol is available from liquor stores everywhere (except in California) and in Mexican border towns like Juarez and Tijuana. For this tincture to work, 190-proof alcohol is essential; anything less than this will result in an inferior extraction.

After the chopped herb is covered, the lid is screwed on and the jar set aside and left untouched for almost two weeks. The remaining liquid is then drawn off and stored in a smaller jar. One-quarter to one-half tea-spoon of this potent tincture is added to one cup warm water for the previously mentioned G.I. complaints.

AGRIMONY
(AGRIMONIA EUPATORIA)

Brief Description

This plant is a member of the rose family. It has foot-long, thin terminal racemes of numerous yellow flowers, five-petaled and roselike, which eventually mature into little round burrs. The basal leaves resemble some-what the shape of mustard greens, and are hairy and pinnate. The stem is between 2-3 feet tall and has smaller, irregular leaves that are usually three-parted. Agrimony is common to the West and Southwest.

Emotional Hypersensitivity Treated

Dr. Edward Bach was a renowned London physician, who discovered through considerable research a small group of natural remedies that helped to treat the mental and emotional aspects of many of his physical-ly sick patients. They eventually became known worldwide as the Bach Flower Remedies and are readily available, usually in fluid extract forms. All of his remedies are prepared from the flowers of wild plants, bushes or trees; none is harmful or habit-forming. They are prescribed, not directly for the organic problem itself, but instead according to the patient's state of mind such as moods of anger, depression, fear or worry. The remedies are designed to bring a calming effect to an otherwise agitated mind.

Agrimony is one of thirty-eight remedies that Dr. Bach frequently used on a number of his patients, who outwardly may have appeared care-free but inwardly were severely tortured individuals. The doctor recalled one such case for which agrimony was typically prescribed. "Man, age 40. He was a courageous person, but restless, high-strung, and suffered from anxieties. He had many family worries, and he drank heavily to gain relief from his mental torture. Agrimony alone was prescribed. After a treatment of two months, he had lost his craving for alcohol and he was able to analyze and resolve his many problems. He had become a normal person again."

The usual method for taking flower essences of any kind morning and evening is by putting an average of seven drops under the tongue or by adding them to water; the therapy generally lasts for a two-week period. They can also be applied topically by adding them to lotions and salves, or to bath water (a very effective method, I might add). The same amount is applied for adults and children alike, and they may also be given to pets.

Something for Burning, Itchy Eyes

A weak tea solution of agrimony leaves makes a very soothing eyewash. In a pint of water, cook one chopped tablespoon of the herb leaves for about 10 minutes. Set aside and let it cool. Then strain and put into a smaller bottle with an eye-dropper top. Tilt the head back, part the eyelids, and put about 5 drops of weak agrimony tea into the eye. It is always surprising to see its success in cases of allergies such as hayfever, where the eyes tend to get red and itchy.

Hives and Moist Skin Eruptions Helped

The same tea made with two tablespoons of chopped agrimony leaves in one pint of water, then cooled, strained and sprayed as a fine mist on the skin every hour or so helps get rid of hives and moist skin eruptions.

Relief for Asthma and Bronchitis

Some years ago when I was doing medicinal plant research among the mountain folks of the Ozarks, I remember one grizzled old-timer taking me out back of his shanty and showing me a bunch of agrimony growing in a waste area. Then we walked up a draw (called a "holler" in these parts, because you can stand at the bottom and easily holler up to someone at the top) where he pointed out some common burdock.

"Anything that's got burrs or stickers on them," he drawled, "is good for what ails a man here," at the same time thumping his chest with a closed fist for emphasis. He spit out some tobacco juice from the plug he had been chewing for several hours and continued talking as we hiked back down. "I make it into a strong tea," he informed me, "and take the stuff straight jest like I do my whiskey. It helps clear out the cobwebs and green scummy stuff from the lungs."

Here's a daintier and more sanitary way of making some of this tea for clearing mucus due to asthma or bronchitis out of the respiratory system. In a clean pan (not one used for slopping the hogs) bring 1-1/2 pints of water to a boil. Then add one full cup of *green*, immature cockleburrs, cover and simmer on medium heat for 10 minutes. Turn off the heat and steep for 25 minutes. Strain one cup, sweeten with honey, and drink while still warm. And, by the way, in case you chew like my informant did, be sure to remove the tobacco plug *before* drinking this tea.

ALFALFA
(MEDICAGO SATIVA)

Brief Description

Alfalfa is a perennial herb commonly found on the edges of fields in low valleys and is widely cultivated by farmers for livestock feed. An erect, smooth stem grows from an elongated taproot to a height of a foot or more. Flowers are blue-to-purple during the summer months, finally producing the characteristic spirally coiled seed pods.

Alfalfa or lucerne was used by the Persians to feed their horses to make them look sleeker and feel stronger. The Arabs designated this common hay feed for livestock, "The Father of All Food." Some modern herbalists have gone even further than this, characterizing alfalfa as being "the Big Daddy of 'em all" in terms of nutritional value, considering that the plant is so rich in calcium that the ashes of its leaves are almost 99% pure calcium.

Prevents Hardening of the Arteries

This has been a discovery of late by scientists rather than traditional herbalists, surprisingly enough. Clinical nutritionists have clearly demonstrated that alfalfa meal, when fed to caged monkeys whose diets included high levels of cholesterol, helped to prevent atherosclerosis and also reduced the serum cholesterol levels.

Based on such medical findings, it's therefore strongly recommended that you take 2 capsules of good quality alfalfa powder with every meal when too much cholesterol might be a problem; it is available in your local health food store.

An Infection Fighter

Henry G. Bieler, M.D., who for years treated many of the great film stars of Hollywood, recounted an episode with alfalfa in his bestseller, *Food Is Your Best Medicine.*

While he was practicing in rural Idaho many years ago, he traveled a great distance to visit a farmer who was suffering from a very bad leg ulcer. The open sore was discharging pus just above the ankle and the entire limb appeared to be dangerously close to becoming gangrenous.

Dr. Bieler inquired if there were any alkaline vegetables around the house, but unfortunately none were available. The only plant available that he could think of was alfalfa, of which the farmer had plenty.

He persuaded the astonished wife to pick the tender young alfalfa shoots, chop them and combine them with equal parts of water and canned grapefruit juice.

The patient was also given canned vegetables, whole grain bread and raw milk in the correct amounts. Eventually, the leg condition healed up completely with the farmer strictly adhering to this dietary regimen.

The rich chlorophyll content found in alfalfa, and other green plants like it, was used by some doctors in major hospitals in the 1940s for treating infections resulting from surgical incisions, bed sores and inner ear problems. In such cases, capsules of Nature's Way Alfa-Max from your local health food store may be of great benefit. Better still, though, would be fresh juice made from raw alfalfa sprouts whipped up in a blender or else run through a juicer. About 4-6 oz. of the juice taken at one time and also applied externally on any surface infection will be of considerable help.

Making Your Own Sprouts

To make your own sprouts, soak a teaspoon of alfalfa seeds in a quart of tepid water overnight. Next morning, rinse the seeds thoroughly with tepid water and drain. Place them in a jar tightly covered with damp cheesecloth.

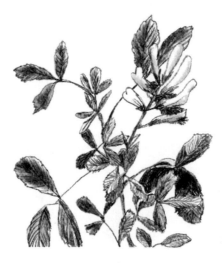

Store in a dark place. Twice a day, rinse the sprouting seeds and drain them well, returning them to the dark after each rinse. After 4 to 5 days, place the sprouts in the sunlight for a few hours to green them, then store in the refrigerator. Use alfalfa sprouts instead of lettuce, since they are far more nutritious.

Control Aid in Diabetes

According to an August 1984 report in the *Journal of Nutrition,* scientists at the University of California at Davis found that alfalfa extracts with a lot of manganese definitely improved the condition of a diabetic who failed to respond to insulin. Two capsules twice or three times daily might be worth trying in instances such as this.

Highly Nutritional

Powdered alfalfa contains vitamins A, B-1, B-6, B-12, C, E, and K-1, niacin, pantothenic acid, biotin, folic acid, etc., as well as many essential and nonessential amino acids. Additionally, it contains 15-25% proteins, major minerals and trace elements like calcium, phosphorus, manganese, iron, zinc, and copper, together with many naturally occurring sugars (sucrose, fructose, etc.).

% RECOMMENDED DAILY ALLOWANCES

Nutrient	Alfalfa (1 oz.)	Parsley (1 oz.)	Kelp (.1 oz.)	Molasses (3 tbs.)	Milk Powder (1 oz.)
Protein	10%	10%	0%	0%	14%
Calcium	75%	43%	5%	51%	38%
Iodine	0%	0%	3300%	0%	0%
Iron	85%	100%	0%	96%	2%
Magnesium	45%	20%	7%	45%	9%
Phosphorus	14%	13%	1%	6%	29%
Potassium	25%	41%	5%	59%	13%
Sodium	0%	3%	4%	2%	4%

Depression Disappears

Probably one of the most unusual recommendations for alfalfa that I've ever run across, recommended its use for clearing up depression, but in a very unusual way. In the autobiography of an ordinary Mormon, *History of a Pioneer: Edward Leo Lyman, Jr. (1881-1958)* (Delta, UT: Melvin A. Lyman, M.D., 1959), is recounted the following item.

"I was old enough to remember many of the things which my father [Edward Leo Lyman, Sr.] taught me. The day he took sick he came up through the field from his farm across my land where I was irrigating in the rain. He stopped to talk to me a little while. My alfalfa looked beautiful and he said to me, 'If you ever get the blues a sure cure is to go out and look at your alfalfa a while.'" I've recommended this bit of sage advice to several farmers who faced foreclosures and were in deep depressions. A couple of them followed it and claimed afterwards just how therapeutic it was to gaze out on their fields of uncut alfalfa hay for an hour or so. They said such greenery seemed to "revive" their drooping spirits.

ALLSPICE
(PIMENTA DIOICA)

Brief Description

Allspice comes from a tall tree that grows prolifically throughout Central and South America and the Caribbean. It is especially abundant on the island of Jamaica, which boasts the best quality to be found anywhere in the world.

The allspice tree has a slim trunk that sheds its soft, light-grey outer bark every year. It branches high above the ground, bearing pairs of lanceolate leaves that are shiny dark-green on top and lighter below. The leaves contain the same aromatic substances as the berries—primarily eugenol, a compound also occurring in clove.

Natural Analgesic for Toothache

A Creole-speaking herbalist from the city of Montego Bay showed me how to make a simple tooth powder to stop any ache or pain. He picked some of the pea-sized berries while they were still green and split them open with a sharp pocketknife, revealing two kidney-shaped seeds inside each one. He put everything together between two pieces of wax paper, and gently tapped the contents with a hammer until fairly well mashed. The top paper was removed and the allspice left in the sun to dry. Another piece of wax paper was put back over and the crude powder pounded a little more finely with the hammer.

This powder was then put into an empty chewing tobacco can. Whenever a toothache occurred, he said, just wet your forefinger, then dip it into this powder and rub it inside the mouth along the gum line to relieve the toothache almost immediately.

Quick and Easy Mouthwash

Madge R., an executive secretary, told me of something she has used from time to time to get rid of bad breath instantly, when no mouthwash is available. At a 1994 National Health Federation convention, she showed me a little piece of aluminum foil wrapped up inside her purse. Inside, she said, was some allspice powder, which she would slip into a small glass of warm water, stir with her finger, and then swish around in her mouth for a minute or so in order to sweeten her breath. She said the pleasant aroma helps to mask bad mouth odor.

ALOE
(ALOE VERA)

Brief Description

Aloe is a perennial succulent native to East and South Africa, but also cultivated in the West Indies and other tropical countries. The strong, fibrous root produces a rosette of fleshy basal leaves. The tissue in the center of the leaf contains a mucilaginous gel that yields aloe gel or aloe vera gel. When Columbus set sail for America, he wrote in his diary, "All is well, aloe is on board!" Aloe was the material used to embalm Pharaoh Ramses II and to preserve the body of Jesus Christ.

Aloe Gel Gets Rid of Warts

A lady from Lubbock, Texas had a wart on her arm the size of a pencil eraser. Each morning she soaked a small piece of cotton in aloe gel and taped it over the wart. Every three hours more gel was added with an eyedropper. Next day, fresh cotton was used and the process repeated. By the fourth day, the wart was beginning to dry up. Two weeks later when the cotton was removed, what remained of the wart came off clean. There was no scar to ever indicate a wart had once been there.

The Medicine Doctors Rave About

Probably no other single herb in modern times has been so well spoken of in regard to its many marvelous healing virtues by members of the medical and dental professions as has aloe vera.

Modern doctors have used aloe successfully for X-ray burns, sunburn, chemical burns, first degree burns, traumatized tissue (after normal and regular cleansing), decubitus ulcers or bedsores, primary candidal dermatitis (skin inflammation caused by infection of the yeast *Candida albicans*), stomal ulcers (intestinal ulcers between the stomach and that portion of the small intestine called the jejunum), herpes simplex, periodontal surgery, insect bites and stings, irritating plant stings (such as from stinging nettle), and other minor dermatological (skin) manifestations.

An oral surgeon from Dallas, Texas reported amazing results in treating facial edema (swelling), immediate denture placement, lockjaw (mouth rinse) and cold sores (mouth rinse).

How to Use Aloe

Aloe vera comes in various forms: the natural gel; prepared ointment, salve or lotion; liquid drink concentrate and encapsulated powder. For a number of minor burns, swellings and inflammations (both internal and external), some of the natural gel from a broken or cut leaf rubbed on or in these afflicted areas will promote rapid healing. For larger inflammations (sunburn), more severe burns (chemical) or sores (herpes), a good ointment, salve or lotion with a high concentration of purified aloe gel may be the best thing to use. In these instances, a simple dressing may be called for. One of the more reliable aloe ointments for heavy duty use may be obtained from AVA of Dallas, Texas (see Appendix).

Internal use falls into several categories. Oral problems can be solved with the natural gel from a broken or cut leaf. For laxative purposes, capsulated aloe vera, found in your local health food store, is good to use. And for all other internal uses, the most healing aloe liquid I know of is an aloe juice concentrate mix (1 oz.=1 qt.; 4 oz.=1 gal.) available only by mail-order from Great American in St. Petersburg, Florida (see Appendix).

Nutritional Properties

Aloe vera contains 96% water, providing water to injured tissue without closing off the air necessary for tissue repair. "The remaining 4% of the pulp," states *Runner's World* magazine for December 1981, "contains complex carbohydrate molecules, believed essential to aloe's natural value as a moisturizer. Substances present include... enzymes, trace sugars, a protein containing 18 amino acids; vitamins; minerals like sulphur, silicon, iron, calcium, copper, sodium, potassium, manganese, and more. The mixture of active ingredients in aloe is called aloin, and is obtained from the gel in the leaf. It's responsible for the plant's healing properties."

AMARANTH
(AMARANTHUS HYPOCHONDRIACUS, A. CRUENTUS)

Brief Description

Not a true cereal, but rather a fruit, it belongs to the same family
(chenopodium) as the edible weed, lamb's-quarter. Looking like a sesame
seed, it has a pleasant, nutty flavor and can be popped like corn or steamed
and flattened into a flake. It requires very little water and fertilizer, growing almost anywhere the common weeds do. It is thought that amaranth
was brought to this hemisphere by those first migrants from the Tower of
Babel, who traveled eastward across China and launched their barges on
the Pacific, eventually reaching what is now western Mexico around 2000
B.C. (In the Book of Mormon they are referred to as the Jaredites.)

Food of the Future

Amaranth seed has been described as "the perfect protein food of the past
for meals of the future," by *U.S. News and World Report* for Nov.25, 1985.
Robert Rodale, publisher of *Prevention* and *Organic Gardening* magazines,
first reintroduced amaranth to this country in the early 1970s after the U.S.
Department of Agriculture showed a lack of interest in it. It is now available in some health food or specialty food stores. Great American (see
Appendix) also offers it for sale by mail-order.

Diarrhea and Bleeding

Amaranth seed and leaves have been used effectively as an astringent for
stopping diarrhea, bloody stools and urine, and excessive menstruation. It
also makes a good wash for skin problems ranging from acne and eczema
to psoriasis and hives. It is an excellent douche for vaginal discharges of
purulent matter, a gargle for sore mouths, gums, teeth and throats, and a
fantastic enema for colon inflammations and rectal sores.

To make an amaranth tea for all these purposes, simply bring 3 cups
of water to a rolling boil. Then add 2 teaspoons of seeds, cover and simmer on very low heat for about 5 minutes. Remove from heat and add 1
teaspoon of leaves (if available) or else just let steep for 30 minutes. Drink
two cups daily for internal problems.

AMARANTH BREAD

This is a delicious bread that has been especially designed for those with allergies to yeast, milk, eggs, butter or sugar. However, it doesn't keep well in the refrigerator so it needs to be consumed in 24 hours or less.

Needed: 3/4 cup warm nut milk (see recipe below);3/4 teaspoon non-acidic vitamin C crystals; 2-3/4 cups amaranth flour, divided; 3/4 cup tapioca starch; 1/2 teaspoon sea salt; 1 tablespoon ground anise or fennel seeds; 1/3 cup extra virgin olive oil; 2 tablespoons hot distilled water; 2 teaspoons Arm & Hammer baking soda.

Preheat oven to 400 degrees F. Combine the nut milk and vitamin C crystals; stir and let stand to dissolve. In a large mixing bowl, combine 2-1/4 cups of amaranth flour with starch, sea salt and ground seeds; whisk together gently.

Next add the liquid with the dissolved crystals and olive oil to the flour mixture. Mix the batter with a wooden spoon. Sprinkle a little of the remaining half cup of flour in a circle centered on a baking sheet. Put the rest of the flour on a piece of wax paper.

Dissolve the baking soda in the boiling water; add to the dough and stir.

The dough will be very stiff. When the water disappears, punch it hard for 10 strokes. Turn the dough onto the wax paper. Roll the dough to coat it with more amaranth flour. Working rapidly, knead for almost 4 minutes. By now the dough will have absorbed enough flour to be more resilient, yet remain soft.

Now gather the dough into a smooth ball, and put it on the wax paper. Pat into an 8-inch round, 1-inch thick at the edges and mounded slightly in the center. To keep the wax paper from sliding around, tape it to your counter or table top. Also a floured bread board can be used in place of this, but the wax paper makes less mess to clean up afterwards.

With a sharp paring knife slash a deep X in the top of the dough. Put immediately into the oven and lower the temperature to 325 degrees F. Bake about 1 hour 10 minutes. Cut inside the loaf for a peek: if uncooked, the dough will appear darker in color; if done it will appear lighter in appearance.

NUT MILK FOR AMARANTH BREAD

Needed: About one-half cup of either raw almonds, Brazil nuts or cashews; 1 cup distilled water; 1/2 teaspoon pure vanilla flavoring; 1/2 teaspoon pure maple syrup; 1 tablespoon green seedless grapes.

Grind nuts to a fine meal in a Vita-Mix food blender. Use the blade recommended for grinding wheat into flour. Then add everything else and blend for 1-1/2 minutes. Stop several times to scrape down container sides with rubber spatula. Add to bread recipe as previously indicated.

AMERICAN CENTAURY
(Sabatia angularis)

Brief Description

American centaury was included in *United States Pharmacopeia* from 1820 to 1870. The plant grows from 1 to 2 feet high. The stem is branched above, square and smooth. Leaves are ovate, about a foot in length, and heart-shaped. The flowers are deep rose-colored with a greenish central star; they are wheel-shaped, 5-parted, and bitter. The flowering herb is used for medicinal purposes.

A Freckle Remover

There aren't very many plants that can do what American centaury can: South Carolina herbalist Mildred Park claims that the flowers and leaves made into tea are great for removing freckles.

She pours two cups of boiling water over 3/4 cup of finely cut flowers and leaves and lets the brew steep for an hour, covered. One or two cotton balls are then soaked in this tea, the excess liquid squeezed out, and then gently rubbed over a small area (the size of a silver dollar) of freckled skin for a minute or so. The process is repeated several times with fresh cotton balls.

She told me that if this is done regularly, it will help to diminish but not entirely eliminate freckles. She thought it could also be used on age spots on older people's hands.

ANEMONE
(Anemone pulsatilla)

Brief Description

This and other anemones belong to the buttercup family. Both have no real petals, just bright sepals ranging in color from cream white to lavender red and 8 or 10 in number. The floral parts possess many yellow stamens, which eventually climax into a conical, silky seed head. The entire plant can grow anywhere from 5 inches to a foot in height. Anemone leaves resemble those of parsley in some ways, but often have a purple stem and a small splash of purple. The herb has a small, dark-skinned tuber of pinkish hue.

Skin Lesions of AIDS Patient Healed

Jerry (pseudonym used to protect privacy) was wheeled by a friend of his to one of my health lectures at a New Age expo in New York City. Afterwards I met with both of them and Jerry confessed that he had developed AIDS but said that he was on a full herbal and nutritional program already under the supervision of an alternative-minded medical doctor. What he wanted to know, however, was what could be used to help heal the numerous skin lesions that were developing all over his body.

I explained how to make an herbal bath from anemone leaves. I told them to add two large handfuls of anemone leaves to a gallon of distilled water and simmer on low heat, covered, for 45 minutes. The liquid was to be strained into a glass container. His friend was to give Jerry a sponge bath morning and evening using some of this tea. I said it always worked well in cases of leprosy and should be of benefit to him. His friend reported back several months later that Jerry's sores were 75% healed by using this treatment on a regular basis.

Saliva Flow Wonderfully Promoted

Many people suffer from indigestion simply because they do not chew their food enough. This means that whatever is consumed isn't being adequately coated with saliva. Moreover, some people's salivary glands don't work well enough to produce sufficient amounts of this important body fluid.

In 1-1/2 cups of hot water, add two tablespoons of finely cut flowering herb. Cover and steep for 30 minutes. Strain and slowly sip one-half cup with a meal. Swish each mouthful around with the tongue to stimulate saliva production, before swallowing. Alternate every 7 mouthfuls of food with some of this tea. You'll be amazed at just how well your food will digest, even without complete chewing of every bite taken.

Malaria Cure

One of the very best remedies for recovery from malaria and from similar dangerous fevers is to make a tea by using equal parts (one teaspoon each) of American centaury and boneset in 1-1/2 pints boiling water, covered, and steeped for 15 minutes. Then uncover and stir in a pinch of powdered goldenseal root, cover again and continue steeping for another 10 minutes. Strain and drink 1 cup of warm tea every three hours.

AMERICAN GINSENG
(see GINSENG)

AMERICAN MISTLETOE
(see MISTLETOE)

ANGELICA
(ANGELICA ARCHANGELICA)

Brief Description

This stout biennial or perennial herb prefers cold and moist places, and is, therefore, quite common to countries such as Great Britain, Scotland, Lapland and Iceland. In the folklore of all North European countries, it's held in the highest esteem as "a protection against contagion, for purifying the blood and for curing every conceivable malady possible."

According to legends, angelica was revealed in a dream by an angel to cure the deadly bubonic plague.

China's Famous "Women's Remedy"

In China, angelica has been used for several thousand years to treat many kinds of female problems. The 10 different angelica species, collectively known by the name of dang-qui (also dong-quei or dong-quai or tang-kuei) are second in China only to ginseng.

Richard Lucas, in his book, *Secrets of the Chinese Herbalists*, described angelica as having "an affinity for the female constitution," being good for treating anemia and weak glands, regulating monthly periods, correcting hot flashes and vaginal spasms (common premenstrual symptoms) and assisting women through the difficult transition of menopause.

Lucas recommended 2 capsules of dong-quai twice or three times daily for severe female problems, with less than this for more moderate conditions. He also mentioned that "since its taste somewhat resembles that of celery, the capsules may be broken open and the contents added to hot soups or broth" without detracting from their flavor.

It has been reported that angelica helped relieve PMS (premenstrual syndrome) and was used successfully instead of estrogen.

A middle-aged woman from San Rafael, California wrote to me a couple of years ago concerning the remarkable transition to menopause she was able to make with this herb.

> During most of my adult life I've never been bothered with the usual PMS problems that other women generally suffer from. So when I entered menopause I thought it would be a snap! Boy, was I ever wrong!
>
> All my internal female organs acted like the devil. I couldn't sleep decently, because I would wake up in the middle of the night with terrific cramps.
>
> A friend referred me to a Chinese herbalist she knew in downtown San Francisco. Because of the difficulty of my case, he suggested I take 2 capsules of don-quai 3 times a day until all my spasms stopped and my organs no longer hurt. Then keep on taking only 1 capsule twice a day throughout the menopause phase until it was finished.
>
> The dong-quai worked like a charm and my miserable feelings disappeared in a little over a week.

Contains Coumarins

The rootstock of this herb has a sweet, spicy, agreeable odor. This is due mostly to the rich presence of many coumarins—white crystalline compounds with a vanilla-like odor. They are valuable in reducing high-protein edemas, especially swelling of the lymph nodes (lymphedema), as well as in treating the psoriasis often accompanying arthritis. The constituent bergapten accounts for its antipsoriatic properties, while other compounds such as linalool and borneol help to explain its antibacterial and antifungal activities. Other constituents include resin, starch and a number of naturally occurring sugars like sucrose, fructose and glucose.

ANISE
(PIMPINELLA ANISUM)

Brief Description

Anise has been popular in the ancient Chinese and Ayurvedic (Indian) medical systems for many centuries. There are several varieties of aniseed, the most common being the ash-colored kind from Spain. Anise belongs to the same botanical family (*Umbelliferae*) as parsley and carrots.

A Multi-Purpose Healing Tea

Imagine having a tea that will get rid of oily skin, improve your memory, calm a nagging cough, produce breast milk for nursing mothers and serve as a natural antacid in place of either Tums or Rolaids for heartburn and indigestion.

All these wonderful things can be accomplished simply by bringing 1 quart of water to a boil. Then add about 7 teaspoons of aniseed, reduce heat and simmer contents down to 1-1/2 pints. Strain and, while still warm, add 4 teaspoons each of honey and glycerine (obtained from a drugstore to preserve syrup tea).

Take 2 teaspoons of this syrup every few hours to relieve hacking coughs, or 2 tablespoons three times daily to strengthen the memory. If using as a tea, omit and drink 2 cups once or twice daily for skin problems, milk needs or to relieve stomach problems.

Great Deodorant for Body Odor

Anyone who has ever had the pleasure of smelling fresh anise knows that the entire plant has a very fragrant odor. Even the seeds, when chewed, help to sweeten the breath. Having said that, it stands to reason that this spice would be useful to mask body odor and bad breath.

What I'm about to relate is weird but nevertheless true. In February 1995 the Grateful Dead, one of rock music's most enduring bands from the 60s, celebrated its 30th anniversary tour in Salt Lake City at the Delta Center, which is close to my office. Fans known as Deadheads started gathering by the hundreds outside the office building where my research center has been located for years. Most of them had long hair (many in tangled dreadlocks) and everyone sported colorful clothes (a few of the men even wore dresses for the occasion).

As I left my building, I had to pass by large crowds of them. It took only a few seconds for my olfactory senses to quickly pick up the undeniable smell they all emitted. (Showers are a luxury for those who live out of a VW bus!) Deadheads either ignore the body odor or else cover it up with scented oils, incense, or "special" herbs.

But as I passed a small group, I picked up a strong licorice scent. I inquired if the pleasant aroma was anise. A man and woman in their 20s both responded that indeed it was. They said they made a tea from the whole fresh plant by simmering two handfuls of chopped herb in one pint of water, and then letting it slowly cook for 30 minutes until only half the amount of liquid remained. This was strained, cooled, and then put into an empty plastic bottle with an aerosol dispenser.

"We spray it on those parts of our bodies," the woman volunteered, "that need it the most. It's the best thing we know of to mask the odor."

"Sure beats the hell out of soap and water or having to bathe," her male partner quipped with typical youthful sarcasm. I thanked them for their information and continued on to my car.

ANNATTO
(BIX ORELLANA)

Brief Description

The annatto tree is a lovely, small flowering tree that grows throughout the Caribbean, Mexico, and Central and South America. It yields large pink flowers that are quite similar to wild roses. But it's the dye from the pulp that surrounds the fifty-plus seeds inside the heart-shaped prickly scarlet fruits that makes the tree commercially important. The Carib Indians, a war-like race, employed the dye to paint their bodies with fearsome designs before going into battle.

Since color makes annatto more important than its flavor, the ancient Maya often employed it as one of their principal coloring materials. Nowhere is this yellowish red dyestuff more evident than in the unique polychrome paintings on the walls and vaulting of a small, three-room building in Guatemala. It is a late Classic Period Maya site in the state of Chiapas.

The striking murals date from the late eighth century A.D. and are the most complete graphic portrayal of Maya life known thus far. Annatto is conspicuous in some of the vivid costumes and elaborate headdresses worn by a number of the jeweled ladies, clashing warriors, dancing lords, and assembled noblemen depicted in varying scenes of an exciting drama. These rare paintings gave me, as an anthropologist, invaluable ethnographic data and insights into Maya social order, styles of dress, types of ceremonial processions, and daily activities. But it also made me realize that these ancient artists relied on spices like annatto more for coloring purposes than for culinary reasons.

Dispels Intestinal Gas and Heartburn

Annatto is exploited to its fullest in the cooking of the Caribbean and Latin America, used primarily for its beautiful color instead of its gentle flavor.

However, it is of some medicinal importance in allaying heartburn and gas that result from the consumption of extremely spicy foods.

It is an ingredient in the spicy sauce that is served over the Jamaican national dish of ackee and salt cod. In Mexico, annatto seeds are ground with other herbs and spices, among them cumin and oregano, for a seasoning mixture that not only has a fragrant and flowery taste, but also helps to prevent intestinal gas from eating beans or heartburn from the consumption of chile peppers.

Indigestion Cleared Up

If you occasionally suffer from indigestion from certain types of food, then you ought to think about an annatto additive. Annatto helps remedy the sometimes difficult digestion of the following foods: legumes, grains, rice, poultry, fish, pork, beef and lamb stews, soups, okra, pumpkin, bell peppers, garlic, onions, tomatoes, curries, spice mixtures, shellfish (especially shrimp), chili sauces, egg dishes, sweet potatoes, and plantains.

Beautiful Rice

Here's a way to really spike up ordinary cooked white rice.

ANNATTO RICE PILAF

Needed: 1-1/2 cups long-grain rice; 4 tablespoons annatto oil; 2-1/2 cups chicken stock; and sea salt.

Rinse and drain the rice. Heat the oil in a pan. Add the rice, stir and cook a couple of minutes until rice is translucent. Add stock and salt to taste. Bring to a boil, then simmer, covered, until the liquid is totally absorbed (about 18 minutes). Let stand 12 minutes before fluffing up with the tines of a dinner fork. Delicious with spicy chicken dishes. Serves 4-6.

To make annatto oil, heat 1 cup grapeseed oil in a small saucepan. Add 2 oz. annatto seed and cook, stirring, until the oil turns a deep orange color (somewhere between 2 and 5 minutes). Timing depends on the potency of the seeds. Once the color is rich and deep, remove the pan from the stove. Cool, strain, and store the oil in a glass decanter in the refrigerator; it will keep indefinitely.

APPLE TREE BARK
(Pyrus malus)

Brief Description

Most indigenous cultures have discovered that bark is a very useful source
of some wonderful medicinal compounds. Many of the brews created by
native folk healers in the past have come from the bark of different trees.
Several times, as I've travelled through the tropical rain forests of Central
and South America, the teas made from the bark of trees by friendly witch
doctors or shamans have proved more effective to me in curing fevers like
malaria or dysentery than have the prescription pills my pharmacist issued
before I left home.

This has led me to consider the barks of some of our ordinary fruit
trees with regard to possible medicinal applications. I have looked especially at the apple tree, since its fruit is so popular. Certainly a heavily laden
apple tree with drooping branches in the orchard of Sir Isaac Newton at
Woolsthorpe, England, played a significant role in 1666, when a single fruit
dropped down upon the man's head and started a chain of thought which
eventually led him to propound the theory of gravitation.

An Old-Fashioned Remedy That Works

Imagine my surprise, however, when I soon discovered that there was
hardly anything on apple tree bark in the common herb books around. But
I was in luck when I came upon the first edition of the all-time herb classic *Back to Eden* by Jethro Kloss, which came out in 1939. This great
Seventh-Day Adventist herbalist helped to heal thousands of sick people
with his natural cures.

Apple tree bark was one of his most standard remedies, which he
claimed to have a wonderful "tonic" effect upon the system. Due to some
of his archaic medical terms, I've rephrased into modern medical jargon
many of the health problems he used the bark for. He prescribed it for the
following: fevers; gall bladder attacks (due to excess bile production or gall
stones or both); delayed menstruation; indigestion; nausea and vomiting;
liver and spleen disturbances; abdominal cramps; kidney stones and
Bright's disease (both kidney problems); dysentery; boils; insect
bites/stings; rabies; and toothache.

In all instances, he used a tea made from the fruit bark for all of these
complaints. Bring one quart of water to a boil. Add 2-3 heaping tablespoons of finely chopped or shredded apple tree bark. Cover and simmer

on low heat for approximately 12 minutes; remove from heat and steep for an additional 38 minutes.

Cool, strain, and store in the refrigerator in a clean jar. It is taken in one-cup amounts, warm or cold, depending on the condition itself.

fevers (warm)

gall bladder attacks (warm)

delayed menstruation (warm)

indigestion (warm)

nausea and vomiting (cool)

liver and spleen (cool)

abdominal cramps (either warm or cool)

kidney problems (either warm or cool)

dysentery (warm)

boils (cool)

insect bites/stings (cool)

rabies (cool)

toothache (warm).

In some cases, the tea may need to be used in the form of poultices applied directly to the skin in order to bring immediate relief. In other instances, it may be necessary to use *both* external poultices and internal tea to bring about satisfying relief to annoying problems.

I should mention that the descendants of Jethro Kloss published "The Authentic Kloss Family" edition of *Back to Eden* (Loma Linda, CA: Back to Eden Publishing Co.) in 1981. The "Acknowledgements" include an expression of appreciation to me for my contributions made in the form of numerous annotations scattered throughout the bulky volume. It is, therefore, understandable that I should harbor very special feelings for Jethro Kloss.

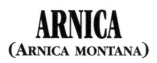

ARNICA
(ARNICA MONTANA)

Brief Description

Arnica is an aromatic perennial with a creeping rhizome, producing a basal rosette of 4-8 downy leaves 1-1/2 to 2-3/4 inches long in the first year. The flowering stem is usually unbranched, somewhat hairy, and almost 12 to 24 inches high, with only 1-2 pairs of opposite leaves. The flowers are golden yellow, daisy-like in appearance and show up in mid-summer to early autumn.

Arnica prefers the central and northern regions of the northern hemisphere, especially favoring sandy acid soils, rich in humus, and in sunny positions.

Goethe's Secret Heart Remedy

Johann Wolfgang von Goethe (1749-1832) was one of Europe's greatest literary figures who exercised dominant influence on the development of German literature.

But in his declining years, this great writer began to suffer frequently from angina pain due to hardening of his heart arteries, otherwise known as arteriosclerosis. A number of things were tried, but none of them brought relief. Finally he decided to try some arnica tea and was pleasantly surprised to see just how well it worked in eliminating the pain. Goethe had his housekeeper make tea every day for him by adding two teaspoonfuls of arnica flowers to 1-1/2 cups of boiling water; this would steep for ten minutes, be strained and then given to him to sip slowly. It never failed to work.

Important Homeopathic Remedy for Sports Injuries, Sprains, Bruises, Shock, Wounds, and Leg Ulcers

Arnica is often the first remedy of choice by homeopathic and naturopathic practitioners in many cases of sports injuries that may include severe sprains, ugly bruises, nasty wounds, and even shock. It is also a likely treatment preference for diabetic leg ulcers. When used topically it can be applied as a tincture, ointment or oil, but should only be used if the skin is unbroken.

To make the tincture, just combine three tablespoons of crushed arnica flowers in two cups of alcohol. Let this mixture stand for two weeks, shaking twice daily (preferably during a full moon). Then strain and pour the liquid into a bottle suitable for long-term storage. Use a diluted solution of about one teaspoon of tincture to a cup of warm water. Soak a small clean cotton cloth in this solution, squeeze out the excess liquid, fold into a small compact square and place over the bruise and leave there for 15 minutes. Repeat the process several times.

To make a simple but effective ointment, just pulverize two tablespoons of *dried* arnica flowers to powder; mix with eight tablespoons of melted petroleum jelly or Crisco. Add several drops of gum benzoin or a tincture of benzoin to help keep the ointment from turning rancid. Then liberally apply to any old wounds, leg ulcers or herpes sores that refuse to heal.

Opera Star Discovers Arnica Tea

A famous German opera star some years ago discovered the virtues of warm arnica tea for clearing up her sore throat and laryngitis. She simply added 10 drops of arnica tincture to a glass of warm water, gargled with it, and in just a few minutes her throat felt as good as new, enabling her to go back on stage and sing some more.

ARROWROOT
(MARANTA ARUNDINACEAE)

Brief Description

During my time in the Philippines in 1994, I became acquainted with this herbaceous perennial. There it was called *bamban* in the native Tagalog dialect. It is very common in the secondary forests, particularly along streams; it grows at low and medium altitudes from the Batanes Islands and northern Luzon to Palawan and Mindanao.

The stems are between 6-1/2 and 10 feet tall, several growing in a cluster, smooth, and widely branched. The leaves are thin, smooth and ovate. Creamy flowers adorn the ends of the slender branches. The creeping rhizome of the plant bears cylindrical tubers that curve upward and are somewhat fleshy; these are covered with large, thin scales that leave circular scars.

Starch is extracted from the rhizome, washed, beaten to a pulp in a wooden mortar, stirred in clean water, and then the fibers are wrung out manually.

The squeezing produces a milky fluid that is strained, permitted to settle and then drained. Following this the starch is dried in the sunlight. When the dried powder is mixed with water it acquires a definite jelly consistency.

Fear-Induced Diarrhea Immediately Stopped

One of the most amusing tales I've ever heard was related by Peter Benchley, author of the popular novel *Jaws*. A couple of years after the release of his novel, he and a friend were scubadiving in the Bahamas, examining a pile of old cannons on a reef.

"I wasn't worried about sharks," Benchley related. "The reef sharks of the Bahamas generally are shy and averse to scuba divers and the odds were long against a tiger shark, a more dangerous species, being in the neighborhood. As for the great whites, well, the possibility of encountering a great white was so remote as to be nonexistent."

Great whites, he noted, preferred cold water; the water he and his companion had been swimming in was bathtub warm. Great white sharks like deep water; their water was shallow. Great whites are "drawn to seal colonies or to the carcasses of dead whales, where food is abundant"; but where Benchley and his friend were swimming that day, there was "nothing worth eating."

He really wasn't paying much attention to the sudden and strange antics of his friend in the distance. The other pointed with some urgency and Benchley merely waved back and kept swimming towards the reef to get a closer look at some of those old cannons laying on the ocean floor. "The next sound I heard," he later recalled, "was the 'thrum' of his fins churning the water as he hurried back to the boat. Strange, I thought." But he casually dismissed it as well.

When he had reached the end of the reef, he began to turn back. Suddenly sensing another presence nearby, he raised his head and looked straight into the pointed snout and the black eye of a 25-foot great white shark. The huge torpedo shape of the gunmetal gray body with its rounded protrusions near the tail, filled him with such terror that it seemed like every muscle in his body momentarily froze.

Recalling this hair-raising moment in his life some years later, Benchley joked that he could have easily pictured what the likely newspaper headlines might have been: "*Jaws* Author Becomes Tasty Meal for Hungry Great White!" However, he wasn't the only one who reacted with fear. Believe it or not, the awesome and fierce-looking shark directly in front of him also temporarily froze. Man and fish just looked at each other in silent astonishment.

Then, without any obvious explanation and to Benchley's amazement, the great white suddenly wheeled about in the deep water, "voided its bowels, and disappeared in a nasty brown cloud."

Benchley continued with his thrilling narrative: "I didn't move. I was too breathless and grateful and stunned. Did that actually happen? Could the most fearsome predator on earth, the largest carnivorous fish in the sea, have fled from a puny human—from *me*—like a startled rabbit?"

Once the element of surprise had vanished, Benchley set a new record in scubadiving, ascending from the ocean floor to the surface and into his boat in less than 25 *seconds!* He lay down on the deck hyperventilating like crazy; his pulse soared near 300 and his skin became a necrotic gray. It took a while for his heart rhythm and natural color to return to normal.

But the nervous distress it produced on his gastrointestinal system took considerably longer to cope with. He found it helpful to stir a tablespoonful of arrowroot powder in some fruit juice and drink that every few hours. Within a few days the diarrrhea was gone and his average bowel function restored again.

Wonderful Dressing for Erysipelas and Sunburns

During the time that Benchley and his friend spent in the Bahamas, they managed to acquaint themselves with some of the local customs and sample a variety of highly seasoned dishes common to islands in the Caribbean. One interesting thing they noticed was how often the natives utilized arrowroot for medicinal as well as culinary purposes.

The starch was made into the form of a poultice and laid on the skin of some who suffered from erysipelas, an intense inflammation of the superficial skin and subcutaneous tissues caused by infection of the blood with group A streptococci. The poultice would then be left on for about 25 minutes before being replaced by a fresh one. Bahamians would also rub some of the arrowstarch on sunburns to help keep them from peeling as badly and to lessen their pain.

ARTICHOKE
(Cynara scolymus)

Maurice Messegue, Europe's greatest herbalist, says that the part of the artichoke we are in the habit of eating is the least active, while all the rest of it, which is unbelievably bitter, is actually the most nutritious and therapeutic for you. "For myself," he states quite emphatically, "I use every bit of the artichoke and encourage others to do the same!"

Two vegetables are called artichokes, but have absolutely no relation to each other. We distinguish them as the globe artichoke and the Jerusalem artichoke. The former is a green vegetable somewhat like a tiny cabbage, except that its leaves are smaller and thicker. The latter isn't even an artichoke, nor has it anything to do with Jerusalem. It came here from South America and first was called "girasole" from its likeness to the sunflower. Later this was corrupted into "Jerusalem." The tubers are pleasant enough to consume, but have no medicinal value.

A Terrific Cholesterol Manager

To make your own special leaf tincture for better managing the problems of too much cholesterol, slightly crush and soak about 5-1/4 cups of artichoke leaves in 2 pints of alcohol for 10 days. Strain and take one tablespoon twice daily in between meals. This should help keep cholesterol from accumulating in fatty globs within the body.

Volume 5 of *Experimental Medicine & Surgery* for 1947 confirmed the artichoke's cholesterol-fighting properties. Laying hens and human subjects manifesting early signs of atherosclerosis had their blood cholesterol contents lowered by administration of artichoke powder. Cynarin is the compound within artichokes that protects man and beast alike from hardening of the arteries and keeps serum triglyceride levels very low.

Brain Food to Make You More Alert

To increase your mental powers, pull an artichoke to pieces, leaf by leaf, and put into a jar with barely enough water to cover. Set a saucer on the jar and stand it in a pan of boiling water for 2 hours, adding more water to that in the pan as it boils away. Remove the jar from the pan and strain the contents, squeezing the leaves well. Three to four tablespoons of this infusion should be taken 3 times a day.

Artichoke leaves also seem to be pharmacologically active in the brain and in portions of the central nervous system. According to *Nutrition Reviews* for April,1978, the leaves contain "several active compounds similar to caffeine." A new kind of herbal combination called Artichoke/ Garlic may be obtained through the mail from Old Amish herbs in St. Petersburg, Florida (see Appendix). Recommended intake has been 2-4 capsules per day with meals as necessary.

Remedy for Liver Problems

Certain acids in artichokes definitely help to activate liver function. Scientific literature indicates a definite improvement in liver problems when artichoke is used regularly.

A Quick Three-Minute Salad

Ever in a hurry and don't have much time to fix yourself something to eat? How about whipping up an instant artichoke salad? Prior to this, when you have more time on your hands, cook some artichoke hearts until tender; drain, then marinate in apple cider vinegar in the refrigerator until needed.

Cut a plump, ripe tomato in quarters or slices. Arrange around marinated artichoke hearts on pieces of chilled Romaine lettuce. Spoon some cold yogurt over them, sprinkle with a dash of kelp and eat with delight.

ARUM
(ARUM MACULATUM)

Brief Description

Due to the obvious sexual symbolism of the very erect spadix of this attractive plant, almost all of its European common names have some sexual connotation: Lords and Ladies, Kings and Queens, Parson and Clerk, Friar's Cowl, and Cuckoopint. It doesn't take much imagination to discern this somewhat embarrassing association with sexuality.

The flowering organs are enveloped in a sheath-like leaf called a spathe, within which rises a long, fleshy stem or column called the spadix, bearing closely arranged groups of stalkless, primitive flowers. At the base are a number of flowers each containing a pistil only. Above these is a belt of sterile flowers, each consisting of only a purplish anther. Above the anther is a ring of glands, terminating in short threads. The spadix is then prolonged into a purple, club-like extremity.

The bright leaves, conspicuous by their glossiness and purple blotches, and their arrow shape, are some of the first to emerge from the ground with the advent of spring. Arum yields large tubers that are edible and nutritious, but more about them later.

Homeopathic Remedy for Sore Throat

In England medical herbalists are licensed to diagnose, prescribe, and even do minor surgery when the occasion warrants it. Many of the herbal preparations they employ are prepared through an elaborate system known as homeopathy. A simplified method of duplicating the same tincture in your home for hoarseness and sore throat is as follows: mix 1/2 teaspoon of powdered arum root with 3/4 cup alcohol and let stand for ten days, shaking at least once per day.

Afterwards, strain and pour the liquid into another bottle suitable for storage in a cupboard. Put about ten drops in 2 oz. of distilled water and gargle vigorously with the solution. Repeat every hour as necessary.

Good Treatment for Ringworm

One medical herbalist from Liverpool, England, shared with me some years ago her ointment for successfully eradicating ringworm from the skin. She took one half of an arum tuber (similar to a potato) and finely grated it; then she gently simmered the root material in about two-thirds cup of goose lard (melted Crisco may be substituted) for 15 minutes on *very low* heat so as not to cause burning or smoking of the fat itself. This was then permitted to cool.

After it had sufficiently set up, some of this arum ointment was then applied locally to the skin or scalp where the ringworm was the worst and left there for 24 hours before removal. Repeated applications may be necessary before it's completely gone. This same ointment is very good for helping to promote the healing of herpes sores and bedsores.

ASAFOETIDA
(Ferula asafoetida)

Brief Description

Asafoetida is the resinous exudation from two species of the giant fennel. Another common name for it is devil's dung; this is because of its extremely foul odor. A true story from the early Mormon pioneers best illustrates just how bad the smell can be. The following is excerpted from the book *Voice in the West: Biography of a Pioneer Newspaper* by Wendell J. Ashton (New York: Duell, Sloan & Pearce, 1950; pp.154-155) and used with permission.

> Back at his father's house, [young George] Lambert passed up breakfast. His pre-cooked meals in the vacant house had taken away his appetite. The youth's father was concerned. He told the lad he would take sick if he did not eat. Further, the father suggested that George take some asafoetida. It would help his appetite. It...had a powerful odor, and tasted like garlic. George knew that it was used as a horse medicine. Anyway, he broke off a piece and put it into his mouth and began chewing.
>
> The deed could have been disastrous in his relations with Michael Grace. Immediately George's breath put the family in an uproar. His father explained that he meant for the boy to take asafoetida pills, not the straight stuff. The stench was terrific.
>
> Returning to the paper mill, George delivered the mended machinery parts to Grace. The dapper superintendent looked up, startled. "What is that smell? he gasped. Several mill workers standing nearby chorused, "It isn't me," and scurried away.

Grace became frantic. He darted in one direction and then another in an attempt to find the source of the smell. He seemed to think it came from outside or from under some machinery.

[The Irishman bellowed out:] "Begorra! Jarge, I don't know how ye stand it! It's killing me. It must come from the divil's own stink factory. But how in the divil it gits in here I dunno. I nivver smelled it until you kem in."

Grace was getting near the source of the smell.

With brave words, George admitted, "I'm used to it; in fact, I'm the cause of it. I have been taking asafoetida, and that is what you smell."

"How did you step in it?" Grace retorted.

"It is a kind of gum, and I didn't step on it at all, but took it as a medicine."

"Arrah, Jarge, ye don't mean it! Ye don't mean ye put it in yer mouth!"

"Yes I did," George confessed, "and chewed it."

"Then hiven have pity on ye! I wonder ye don't turn inside out and then go and wash yourself in carbolic acid. I'd rather chew dung and let a polecat [skunk] do my laundry work than go near such a foul stench."

George volunteered to leave the plant until he could rid himself of the smell. He ate most anything he could get his hands on in an effort to chase away the odor. He washed out his mouth, picked and scrubbed his teeth, and chewed gum and sagebrush. After about a week, the stench had almost faded.

Stomach Pains Cured

Toward the end of 1981 business took me to Arizona. One weekend found me in Yuma where I read the local paper, the *Daily Sun*. My attention became more focused when I perused Ann Landers' column.

"An Old-Timer in N.Y." told of a medical doctor many years earlier prescribing some asafoetida "for my brother's severe stomach pains." Though no further details were given, other than "it helped" him, it was undoubtedly taken in the form of a tincture because of the nauseating taste. Decades ago natural-minded doctors would recommend 15-20 drops of the tincture in 6 fluid ounces for severe stomach pains and similar gastrointestinal distresses. To make the tincture, put 2 oz. of the brown root gum powder in 6 oz. alcohol; let stand for 2 weeks and shake once daily. Strain and pour the liquid into another bottle suitable for storage.

Prevents Insect Bites

When I was in New Orleans for a health convention in April 1986, I read *The Times Picayune* and found the comic strip "Hagar the Horrible" by Dik Browne funny and especially interesting because of my line of work.

The red-bearded Viking Hagar is leaving on another boat trip with his warriors. His heavy-set wife comes down to the pier with something in her hand. "Wear this asafoetida bag," she tells him. "It will protect you from all harm."

As she ties it around his neck, Hagar grumbles that it stinks!

Her response is: "It's supposed to...that's its power! It'll ward off evil spirits, plague, demons, devils, monsters and all dangers!" Then, in the last panel, as her husband slowly walks on board his ship stinking to high heaven, she flashes a conniving smile and silently thinks to herself, "Including flashy redheads."

These repelling features of the dried root latex stayed with me for several years, probably because of the cartoonist's humor. Shortly thereafter I was in the Florida Everglades, where mosquitoes are rampant. I remembered Dik Browne's comic strip, and wondered if some asafoetida might work as well with annoying insects.

I procured some lumps of the dried gummy resin and kept them stored in an empty pipe tobacco can to retain the foul aroma. I also took some cheesecloth and string. When I reached my destination, I fashioned a little bag from this material and inserted a couple of small pieces of asafoetida. I drew the ends together, tied them with a length of string, and hung it around my neck so that it reached almost to my breastbone. I put my shirt back on and went forth to do my research.

Although my other two colleagues suffered terribly from the swarming hordes of mosquitoes, I was left virtually untouched except for a few bites on my lower extremities where the effect of the gum smell was somewhat weaker. I have since used it equally successfully to repel gnats. I highly recommend asafoetida as the *ultimate* insect repellant, especially if some slivers of raw garlic clove are included with it!

Headache Remedy from Kazakstan

Kazakstan was a constituent republic of the former Soviet Union, but is now an independent nation. It is in Central Asia bounded by Russia on the north, China to the east, the former Kirgiz and Uzbek Soviet republics on the south, and the Caspian Sea and a small portion of the former Soviet republic Turmen to the west.

Before the advent of Communism, the Kazaks were traditionally pastoral nomads, dwelling the year round in portable, dome-shaped tents (yurts) constructed of dismountable wooden frames, covered with felt; they would migrate seasonally to find pasture for their livestock. They bred horses, sheep, goats, cattle, and a few camels. Their diet consisted mainly of milk products supplemented by mutton. Fermented mare's milk (called koumiss) and horseflesh were highly esteemed but usually available only to the prosperous.

In Kazak folk medicine asafoetida was employed for a number of different ailments. The giant fennel from which it comes grows abundantly on its central steppes. Kazak folk healers would make decoctions from pieces of the dried gum and administer them to their patients suffering from excruciating headaches.

I wondered whether this particular remedy might be effective for modern day tension headaches. I advised several executive secretaries to put 1/8 teaspoon crumbled dried asafoetida in 1-1/2 cups hot water and let simmer for 15 minutes before drinking. In *every* case, they reported back on how quickly and easily their headaches had disappeared, showing me just how reliable folk medicine can be.

Preventing Snakebites

Some years ago the former Soviet Union became entrenched in a bitter and costly war with Afghanistan. A former Russian soldier, who served in that conflict and later emigrated to America, told me that the Afghan rebels would rub small chunks of asafoetida over their boots to keep away deadly snakes or vipers that lurked in the rocks of the treacherous mountainous terrain in which they lived for years.

Culinary Agent

Asafoetida is very popular for flavoring Indian vegetarian dishes since the awful odor disappears with cooking. The ancient Romans used it for flavoring sauces and wine. Ground asafoetida is the most convenient form to buy; in order to accommodate the strong flavor, use in minute quantities. A tiny pinch is just the right amount to use for any dish.

RICE WITH PINE NUTS AND MUSHROOMS

The Romans stored asafoetida in jars with pine nuts and used a few crushed nuts to flavor dishes. This particular version of risotto is a modern-day application.

Needed: 4 tablespoons unsalted butter; 4 oz. mushrooms, sliced; salt; freshly ground black pepper; 1 oz. pine nuts; 1-2/3 cups long-grain rice, cooked; a small pinch of asafoetida; 2 tablespoons finely chopped parsley.

Melt butter in frying pan, add mushrooms, and gently sauté over medium heat until lightly browned. Season to taste. In smaller frying pan, roast pine nuts, shaking pan back and forth every so often until they are very lightly browned. This will take about 3 minutes.

If necessary, reheat rice to warm through. Fold mushrooms, pine nuts, asafoetida, and parsley into rice and taste for seasoning. Serves 4.

ASH
(Fraxinus americana)
(Also see PRICKLY ASH)

Brief Description

The ashes comprise a large genus of deciduous trees valued for many different reasons. Practically all ashes have been planted for use in landscaping because they make excellent shade trees. A dozen varieties of European ash are cultivated. Native favorites for landscaping include white (F. americana) and green (F. pennsylvanica) ash in the eastern and central U.S. and velvet ash (F. velutina) in the Southwest.

Ash is a tall, handsome tree readily distinguished by its light-gray bark (smooth in younger trees but rough and scaly in older specimens) and by its unusual leaves. The large compound leaves are divided into 4 to 8 pairs of lance-shaped leaflets, tipped by a single one. This unique arrangement imparts a light feathery quality to the foliage in general. The leaflets have sharp-toothed margins and are about 3 inches in length.

Ash is the toughest and most resilient of all timber wood. In ancient times it was used for spears and bows. An ash joist will endure more weight before it snaps in two than one made from any other tree. It matures more rapidly than oak and is valuable as sapling wood. It has often been used to make higher quality handles for axes, hatchets, and shovels, as well as for wood ladders.

An Old Frontier Remedy

Settlers in 18th and 19th century America relied extensively on white ash to effectively treat a number of different problems such as: mastitis or breast inflammation; splenitis or enlargement of the spleen; a common form of eczema known as allergic or atopic dermatitis; gout and arthritis.

An infusion of white ash bark was the standard form used for treating these problems. One heaping tablespoon of the dried, chopped bark was added to one pint of boiling water, covered, and simmered on low heat for about ten minutes, then removed and allowed to steep for another 45 minutes. One cup of the strained tea was taken on an empty stomach a couple of times a day for internal problems; the skin was washed or a compress made for external purposes. If the powdered bark was used, only 1/2 teaspoon was added to 2 cups of boiling water and steeped 15 minutes before straining and drinking. The powder could also be mixed with a small amount of hot water and made into a paste to apply to the skin or around swollen breasts.

Expels Intestinal Parasites

An old frontier remedy for getting rid of scours and pin worms in horses and cattle called for some white ash bark to be burnt to ashes. This made a rather strong lye which was them mixed (1/2 pint) with one pint of luke-warm water and given to such animals two or three times daily.

The same remedy for humans calls for 1/2 teaspoon of burnt bark ashes stirred into 8 fluid ounces of warm water and then taken on an empty stomach for similar reasons.

ASHWAGANDHA
(WITHANIA SOMNIFERA)

Brief Description

Thanks in part to several best-sellers by Deepak Chopra, M.D. such as *Quantum Healing* (New York: Bantam Books, 1989) and *Perfect Health* (New York: Harmony Books, 1990), the ancient healing art from India known as Ayurveda has become quite popular throughout North America within the last half decade. He explained to me some time ago at an alternative health convention: "Ayurveda is nothing more than the human mind exerting its deepest influence on the body, thereby making us aware of the need to bring it more into balance with nature."

He noted that a number of different herbs and spices are employed in order that the greatest balance between mind and body may be achieved, so that one always enjoys freedom from sickness. One of the plants that helps to achieve this is ashwagandha. The name indicates the peculiar odor of this plant, which smells something akin to a sweaty horse. However, this erect branched shrub with the greenish or lurid yellow flowers, that is prolific in India, Pakistan and Sri Lanka, is esteemed in those parts of the world about as much as ginseng is in the Orient. Its active principles—alkaloids and withanoloids—are somewhat similar to those in ginseng; in fact, both are highly touted longevity-enhancing and sexually-stimulating properties.

Mental Problems Improved

One of the most promising uses for ashwagandha has been in the field of mental health. In the published monograph *Selected Medicinal Plants of*

India (Bombay: Chemexcil, 1992), a study was cited in which this herb was given to 30 mental patients suffering from anxiety neurosis in doses of 40 militers per day (in two equally divided doses) for one month; at the end of that time most of their anxiety disorders, panic attacks and similar mood phobias had pretty much dissipated. Ashwagandha has been used on an experimental basis by several American psychiatrists with some of their patients who've suffered from their own psychoses, generally marked by delusions, hallucinations, incoherent speech, or agitation. The psychotic disorders helped the most were manic depression, alcoholic paranoia, and schizophrenia. Up to four capsules were given daily, in between meals, for 45-60 days with very good results. Learning enhancement and memory retention have also been dramatically improved when ashwagandha (3 capsules), gotu kola (2 capsules), and ginkgo biloba (2 capsules) were taken regularly on a daily basis.

Anti-Tumor, Anti-Inflammatory Effects Noticed

Studies with rats and human volunteers have conclusively shown that ashwagandha is helpful in putting cancer tumors into regression (when used as an alcoholic root extract) and in reducing inflammation in rheumatoid arthritis. The plant's high steroid content has shown more potent action than hydrocortisone in animal and human arthritis. The standard recommended amounts for this and for sports injuries, according to Virender Sodhi, M.D. of Bellevue, Washington, is 3,000 to 6,000 mg. of the root powder or 500 mg. 3 times daily of the alcoholic extract.

ASPARAGUS
(ASPARAGUS OFFICINALIS)

Brief Description

Asparagus was cultivated in ancient times by the Romans. The vegetable is a member of the lily family and grows like a weed on the seacoasts of England and in the southern parts of the former USSR and of Poland, where the tundra steppes are literally covered with this garden delicacy, providing excellent grazing for cattle and horses.

Blemish Remover

For those bothered with blackheads, pimples and general facial and lip sores, this simple preparation might help. Tie 24 large spears into two separate bundles of 12 each. Trim even. Stand butts down in preheated boiling water up to about 1-1/2 inch below the tips. Simmer for half-hour uncovered until tender. Store cooked spears in refrigerator and use in the recipe below. Save the asparagus water for cleansing the face morning and night.

Remedies Kidney Problems

Cooked asparagus and its watery juice are very good for helping to dissolve uric acid deposits in the extremities, as well as inducing urination where such a function might be lacking or only done on an infrequent basis. Asparagus is especially useful in cases of hypertension where the amount of sodium in the blood far exceeds the potassium present. Cooked asparagus also increases bowel evacuations.

Handy Casserole

This has been adapted from *Recipes to Lower Your Fat Thermostat* (see Appendix) with permission of the publisher.

LUSCIOUS-LAYERED CASSEROLE

Needed: 1 cup sliced onion; 1 cup chopped green pepper;1 cup sliced mushrooms; 1/2 lb. sliced potatoes;1 cup thinly sliced carrots;1/3 cup raw brown rice; 1-3/4 cups short parboiled asparagus spears (use those in remedy above); round kelp; 3 1/2 cups stewed, mashed tomatoes (you can replace the tomatoes with onion soup and turn this into a different casserole).

Sauté the onion, pepper and mushrooms in a lightly oiled frying pan set on medium heat. Use either olive oil or lecithin from your local health food store to oil pan and baking dish. Next place sliced potatoes in a 2-1/2 qt. baking dish. Then alternate layers of carrots, rice, onion mixture and asparagus. Finally stir kelp into mashed tomatoes and pour over the vegetables. Cover and bake in preheated oven at 350º F. for 2 hours. Serves 8.

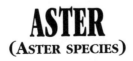

ASTER
(ASTER SPECIES)

Brief Description

Asters are common in open fields from the Colorado Rockies through the heartland of America's Midwest all the way up to New England. Often reaching a height of 3 feet, asters have dense leaves covered with bristly hairs. They bear clusters of flowers at the tips of leafy branches. The flowers themselves are a unique blend of golden yellow in the middle surrounded by violet-purple. These hardy perennials will self-propagate in even the poorest soil if there is adequate moisture to help them survive.

An Ornamental for Bleeding and Diarrhea

Who would ever think by looking at asters that they would be extremely useful in cases of hemorrhaging, excessive menstruation, bloody stool or urine, and diarrhea? But after having experimented with these beautiful wildflowers for several years, I've discovered they make an excellent remedy for these problems.

This is the way I recommend using asters: gather a handful of the top plants, wash them in a colander under running water to remove bugs and dirt, and then steep them in a quart of boiling water for 30 minutes. Pour the liquid through a strainer and refrigerate, discarding the solid materials.

Drink one cup every four hours on an empty stomach for excessive internal bleeding or to curb diarrhea. CAUTION: Be sure to wear gloves when gathering. *Do not* gather from any fields that may have been sprayed, or by railroad tracks or roadsides.

ASTRAGALUS
(ASTRAGALUS MEMBRANACEUS)

Brief Description

Astragalus is a twining leguminous perennial plant that grows 11-1/2 to 39 inches high. The stem has many branches, slanting upward and slightly hairy. The pinnate leaves are alternate and the 9 to 21 leaflets are elliptical-shaped, 1/4 to 3/4 inches long and about 1/3 inch wide. The racemes are axillary and the peduncle slender, with anywhere from 3 to 9 flowers growing at the top. The pod is spindle-shaped, inflated, a little over an inch in length and beaked at its tip. It has 20 to 30 seeds. It grows in grasses or in thickets on hillsides in northwest China, Manchuria and Mongolia.

Medicinal value is in the root. Astragalus root is flexible and long, as large as your forefinger, and covered with a tough, wrinkled, yellowish-brown skin, which has a tendency to break up into woolly fibers. The woody interior is of a yellowish-white color and has a faint sweetish taste that reminds you of licorice root.

Tonic for Physical Exhaustion

There are certain energy-draining diseases that leave a victim's body thoroughly exhausted, such as chronic fatigue syndrome, candidiasis, herpes simplex, mononucleosis, and hypoglycemia. A number of different measures, including dietary, herbal, nutritional and drug, are resorted to by those who are desperately seeking solutions to their problems.

In Oriental medicine one herb stands out as extremely useful as a remedy for this physical weakness: astragalus root. It has been employed by Chinese herbalists for "every sort of wasting or exhausting disease." It seems to work best, however, when used in conjunction with Korean ginseng root (see GINSENG). While both herbs are available in capsule form, they make their greatest impact when administered as a tea.

Bring one pint of water to a boil; add one teaspoon each of dried, cut astragalus and ginseng roots. Cover and simmer on low heat for 5 minutes, then remove and steep for 20 minutes. Strain and drink 1-2 cups before a meal twice daily for badly needed boosts of energy that can last up to 5 hours.

Increase Your Resistance to Disease

Traditional Oriental medicine teaches that astragalus root is a wonderful tonic for the "spleen" and "lung chis." Chi is considered to be the vital energy of the body. Most of the different kinds of chi are usually explained in terms of their "sphere of influence" or part of the body. It should be pointed out, though, that the naming of the chi for the body's organs doesn't strictly correlate with our concept of these organs. When an Oriental herb doctor remarks that astragalus root "tonifies the spleen," it doesn't mean that the effect is on the physical organ that removes foreign bodies and damaged cells from the blood. Instead, it refers to a concept of health and the body's energy in balance.

The "spleen chi" is referred to as the "middle burner," where our body's energy builds. When our "life energy" becomes deficient, astragalus root is believed to increase or supplement it. More interesting is the fact that this herb is said to "stabilize the exterior" of the body, which Oriental herbalists interpret as protecting the system against disease. This equates to our own concept of increasing resistance.

The root works best to reinvigorate the immune system *before* disease occurs; it does not work as well once sickness has set in. Astragalus capsules (3 per day) or the tea (1 cup daily) can be taken on a regular basis for prevention of illness.

Shrinkage of Some Cancer Tumors

In 1987 I attended the 28th annual meeting of the American Society of Pharmacognosy at the University of Rhode Island. I had a chance to meet Dr. Chang-xu Hu from the Institute of Botany with the Academia Sinica in Beijing, China, who was there to deliver a paper on some wonderful immune-stimulating compounds that had recently been isolated from astragalus root.

Over lunch he explained how Chinese research has demonstrated that an extract of the root stimulated T-cell production in sick animals and restored immune function in impaired cancer patients. In some instances, he noted, "malignant tumors showed regression."

He indicated that the root tea displayed the greatest anti-tumor activity, particularly when used in conjunction with other therapies.

ATRACTYLIS
(ATRACTYLODES LANCEA)

Brief Description

Atractylis is the name given to several different species of the genus of medicinal plants known as Atractylodes. In Chinese they are collectively called *zhu*; there is cang zhu (a blue-green variety) and bai zhu (a white type). The bai zhu kind is rarer and considered to be more therapeutic.

The roots of the atractylis plants, when cut open, reveal a beautiful yellow-orange resin clinging to the interstices. This substance can be dissolved in spirits to produce a yellowish tincture, which when further purified produces the botanical drugs atractylol, atractylon, atractylodin, and atractylilodinol. When tested in experimental animals, they demonstrate the ability to increase the body's utilization of glucose, and to lower elevated blood sugar levels.

An Herb for Diabetics

Many people still look for the proverbial "magic pill" (or in this case "magic herb") that will solve all of their problems. Unfortunately there is no such thing as "the magic bullet" for any disease.

Some herbs like goldenseal, garlic, onion, cayenne, and pau d'arco are decidedly hypoglycemic and, therefore, of obvious benefit to diabetics.

They generally treat the symptoms, but do very little in correcting the problem itself. But atractylis differs in this respect: it *strengthens* those major organs directly involved in diabetes.

In Chinese traditional medicine, the spleen, pancreas and liver that are involved in the metabolism of sugar for energy are supported by the heart, lungs and kidneys. The use of atractylis *with* other herbs in something as serious as diabetes, appears to act not so much as a cure, as it does to *strengthen* the chis or vital energies of each of these individual organs.

It therefore should be thought of always as an energy *tonic* and metabolic balancer. Atractylis works best when combined with other herbs such as the roots of ginseng or licorice; it is more of a *formula* herb. Its combination with several other Oriental herbs should be taken routinely when problems like diabetes exist. Three capsules daily with a meal is recommended.

A Guarantee for Stopping Hemorrhages

A number of different herbs has been repeatedly recommended for prolonged bleeding in many of the herbal books available today. But none of them, to my knowledge, specifically indicates atractylis for this problem. I found information in a voluminous work entitled *Zhong Yao Lin Chuang Sheng Yong Yu Zhi Yong* [The Clinical Use of Fresh and Prepared Chinese Herbs] (Beijing: People's Medical Publishing House, 1981).

Some interesting hematologic effects were noted in a couple of experiments conducted on rodents and in humans. When decoctions of atractylis root were administered via gastric lavage to rats, it was discovered that their prothrombin or blood-clot forming times were "mildly elevated." So a tablespoon of a 1:20 solution of the same decoction of this root was given to healthy volunteers three times a day for four days. There was "a significant prolongation of the prothrombin time" observed; this didn't return to normal until almost ten days after administration had ceased. Alcohol-based tinctures had a considerably weaker effect.

What this information tells us is that a tea made from atractylis root and sipped in small half-cupful amounts several times daily on an empty stomach will help to bolster the blood's coagulation ability; this is important for those experiencing continued bleeding, whether it be internal or external. In one pint of water put 1-1/2 tablespoons of atractylis root, cover, simmer for 5 minutes, then steep away from the heat for 30 minutes; strain and drink as previously directed.

AZALEA
(RHODODENDRON SPECIES)

Brief Description

The azaleas common to North America are usually deciduous, while those in Asia are evergreen. Most azaleas grow in damp, acid soils of hills or mountains. The better known garden varieties cultivated by many Americans include the flame azalea of the Appalachians, the pinxter flower and the fragrant white azalea or swamp honeysuckle of the eastern U.S., and the Western azalea common to Oregon and California.

Hispanic Solution to Lice, Ringworm, and Chiggers

Lice are tiny, sluggish, blood-sucking parasites that live on man and beast alike. Ringworm is a contagious disease of the hair, skin, and nails of man and domestic animals that is caused by fungi and shows up on the skin in the form of ring-shaped discolored patches covered with vesicles and scales. Chiggers (also spelled "jiggers") are tiny six-legged larval mites that suck blood from their hosts and cause intense skin irritation.

Elena Rodriquez, an expert *curandera* (folk healer) residing in the southwest, has an effective way of handling all three problems. She showed me how to boil up a handful of azaleas in equal parts (one pint each) of water and tequila (a Mexican liquor), then cover the pot and simmer on low heat for 10 minutes, before setting aside and steeping for another 40 minutes. She strains the liquid, bottles it, and stores it in a cool, dry place until needed.

She explained that the scalp, skin and nails should be routinely bathed with some of this liquid several times a day. She suggests using WISK detergent in place of soap with this azalea tea. Her method is guaranteed to remove lice, ringworm and chiggers in a short time.

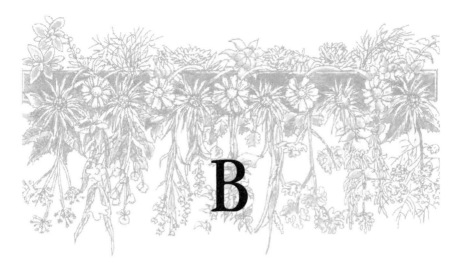

B

BABY'S BREATH
(GYPSOPHILIA PANICULATA)

Brief Description

Baby's breath is popular with many florists as an attractive accompaniment to roses and other cut flowers. It produces a spray of tiny white, pink or reddish flowers on a diffuse array of small branches. Various species of *Gypsophilia* often appear as favorite perennials in outdoor rock gardens.

Bronchitis Treatment from Austria

Dr. Ahron Forschung has been in medical practice in Salzburg, Austria for several decades. His specialty is treating disorders of the respiratory and gastrointestinal systems. Like his other medical colleagues, he was at one time averse to using herbs, but eventually came around to considering a few medicinal plants for some of his more serious cases.

One of the plants with which he has experimented has been baby's breath. In stubborn cases of bronchitis, he found that nothing else works quite as well as a hot tea made from the roots of this garden ornamental. His usual method of preparation is to have the patient boil two heaping tablespoons of the chopped fresh or dried roots in one quart of water on medium heat, covered, for 20 minutes. The tea is then removed from the heat and simmered another 20 minutes before being strained. Patients with bronchial problems are instructed to drink one cup of *warm* tea every 5 hours or in between meals. He claims it works wonders for them in dislodging the mucus and helping them to breathe better.

BALM

(see LEMON BALM)

BALM OF GILEAD

(see POPLAR)

BAMBOO
(Bambus arundinacea)

Brief Description

Some years ago I had the opportunity to visit the Wang Valley in northern Thailand. Taking only minutes to pass through one of the local villages in the region, the *song-tao*, or "two-bench" pickup truck, was well on its way to Kao Pah Nam (Wild Thorn Hill), a craggy spine of limestone clothed in treacherous thorn scrub. Those of us in the *song-tao* had enough sense to lean into the center of the vehicle to avoid having the razor-sharp thorns rake open our flesh.

Reaching our destination, my guides and I filed out of the pick-up truck, impatient to flex cramped limbs, shake off the layers of cold dust, and rub new bruises. From the forest around us came the complacent, comforting cooing of "forest chickens" as the local natives called them. Suddenly, a series of loud explosions silenced the birds and startled me. I inquired about who was setting off the dynamite blasts. My guides seemed rather unperturbed by the disturbance and couldn't figure out why I had suddenly become so excited.

Finally one of them told me in halting English that it was just exploding bamboo. Some local villagers had set fire to an unseen grove of bamboo; the air in the sealed bases of the hollow bamboo trunks expanded until they blew apart, felling the giant stalks. Millenniums ago such explosions were actually the first fireworks known to man. In fact, the very name originally appropriated to it because of such loud explosions was BAMBOOM, later shortened to "bamboo."

A Light Bulb of an Idea Inside Mr. Edison's Head

One of the world's great inventors, Thomas Alva Edison, read in some Oriental medical literature that bamboo tea was a useful aphrodisiac for impotence. He made tea by adding one-half cup cut green bamboo to one pint of boiling water, covering and simmering for 10 minutes, then straining and drinking one cup twice daily. He is reported to have said that there was a "quiver of excitement" (his own words) in a certain part of his anatomy.

But drinking the tea actually gave him an idea for something far more important. When Edison was inventing the incandescent lamp, he had to find an appropriate material for a filament. During the time he was drinking this bamboo tea in 1880, he also learned that finely shredded slivers of this plant served as a firm support for round hemp palm leaf fans. Taking this hint, he collected all available varieties of bamboo from throughout the world, including species from Southeast Asia and Japan. After many experiments, he ascertained that a variety from Kyoto would best serve his purpose. Two years later, he set up a company to produce incandescent lamps from the filaments of Japanese bamboo and illuminated the nights of New York City.

Withstands Radiation

The following medicinal discovery came about more out of my curiosity than anything else. I hypothesized that bamboo tea might be good for those who had been exposed to large amounts of radiation over a long period of time.

The Second World War demonstrated the capacity of this plant to withstand powerful A-bomb blasts. According to one eyewitness in Hiroshima at the time the Enola Gay dropped the first atomic bomb, "A flash over my city on 6 August, 1945, announced the arrival of the most horrible havoc imaginable ...Within a matter of seconds streets and houses collapsed, trees and grasses were charred to bits, and 200,000 souls...one-half of my city's total population...perished...in the wake of the relentless destruction, however, one living thing held out. In the very epicenter, a thicket of bamboo stood through the blast, suffering only one side to be scorched."

When I heard this I wondered if bamboo might not be an effective medicinal agent for those who had had long-term exposure to radiation. After a little experimentation I finally settled on a tea made from the foliage leaves. Some of these stalked blades were cut up into very small pieces, enough to make about a cup of bamboo leaves. These were then simmered in 3 cups boiling water for 25 minutes, uncovered. The tea was allowed to cool before being strained and drunk.

Several people who lived in southern Utah, near the city of St. George, who had been exposed for decades to many of the nuclear bomb blast tests in the adjacent Nevada desert, kindly volunteered to try this tea. They were part of a larger group known as "Downwinders," a name given them by the media because they lived downwind from the direction in which much of the radioactive dust blew every time there was an above-ground test.

Now those who volunteered for my 8-month study had not as yet been diagnosed with cancer. But a number of their friends and relatives, who resided in the same general area, had previously been diagnosed positive and some had already died when my research began. In the time that these few volunteers drank two cups of bamboo tea 3 to 5 times a week, none of them experienced an occurrence of cancer. Even after my research ended (8 months), several families still continued drinking the tea on their own.

From what I could tell, those who stayed with the bamboo tea for at least a year or more seemed to be at *lower risk* for developing cancer related to the nuclear blasts in the desert. Bamboo tea afforded them some kind of reasonable protection in that it either delayed tumor development or else helped to flush radioactive isotopes from their body tissues.

BARBERRY
(BERBERIS VULGARIS)

Brief Description

This stout shrub has yellow wood and spiny, hollylike leaves that are arranged in fives or sevens. Flowers appear in little grapelike bright yellow clusters, blooming in late spring to early summer; afterwards they ripen into slightly inflated berries, which turn a dull purple in higher elevations and dull brown in the desert. The berries taste about 90% "yeecch" and only 10% "yummy."

The stems grow from 3 to 9 feet tall and the plants generally form irregular bunches, The most distinguishing feature of *all* barberries is the bright, almost fluorescent yellow rootwood; the golden hue is due to a nasty-tasting alkaloid called berberine (which also occurs in goldenseal root).

Navajo Healer Blesses Flag and Cures Fevers

Ross Nez of Teesto, Arizona is one of a dwindling number of Navajo "singers" or shamans. For years he has used medicinal herbs to cure diseases in hundreds of Navajo patients. One of his favorite remedies is barberry root bark for fevers of all kinds. Ross digs around the base of a bar-berry shrub, uses his pocket knife to cut away a few of the roots, but leaves the rest so the bush won't die. He then scrapes away slivers of the outside bark until there is the equivalent of one-half palm full. This he throws into an old coffeepot partly filled with about 1-1/2 pints hot water and lets the mixture percolate on low heat for about 20 minutes. Then he strains the tea and gives one cupful to a patient stricken with fever. He repeats this every four hours and makes sure it is taken on an empty stomach. He swears it has never failed to work for him in all the years he has been a practicing medicine man.

Nez achieved unintentional media fame in early February 1995 when he was invited to bless a Navajo flag that was carried into space aboard the shuttle Discovery by Bernard Harris, a physician, who grew up on the Navajo reservation and who was to be the first African American to walk in space. Navajo President Albert Hale sanctioned the flag's blessing after being reassured by Harris and the rest of the Discovery astronauts that the shuttle's orbit would follow the route of the sun. Hale told reporters that Nez's blessing of the flag was a "symbol of our nation and reminded us of how we must live in balance with Mother Earth to survive."

Harris watched as Nez, the medicine man, poured a little corn pollen from a deerskin pouch he carried and tossed it into the wind in the hopes that it would bring goodness for the astronaut and the tribal flag he would soon be carrying into outer space. At the same time Ross started "singing" a typical Navajo blessing prayer in a low, monotone chant that lasted for several minutes.

Tea for Constipation, Hangover and Hepatitis

Nez informed me that the same tea he used for curing fevers was also effective for promoting bowel movement in cases of constipation, in clearing up alcoholic hangovers, and in returning the blood to normal in those with a history of hepatitis. Half-cup doses every 6-8 hours was what he recommended.

BARLEY GRASS
(HORDEUM VULGARE)

Brief Description

Barley is an annual cereal plant cultivated by man since the very beginnings of civilization. It was known to the ancient Sumerians, Egyptians, Chinese, Greeks and Romans. Barley remained the chief bread staple in Europe as late as the 16th century. It has a wide range of cultivation and matures even at high altitudes, since its growing period is short; however, it can't withstand hot and humid climates.

Today barley is typically a special-purpose grain with many varieties rather than a general market crop. It's a valuable stock feed (often as a corn substitute) and is used for malting when the grain is of high quality. It's also a minor source of flour and breakfast foods. Pearl barley is often used in soups. In the Middle East a limited amount of barley is eaten like rice.

Gluten Allergies Abated with Barley Chlorophyll

Celiac disease is an internal physical condition brought about by gluten intolerance. Barley grass contains no gluten and can be used safely to combat the symptoms of this allergy. The immune system mounts a defense against things it can't tolerate; the chlorophyll nutrients in barley grass dilute and enhance the elimination of the offending substance in the digestive tract that is produced by the immune system.

Several alternative-minded allergy specialists in southern California have been recommending a unique powdered drink containing barley to many of their allergy-prone patients. The product, called Kyo-Green, contains the concentrated juices of young barley and wheat grasses, brown rice shoots, an algae called chlorella, and giant seaweed called kelp (dubbed "redwoods of the ocean" by marine biologists for their towering heights). These doctors recommend that their allergic patients take one rounded teaspoon (2.5 grams) of the powder and add it to 6 or 8 fluid ounces of distilled water. After it is properly stirred the resulting emerald-green drink is taken on an empty stomach for maximum efficiency.

Energy Booster Par Excellence

Stanley Hirsch is a high school coach in southern California. He said he has routinely given glasses of barley grass juice powder (1 teaspoon) mixed with tomato or V-8 juice (7 fluid ounces) to his star athletes before a major competition or game in order to "boost their energy levels dramatically." He noted that "every one of my kids who've drunk their Kyo-Green and tomato concoctions have done well" in their respective sports. (See the Appendix under Wakunauga of America for more information on Kyo-Green, which can be purchased at most health food stores or nutrition centers.)

BASIL
(Ocimum basilicum)

Brief Description

Basil is cultivated worldwide as an annual plant. Many varieties have different compositions and flavoring characteristics. The herb is strongly affected by environmental factors like temperature, geographic location, soil and amount of rainfall. Its thin branching root produces bushy stems growing from 1-2 feet high and bearing leaves of a purple hue, and two-lipped flowers, varying in color from white to red, sometimes with a purple tinge.

A Multi-Purpose Health Tea

Maurice Messegue, a world-renowned French herbal folk healer, swears by basil as an excellent nightcap tea for restlessness and migraines. He also recommends the tea to promote more milk in nursing mothers, and as a useful gargle for *Candida albicans* or yeast infection of the mouth and throat. It's also very good for women to take before and after childbirth to promote blood circulation.

The steaming tea is also good for a patient with fever to inhale while covered with a blanket. Cool basil tea is good for all kinds of eye problems, both as an eyewash and internal tea.

Obviously fresh basil leaves and unground seeds are the best to use when making a tea. If such is obtainable in your immediate area, bring 2 pints of water to a boil and add 15 basil seeds. Cover and reduce the heat, slowly simmering for about 45 minutes. Remove from heat and add 1-1/2 handfuls of fresh or half-dried basil and steep for another 25 minutes or so.

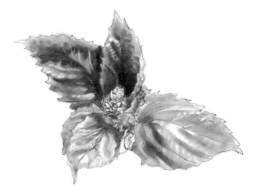

Drink or gargle with this tea on the average of 2 cups per day as needed. When lukewarm, the strained tea can also be used to bathe the eyes.

If ground basil is all that's available, another form of tea can be made and used for most of the previously described problems *except* as an eye-wash. Bring 3- 1/2 cups of water to a boil; remove from heat and add 1-1/4 level teaspoons ground basil. Cover and steep for half an hour. Sweeten with a touch of pure maple syrup and drink on the average 1 cup twice daily.

Magical Headache Reliever

Ever had a headache and needed a simple relief remedy? It's easy to pre-pare. Just take a level teaspoon of dried, ground basil and put into 1 cup hot water for 10 minutes, then strain. When the liquid is cool, add 2 table-spoons Tincture of Witch Hazel that's been previously refrigerated for a while. You can get the Witch Hazel tincture at your local drugstore or supermarket pharmacy section. Apply the solution as a compress to the forehead and temples, for relief you wouldn't believe possible!

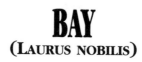

BAY
(LAURUS NOBILIS)

Brief Description

Bay laurel or sweet bay is a small evergreen shrub or tree native to the Mediterranean region and Asia Minor. It has been admired for its beauty and aromatic leaves since Greek and Roman times. The leaves are leathery, lanceolate, pointed and experience maximum oil content increases during early and mid-summer only. Several botanicals are known by the name of "bay"—i.e., West Indian bay (*Pimenta racemosa*) and California bay (*Umbellularia californica*). Hence, the term *bay* in the existing herb litera-ture can mean any one of these botanicals, among others.

Anti-Dandruff Rinse

Bay makes a terrific anti-dandruff rinse. Simply bring a quart of water to a boil. Remove from heat and add approximately 3 level teaspoons of crum-pled bay leaves. Cover and let steep for 25 minutes. Strain and refrigerate tea. When washing your hair, first rinse all soap out with ordinary water. Then pour some liquid bay tea on your head and massage well into the scalp. Follow with a few more ounces of the same cool tea, working it in well with your fingertips. Leave in the hair for about an hour or so, then rinse out. Should keep dandruff from occurring if used faithfully each day.

Bronchitis and Cough Remedy

Use boiled bay leaves as a poultice applied directly on the chest and covered with a cloth to relieve bronchitis and hacking cough.

Benefit to Arthritic Pain

Oil of bay may be rubbed on arthritic aches and pains, muscle sprains and tendon swellings for relief. To make the oil, simply heat some of the leaves in a little olive oil over very low heat for about 20 minutes without actually cooking the oil too much or causing it to burn and smoke. Set aside and allow the leaves to further simmer for a while. Strain and use the oil as needed for these conditions and others like lower backache, varicose veins and so forth.

BAYBERRY BARK
(MYRICA CERIFERA)

Brief Description

Wax myrtle or bayberry is an evergreen shrub native to the eastern U.S. from New Jersey to southern Florida and west to Texas. It also grows in the Bahamas, West Indies and Bermuda. The fruit is a grayish-white, round drupe-like nut covered with a waxy crust. The medicinal properties are similar to those of wild oregon grape root or barberry (*Berberis vulgaris*).

Cures, Prevents Varicose Veins

Mike Tierra, a practicing California herbalist, recommends bayberry for "relieving, curing and preventing varicose veins" as a fomentation. It is made by dipping a moisture-absorbent towel or cloth into some bayberry tea and applying the towel over the affected legs as hot as can be tolerated without burning. The towel is covered by dry flannel cloth and a heating pad or a hot water bottle is placed on top of this. A plastic covering can be used to protect bedding if applied overnight.

Reduces Fever, Expels Parasites

To make a potent tea for using externally for varicose veins, and internally for raging fevers, intestinal parasites, and liver and kidney problems, simply bring 1 quart of water to a boil, then add 2-3 tablespoons of chopped bark, cover and simmer on low heat for 5 minutes. Remove and let steep for an additional 40 minutes. Strain, sweeten with honey or pure maple syrup and drink. Take about 2-3 cups per day as needed.

An Aid in Women's Complaints

Two to three cups of tea per day, consumed orally or used as a douche, are of value in stopping bleeding of the lungs, bowels and uterus, in treating prolapsed uterus, excessive menstruation and vaginal discharge. Also it's a darned good laxative, either in capsules (3 at a time) or tea (1-2 cups daily).

BEAN
(PHASEOLUS VULGARIS)

Brief Description

"Kidney bean" is occasionally used to designate all kinds of beans. Here it is used in a very limited sense to specify only the large, purplish-brown, characteristically kidney-shaped field bean. An average kidney bean is usually a half-inch long and red in color.

The plant on which such a bean grows is a twining annual that originated in South America; it is still the predominant bean cultivated throughout the Americas. The leaves of the kidney bean plant are alternate, each leaf consisting of three broad-ovate to rhombic-ovate, entire, pointed leaflets. The white, yellow or purplish flowers grow in sparse, axillary clusters. The bean itself is contained in a green or yellow pod.

A Diabetic Tea That Really Works

Kidney bean pods are really effective in lowering elevated blood sugar levels without disturbing already low blood sugar levels. In other words, the pods can be safely used by diabetics *and* hypoglycemics alike! It won't do much for the latter, but certainly won't upset them either.

Since a large amount of the pods would have to be consumed each day by a diabetic to do any good (about 16 lbs.), it is obviously more practical to make a tea instead. The pods should be picked before the beans inside ripen, and *fresh* pods are more effective than dried ones by 8 to 1.

Bring 3 quarts of water to a boil, toss in five handfuls of coarsely cut kidney bean pods, and cook uncovered for 3 hours. Strain and drink 3/4 quart a day with meals.

Good for Arthritis, Gout, and Sciatica

The same tea is also very useful in removing uric acid crystal from body tissues and joints. Once these toxic accumulations are flushed out of the system, then many of the painful symptoms of arthritis and gout soon disappear. Kidney bean pod tea is also helpful in easing the pain that accompanies sciatica.

BEARBERRY

(see UVA URSI)

BEARDED DARNEL
(LOLIUM TEMULENTUM)

Brief Description

One of the great parables in the New Testament contains an indirect reference to bearded darnel. In Matthew 13:24-30 we find this little story:

> The kingdom of heaven is likened unto a man which sowed good seed in his field. But while men slept, his enemy came and sowed tares among the wheat, and went his way. But when the blade was sprung up, and brought forth fruit, then appeared the tares also.
>
> So the servants of the householder came and said unto him, "Sir, wilt thou then that we go and gather them up?" But he said "Nay. Let them grow together until the harvest. And in the time of harvest, gather ye together first the tares, and bind them in bundles to burn; but gather the wheat into my barn."

The "tares" here are nothing more than bearded darnel, which close-ly resembles wheat in many ways, but only in the early stages of growth. Darnel is common to Israel and Syria and grows right up along with plant-ed wheat. But bearded darnel can't be distinguished from normal grain until the ear appears; this proverbial tare resembles wheat in form, but is smaller and dark in appearance.

Both darnel and wheat belong to the same class and order of grass-es. They are easily distinguished when in flower: darnel has one glume and its florets have their backs next to the rachis or common stalk; wheat has two glumes and its florets have their edges next to the rachis.

Skin Wash for Herpes and Bedsores

When taken internally for very long or in large amounts, bearded darnel can cause hallucinations or mild convulsions. But externally, it is terrific for some skin problems. Bring a quart of water to boil and add three level tablespoons of bearded darnel seed. Cover and simmer on low heat for 25 minutes. Steep an additional 40 minutes.

Bathe herpes lesions, genital sores and bedsores with this tea 4 or 5 times every day. In fact, two cotton balls can be pressed together and thor-oughly saturated in some of the tea, with excess liquid being gently squeezed out. Then they can be laid on top of a sore and taped in place for several hours before changing them. Healing is rapid with this procedure.

Medical Treatment for Dizziness and Insomnia

Some Near East doctors will occasionally prescribe bearded darnel tea for treating dizziness and insomnia. The tea is given only, however, in small amounts (1/4 to 1/2 cup) and not for very long (10 days at the most). But this should only be done under medical supervision.

Bearded darnel is common to wheat fields throughout the world, including those of the U.S. and Canada.

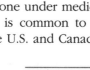

BEDSTRAW

(see CLEAVERS)

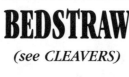

BEE BALM

(see BERGAMOT)

BEECH
(FAGUS GRANDIFOLIA)

Brief Description

The American beech is a magnificent tree with a trunk circumference that can reach almost 4 feet in diameter and a towering height of more than 100 feet. Its green leaves, 2 to 5 inches in length, turn brightly silky before they mature, beautifully yellow in the autumn. Its closely clasping, bluish or light gray bark, frequently blotched in the autumn, is smooth. During winters the American species can't be mistaken for any other native tree on account of its slim, distinctively cone-like, scaly buds about an inch in length.

Both the pollen-rich male flowers and the pistillate female blossoms grow on the same tree, the latter in pairs where the upper leaves lift from the twigs. These mature in the autumn into small, hairy, four-part burrs, readily opened by the thumbnail to reveal two tiny, brown, triangular, concave nuts eagerly sought after by noisy birds and squirrels, as well as hungry humans. Deer like to nibble the buds, twigs, foliage, and bark.

Bach Flower Remedy for Intolerance

A renowned British physician, Dr. Edward Bach (1886-1936) originated the concept of flower remedies, based on earlier studies from several centuries before him. His plant sources were employed to treat the mental and emotional side of illness, rather than the actual disease itself. The beech remedy was intended for persons who are intolerant of others, and always passing judgments upon them without due cause. Seven drops under the tongue twice daily or in water for up to two weeks is the standard therapy.

Treatment for Frostbite, Scalds, and Burns

Early Native American tribes in the eastern United States and Canada relied on beech leaves as effective treatments for frostbitten fingers and toes and injured skin that had been accidentally scalded with hot liquid or else burned by fire.

The equivalent of three tablespoons of fresh or dried beech leaves was put into about 2-1/2 cups boiling water and simmered over a low campfire for 30 minutes or longer. Native Americans and early fur trappers and explorers then strained and cooled the tea before dipping their fingers or toes into the liquid. Scalds and burns were frequently washed or else cloth poultices of the tea were applied.

Diaper and Poison Ivy/Oak Rash Cleared Up

Some Native American tribes of the early 19th century, such as the Rappahannocks, would cut bits of the tree bark from the north side (which was usually darker) and steep them in 2 cups of slightly salted hot water until the liquid was well-colored. They used this to bathe parts of the body afflicted with poison ivy/oak inflammation. Squaws would often bathe their babies to clear up diaper rashes.

Good Gangrene Remedy

Beech tree roots are sometimes subject to a parasitic growth, which has a horrible taste when fresh but goes away when dried. If this is made into a strong tea and applied locally to gangrenous ulcers, it will soon arrest the infection.

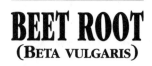

BEET ROOT
(BETA VULGARIS)

Brief Description

Garden beet is undoubtedly a native of the Eastern Mediterranean countries, but it grown the world over. It is a small, red type, probably developed by selection from a larger stock beet. There are two general subtypes: the long, tapering turnip-rooted type and the short or fat ball type. They vary somewhat in interior color. The ideal color, though, is a full dark red with no white stripes.

Food Chemotherapy for Cancer

For several years now I've served as editor of an annual publication, *Folk Medicine Journal*. It covers all manner of alternative medicine topics, but from a strictly "hands-on, do-it-yourself" approach. In the first volume was an English translation of an original article representing the research of a Hungarian physician, Dr. Alexander Ferenczi, which he conducted on hundreds of patients between 1955 and 1959.

What was so remarkable about his work was that he used an ordinary food for the remission of many different types of cancer. This "beet root chemotherapy" has been used with amazing results since then by other qualified doctors. I've excerpted some of the more important points from his original research report.

"Since October 1950, we tested in our department [for Internal Diseases at the district hospital in Csoma, Hungary] the tumor-inhibiting action of beetroot...We gave this to [cancer] patients raw, finely grated, 200-250 grams [7-8.5 ounces] spread over the day after meals...If the patient could not take it in this way, the grated beetroot was pressed by means of a handpress...1 kilogram [2 1/4 lbs.] beetroot yielded approximately 300 milliliters [about 1/2 pint] juice, which the patient also took, spread over the day after meals.

"...I tried the above mentioned treatment also on other patients. Naturally, all the patients were inoperable...and other forms of treatment ....were ruled out. Up to now, I had 22 patients of this kind: ten with tumor of the lung, four with cancer of the stomach, two with cancer of the breast, one with metastasis after an operated cancer of the lip, one with cancer of the prostate, one with cancer of the uterus, one with cancer of the skin... The treatment with beetroot was started on many more patients; however, only a few were able to continue the treatment over a longer period. Those suffering from cancer of the liver or stomach in particular were not able to tolerate continued consumption of the [fresh] beetroot.

"The result was that out of 22 patients , 21 showed an improvement, manifesting itself by a shrinking of the tumor, a gain in weight of 3-11 kilograms [6.5–24-1/4 lbs.]...and also an improvement in appetite and general state of health. Unfortunately, after three to four months, the patients stopped taking the beetroot whereupon after two to three further months, their condition started to deteriorate.

"Experience gained up to now points to the fact that beetroot contains a tumor-inhibiting (anti-cancerous) active ingredient. However, for the present, no clue has been found as to the nature of this active substance. One thing is certain: beetroot is fairly stable because it acts when taken orally; therefore, digestion does not harm it. The very apparent red color may suggest that the active substance is the coloring matter. Treatment with beetroot presents several advantages over the rest of the medication used in the treatment of cancer. Firstly, because it is non-toxic and one can administer red beetroot in unlimited quantities. Also, there are unlimited supplies of beetroot at our disposal. We have therefore endeavored to administer to the patient this active substance in the most concentrated form and in the largest quantities possible..."

There is only one source in the United States for the *concentrated form* that Dr. Ferenczi employed in his many successful cancer treatments. It is organic beet root juice powder available in bulk from the following company: Pines International, P.O.Box 1107, Lawrence, KS 66044 (1-800-642-PINE). One level tablespoonful in 8 fluid ounces of water or juice of some kind (liquid chlorophyll is the best) every morning before breakfast will dramatically increase a person's resistance to cancer. However, in the event that some kind of cancer is already present, then this amount should be doubled or even tripled each day, but always taken *with meals* and never on an empty stomach. Due to the increased intake, the stomach or liver may reject some of it unless accompanied by other *solid* food.

BELLADONNA
(ATROPA BELLADONNA)

Brief Description

Belladonna is also called "deadly nightshade" for its potentially poisonous properties if used without wisdom and experience. This perennial has a leafy, smooth, branched stem that can reach up to six feet in height and is attached to a thick creeping rootstock. The leaves are dull green, of unequal-sized pairs that are 7-1/2 inches long, bearing solitary bell-shaped purplish-brown drooping flowers that are about three-quarters of an inch in diameter in their axis. They appear from the middle of summer to early fall, followed by shiny black berries.

Reduces Pain

Belladonna was first mentioned in a medical book composed by the Roman physician Galen. He employed it for relieving the medical condition that doctors now refer to as heart arrhythmia. Some centuries later Dioscorides prescribed it in his own ancient herbal for problems that are known as erysipelas, shingles, migraines, heartburn, and acid indigestion. In one of the first published herbals, *Grand Herbier* (printed in Paris in 1504), several French doctors lauded belladonna's virtues as a strong sedative for insomnia. In his voluminous work *The Herball or Generall Historie of Plantes* (London: 1633) author John Gerard advocated it for gout and what would now be called rheumatoid arthritis.

The rootstock and leaves are employed for reducing pain in the afore-mentioned maladies. But because of the plant's extreme potency, it is usually administered in the form of a fluid extract that requires only a very small dosage to effect the strong relief desired. To make this combine 3 oz. powdered rootstock and 1 oz. powdered leaves of belladonna in 10 fluid ounces of rum or Scotch whiskey. Add 4 fluid ounces of distilled water to dilute the alcohol a little. Let this mixture stand in a jar for about a dozen days, shaking twice each day. Then strain and pour the liquid into several smaller, dark-colored bottles. Use only 5-8 drops at the most beneath the tongue. **NOTE: There should be medical supervision from an expert trained in herbal medicine when this is undertaken.**

For external purposes, a liniment rub of belladonna is rubbed into the skin for relieving aches and pains. Two ounces each of dried, or eight ounces each of fresh, pulverized rootstock and leaves are put into a quart bottle. Add a pint of gin, brandy or vodka and set aside for almost two weeks, shaking the bottle contents twice daily. The liniment will have a cooling effect when applied to the skin and bring relief in less than five minutes. Apple cider vinegar may be substituted for the alcohol with near similar results.

Famous Homeopathic Treatment for Scarlet Fever

Samuel Hahnemann (1755-1843) is generally credited with developing that peculiar philosophy of health and formal system of drug therapeutics known as homeopathy. It seeks to treat an illness by creating a second set of symptoms similar to the ones manifested by the disease itself. In other words, "fighting fire with fire." Belladonna was widely employed by Hahnemann and those who followed him as a successful cure for scarlet fever, a generally fatal children's disease. This homeopathic remedy eventually came to be used by many orthodox medical doctors right up to the end of the 19th century.

BERGAMOT
(MONARDA CITRIODORA)

Brief Description

Bergamot is common to Georgia and Tennessee, but grows as far north as Michigan and the Canadian province of Ontario, and as far west as Nebraska and South Dakota. It is also frequently known by the common names of Oswego tea and bee balm. This plant is a member of the mint family. At the time of the British occupation of the eastern United States, many early colonists took to drinking this tea instead of that imported from England.

Bergamot yields an aromatic odor closely reminescent of the garden herb thyme. This is due to the presence of an important constituent, thymol. Its showy flowers are scarlet and appear stunning atop the stem. They are supported by leafy bracts, the leaflets being pale green with a touch of red intermingled. The hard stems grow almost two feet in height and are square and grooved.

Quell Nausea and Vomiting

Some years ago I met a man named Zeke Jones at the Alice Lloyd College in Pippa Passes, Kentucky, where a seminar devoted to Appalachian folk medicine was being sponsored. Zeke was there to share with those in attendance some of his own "tried and true" remedies.

He told us how he used bergamot tea to stop nausea and vomiting sensations in pregnant women suffering from morning sickness, or in those who had eaten something that didn't agree with them. To one pint of boiling water he added a half-handful mixture of cut flowers and leaves. He covered the pot and set it aside to steep 30 minutes. Then he strained the liquid and gave his sick patients 1-2 cups to drink at a time. Usually it took no more than a couple of minutes for the "upchuck feeling" (as he humorously called it) to pass.

Fevers and Colds Disappear

There are several herbs effective in relieving the miseries of a fever or cold; bergamot is one. According to our backwoods "doctor" Zeke, one or two cups of the warm tea will make a person rest better and feel better in no time at all. It works just as well for influenza, but I would recommend the addition of vitamins A (50,000 I.U.) and C (5,000 mg.) each day *and* plenty of rest until the person was well.

Deafness, No; Migraine, Yes

As with so much of folk medicine, there is always going to be much that has medical merit and some interwoven with the rest that is more lore and legend than anything else. This was true in Zeke's case: he claimed that his "best cures" using bergamot came when he applied hot/cold packs of the boiling/cold tea to the forehead for "long-standing deafness." He would alternate the packs every few minutes, keeping a dry cloth or towel over the wet ones to retain the heat or cold longer.

Well, I experimented with this little remedy on some hard-of-hearing senior citizens I know. While it didn't do anything for their acquired deafness, it sure helped to clear up some of their migraine headaches.

BETONY
(see WOOD BETONY)

BILBERRY
(VACCINIUM MYRTILLUS)

Brief Description

In one of my other encyclopedias devoted to nuts, berries and seeds, I devote some space to this useful plant, which I have listed under its more common name of huckleberry. Bilberry is widespread, but prefers the acid soils of marsh lands, bogs, and coniferous forests to more alkaline ground.

This low-growing, deciduous shrub seldom gets above 20 inches tall. The branches are green and angular. The leaves are oval-shaped, slightly dentate, and bright green. The flowers are bell-shaped and greenish-pink. The fruit that is used for medicinal and eating purposes looks as if it has been in a fight: it's black-and-blue all over!

Stop Diarrhea in a Hurry

Zeke Jones, the backwoods healer previously mentioned in my discussion of bergamot, spoke at a symposium some years ago that highlighted folk medicine remedies. He told the sizeable gathering that consuming just a half-handful of raw bilberries would stop diarrhea "before nature sent you scurrying off to the outhouse again." I've heard this same thing from mountain folk in other states; when there are enough verifications like this, you can almost depend on the remedy to work.

Tea Helped Her Momma's Diabetes

Zeke's wife, Agnes, told some of us later that she made a tea (2 cups boiling water) from bilberry leaves (2/3 cup), covered and steeped it (25 minutes), then strained the liquid and gave it to her mother (2 cups daily). "Sure helped with momma's diabetes," she said with obvious satisfaction.

Wound and Ulcer Healings Scientifically Proven

Scientific research backing up some of the claims made for a particular plant in folk medicine is always reassuring. For several centuries now many common people throughout Italy have been utilizing bilberry as a tea and poultice to help heal stomach ulcers and exterior wounds. But it wasn't until the late 1980s that such a popular remedy could be medically verified.

Two scientists, A. Cristoni and M.J. Magistretti, conducted some experiments using extracts of bilberry on rodents at the Inverni Della Beffa Research Laboratories in Milan, Italy where they then worked. A report of their study was eventually published in the Italian pharmacological journal *Il Farmaco* (42:29-43, February 1987), from which the following summary information has been taken.

The two men deliberately induced ulcers and wounds into a number of rodents in order to test the validity of the curative claims made for bilberry. They then administered extracts of the herb by gastric tube while rats were confined in small strait jackets to keep them from wiggling around. After several days, the animals were killed and their stomachs carefully examined. Those which received the bilberry on a daily basis showed remarkable healing of their chemically-induced ulcers. As for the rats suffering from external wounds, they were given daily topical applications of the same bilberry extract for three days. Results were a more rapid healing of the wounds than usual, which amazed both men. Clearly the empirical use of bilberry is medically validated.

BIRCH
(BETULA ALBA)

Brief Description

White birch grows to about 70 feet in height and is found mainly in the northern U.S., Canada and northern Europe. It has white bark and bright green leaves that are minutely hairy. Black birch averages 60-85 feet in height and occurs from Maine to Georgia and west to Michigan. The bark is brown when the tree is young, dark gray later and is horizontally striped. On older trees the bark is more irregularly broken. The leaves are ovate, pointed and alternate in pairs on the tree.

An Unbeatable Remedy for Wounds and Sores

Birch is practically unexcelled in tree bark remedies for successfully treating psoriasis, eczema, herpes, acne and similar chronic skin diseases. A tea was once made by boiling the bark that eastern U.S. Indians used on the skin either as a poultice or ash to treat burns, wounds, bruises, eczema, and sores. A similar tea can be made by bringing 1 quart of water to a boil, reducing the heat, adding 3 tablespoons dried bark, covering and simmering for about 10 minutes. Remove from heat and steep for an additional hour. Clean muslin cloth soaked in the strained solution, lightly wrung out and then laid on the afflicted skin makes a good poultice.

In the November 1979 issue of the Soviet medical journal *Vestnik Khirurgii Imeni* was a report of superficial, deep and cavity wounds being successfully treated in 108 patients with a 20% tincture of birch buds in a 70% alcohol solution. To make your own tincture, combine 4 oz. (approx. 8 tablespoons) of powdered or cut birch or fresh birch buds (if available in your area) with 1 pt. of vodka. Shake daily, allowing the bark or buds to extract for about 2 weeks. Let the materials settle and pour off the tincture, straining through a fine cloth or filter. Apply as often as needed to wounds and sores alike.

A Native American Enema

In his "Uses of Plants by the Chippewa Indians," published in the *44th Annual Report of the Bureau of American Ethnology* (Washington D.C.:Smithsonian Institute, 1926-27), ethnologist Frances Densmore mentioned that Chippewa medicine men in the early part of the 19th century "understood the administering of both nourishment and medicine by means of an enema." The primitive enema device itself was composed of a deer bladder into which the proper medicine was inserted, "then a short piece of hollow rush was tied to the opening by means of a strip of wet slippery elm [with] the rush projecting about an inch." This was then inserted into the patient's rectum and the liquid medicine dispensed.

Chippewa shamans used the enema to promote a laxative effect in their patients suffering from constipation or else to stop watery stools in those suffering from diarrhea. The equivalent of 1-1/2 tablespoons of birch bark was boiled in 1-1/2 pints of water for 15 minutes; when the liquid was lukewarm, it was administered through the rectum to promote active bowel movement. Or, if diarrhea was the problem, then equal parts (1-1/2 tablespoons) of birch and ash barks were boiled in the same amount of water for 15 minutes, then allowed to cool before also being given as an enema.

Newly Discovered Cancer Treatment

A chemical found abundantly in the bark of common birch trees seems to be highly effective in the treatment of melanoma. So reported *The Orange County* [Calif.] *Register* in its March 22, 1995 edition. Researchers quoted about the amazing breakthrough said they had been experimenting with it on animals for quite some time and were pleased with the success in the tree bark's ability to turn back this often fatal and aggressive type of skin cancer.

Scientists expect to begin clinical studies on humans sometime in 1996. They attribute the bark's cancer-fighting properties to a substance known as betulinic acid. John Pezzuto, head of the Department of Medicinal Chemistry and Pharmacognosy at the University of Illinois at Chicago, described his team's incredible discovery at the 86th annual meeting of the American Association of Cancer Research in Toronto.

"The activity of the compound is very remarkable," he noted. "It certainly is the most promising discovery among more than 2,500 plant extracts we've studied."

Not only is it fantastic in stopping skin cancer, but it's also quite safe and relatively inexpensive. Tests on lab mice indicated it had no significant side effects, even at high doses. In addition, Pezzuto told the astonished audience how he and his colleagues scrounged enough birch bark from a yard where firewood was being sold to make more than 100 human doses of betulinic acid!

Based on that evidence, birch bark tea may be one of the more reasonable alternatives in treating existing melanoma. However, if an individual elects to do this, he or she should inform the attending physician of such plans well *before* the system has been nuked to death by cobalt radiation or poisoned into extinction by potent chemotherapy drugs.

Bring a quart of water to a boil. Add the thin shavings of 1-1/2 cups of birch bark. To get the shavings, scrape the tree with a sharp knife or else plane the side with a hand-held wood plane. Simmer 4 minutes on low heat and steep away from the stove burner for another 40 minutes. Strain and drink 3 cups daily—morning, noon and night—on an empty stomach.

Chaga, a Russian Folk Remedy for Cancer

Chaga is the Russian name given to a type of fungal growth that appears on the outer bark of birch, beech and other trees. The tree "mushroom" is rough, dry, porous, and crusty, with deeply cut and crooked separations having the appearance of dull charred wood on the outside. The surface is almost black in color. When this growth is sawed off the tree, it's almost as if the tree was undergoing some kind of cosmetic surgery for the removal of a huge wart.

Chaga was popularized in the novel *Cancer Ward* by famed Russian author Aleksandr Solzhenitsyn. Published in 1968, it concerned the complex social microcosm within a government-run hospital. Both in the fictional account as well as in real life, cancer patients who wished to recover from their disease would make an extract of the fungus *only* by *prolonged* decoction and *not* steeping it as in making tea. What this meant was that the fungus would be gently *simmered* in plenty of water on low heat for several hours, with extra water being added as necessary. The strained liquid would be taken 3 to 5 times daily.

Clinical investigations into Chaga in Poland, the former Soviet Union, and the United States showed that this simple preparation made hard tumors softer, smaller and less painful, with patients sleeping, eating and feeling a lot better than they did before.

BIRD-OF-PARADISE
(STRELITZIA REGINAE)

Brief Description

Bird-of-paradise is a popular cut flower widely favored by florists across the country in creating modern flower arrangements. Many gardeners and plant enthusiasts also like to keep it as a nice ornamental around the house. The leaves of bird-of-paradise are rather large and can reach almost 1-1/2 feet in length if the plant is kept outdoors in the sun. They have a calfskin leather glove feel and are shaped to a pointed oval. The leaves grow on sturdy stalks reaching anywhere from a foot to over 2 feet in length. Generally speaking, a typical bird-of-paradise can reach the average height of a small, four-year-old child.

The real distinction of this plant, however, is its bird-like flower. The plant flowers from about the age of six. The flowers grow on a long stalk, which can grow to almost 30 inches indoors. In the beginning, bird-of-paradise produces a nearly horizontal beak-shaped bract. From this, bright orange flowers with violet tongues grow vertically. The effect is that of a brilliantly colored, crested bird. This plant should not be confused with another bird-of-paradise (*Caelsalpinia gilliesii*, which is occasionally sold as *Poinciana gilliesii*), which is an outdoor shrub.

Inspired Relief for Wasp Sting

In the middle of Los Angeles International Airport there is a large restaurant suspended in mid-air by several huge semicircular concrete arches. In some ways the structure reminds one of a daddy-longlegs spider, only with fewer legs. The outside entranceway is surrounded by a number of bird-of-paradise flowers.

During an arrival at this particular airport, I had the misfortune of making an unexpected and rather abrupt contact with a yellowjacket wasp, who decided to punish me for trying to swat him with my rolled-up newspaper. He stung me on the back of my hand and then flew off. I cursed him and my bad luck and quickly looked for something to soothe my injury.

As I meditated on my unhappy state of affairs, the thought suddenly occurred to me to take some of the flowers from a nearby bird-of-paradise plant and chew them thoroughly before putting the flower-and-saliva mass on my injured hand. I did so and kept it there for a while; soon the throbbing pain and incredible itching went away and the swelling went down.

BIRTHWORT
(ARISTOLOCHIA CLEMATITIS)

Brief Description

Both the common and Latin scientific names of this plant indicate it was once held in high esteem for childbirth. William Turner (1520-1568), a distinguished physician and graduate of Cambridge University, was the first one to give the herb its common name of birthwort in *A New Herball*

(London:1551). This "father of English botany" claimed that nothing surpassed the herb for inducing easy childbirth.

Birthwort is more common to, and, therefore, has enjoyed greater popularity in, Europe and Great Britain. But it is also found in the temperate parts of North America and in the warmer south of Japan. It prefers thickets, vineyards, and the weedy perimeters of fields.

The creeping underground stem produces upright shoots, 1-1/2 to 2 feet high, with pale green, deeply incised heart-shaped leaves. Clusters of yellow, elongated tubular flowers arise in the leaf axils. Pollination is by flies, which crawl down the long floral tube and are kept trapped by hairs pointing downward; once these insects have finished their job of pollination, however, the hairs turn upward releasing them from their temporary captivity.

Ideal Solution to Drug-Resistant Bacteria

The journal *Science* (249:22) reported in its July 1990 edition that "the widespread use of antibiotics—in humans and in animal feed—has fostered the rise of drug resistance among harmless and harmful bacteria alike." This is precisely what killed famed Muppeteer Jim Henson in May of the same year. Healthy to all outward appearances, the creator of "Miss Piggy" and "Kermit the Frog" was stricken by a particularly virulent strain of group A streptococcus, and all the valiant medical efforts proved to no avail.

But what baffled doctors the most was how a common organism that gives rise to strep throat, impetigo, and scarlet and rheumatic fevers in children was suddenly causing an acute, fatal disease in otherwise healthy adults like Mr. Henson. The answer, of course, lay in a whole new breed of bacteria and viruses that have developed astonishing resistance to most synthetic antibiotics. The CBS News television program "48 Hours" devoted an entire hour to this very theme on its May 4, 1994 broadcast, which was appropriately entitled "In the Danger Zone."

A friend of mine, a practicing physician who is a member of the prestigious Royal College of Surgeons in London, wrote to me some time ago concerning an interesting case. Because it involved herbs, he thought I might find his information useful to my own research. He requested total anonymity; however, highlights of the difficult case he and his staff attempted to treat are essentially these:

A 38-year-old Caucasian woman entered his facility suffering from what was eventually diagnosed as a very serious case of necrotizing fasciitis bacteria—otherwise sensationalized in the media as "flesh-eating bacteria." This "super germ" group A strep bacteria had already consumed 5% of the woman's upper thigh, including skin, flesh, nerves, and raw muscles.

"It looked like a bloody shark had taken a very big bite out of the woman's leg," he wrote. "We decided then and there we had better work fast and damn well hope that our drugs worked before she succumbed entirely to this fast-moving disease." But "the harder we worked with our [conventional] drugs" the worse it got.

The patient's condition had reached a point, he noted, "where I was ready to do anything to save her, even if it meant swallowing my pride and consulting with an herbalist from the countryside." Which is precisely what he did. The older woman from a nearby town, who had practiced the botanical arts of healing for over four decades, suggested that he and his team of doctors try using some sodium salt of aristolochic acid on their patient. She recommended a particular homeopathic dilution of Aristolochia (birthwort) that was 12x potency. "We also managed to obtain by air post [mail] a proprietary preparation called Tardolyt that is manufactured by Madaus" [a huge German pharmaceutical firm].

They saturated the area of rapidly spreading infection with both solutions. "I tell you, we were extremely relieved to see the infection cease within hours," he confessed. My friend concluded by saying that this "birthwort seems to work in even the most stubborn cases of infection" where all other conventional drugs have failed.

BITTERS

(also see GENTIAN and WORMWOOD)

Brief Description

There is an old saying common to some of the herbals published centuries ago in England and Germany that " the more bitter a plant is, the better it must be for you." A number of herbs contain bitter principles as their chief constituents; these, in turn, pretty much determine the medicinal actions of those plants once they're ingested.

But just because the awful flavor may not agree with your taste buds doesn't mean it's necessarily bad for you. In fact, some of the worst tasting plants make the best digestive aids, because they stimulate gastric juice secretion which helps in the breakdown of foods. Bitter herbs also have a wonderful tonic action and can stimulate important glandular secretions.

Improved Cardiac Function Observed

Some German cardiologists and internists who have incorporated botanical extracts into their practices on a very limited or expanded basis, have discovered that certain bitter herbs, when administered to some of their heart patients, had them showing definite improvements in their overall cardiac functions.

Particularly useful were a fluid extract of gentian and a tea made from blessed thistle. These were especially helpful where low blood pressure or slow or irregular heart beats prevailed. These herbs had a way of "jump-starting" heart action.

Gastritis Helped

Hans Pfleiger, a postal clerk in Salzburg, suffered from acute gastritis. No regular medical treatment seemed to help him. But one doctor at Vienna University Hospital, more open-minded than his colleagues, wasn't averse to recommending different herbs when everything else failed.

He advised his patient to drink a cup of either centaury or wormwood tea with every meal, and promised his patient that his condition would improve. Hans boiled 1/2 pint water before eating and added 3/4 level teaspoon of either herb, but *not* both at the same time. He reduced the heat, covered and let simmer for 3 minutes and steep away from the stove 30 minutes. He then strained the tea, sweetened it with a little honey or sugar and drank it with every meal.

Within days he was noticing a big difference in how he felt, and reported back happily to his doctor just how great the remedy had worked for him.

My own experience with bitters has taught me that angelica, blessed thistle, calamus, and gentian are the four best herbs for any kind of chronic stomach condition. To this list, I probably should add a fifth, yarrow. For acid indigestion, heartburn, colic, and intestinal gas, they are all terrific by themselves and need not be combined necessarily.

Great Remedies for Gall Bladder Problems

These five herbs are absolutely wonderful in promoting normal gall bladder function. Old Amish Herbs of St. Petersburg, Florida makes a great "Bitters" that works well for sluggish liver, indigestion, and gall bladder problems. (See Product Appendix for further information.)

BLACK ALDER
(ALNUS GLUTINOSA)

Brief Description

The first word in the common name of this wet environment tree really is a misnomer, since it doesn't correctly describe the actual color of the bark, which is more of a reddish-yellow. But the reference to "black" probably comes from the fact that the bark yielded either a black or red color when it was used to dye wool in Great Britain.

For several centuries the tree bark has been preferred throughout Europe in the manufacture of expensive cigar boxes for wealthy gentlemen because of its reddish color, cedar-like and slightly aromatic wood. In fact, I was told some years ago by a London cigar emporium owner that many of his rich clientele claimed that such black alder boxes actually improved the flavor of their favorite Havanas or Dutch Masters when smoked after an enjoyable meal.

Sore Throat Cured

Lyle Hampton of Lancashire, England informed me some years ago in his quaint Cockney accent what he did for a very bad sore throat. "I had me self a nasty cold. And me throat got so swollen up that I could barely swallow. So's I consult with an old bud of mine at the local pub. And he tells me, 'just make yourself a good shot of black alder bark, gargle with it, and you'll feel fit as a fiddle.' So's I take his advice, boil me self up some of this bark, and did like he says. I tell you, sir, it cleared me throat up in nothing flat!"

BLACKBERRY
(RUBUS VILLOSUS)

Brief Description

The genus *Rubus* consists of roughly 400 different species of deciduous or evergreen shrubs or vines that can be either erect or trailing, thorny or thornless, a few inches or many feet in height, and of a wide variety in color and even taste.

But the berries of all of them are pretty much similar in appearance—each one is made up of innumerable tiny, fleshy and juice-rich little globes. In the middle of each of these is a seed, readily detached from its light-colored, stem-attached centers and five-petaled hulls. They come off in the hand in a fragile, hollow completeness in which each part has rounded from its own ovule.

The colors range from ink-black to black-purple, black-red, and purple in those specifically designated as blackberries.

A Famous Conservationist's Diarrhea Remedy

The late Dr. Stanley A. Cain was a pioneering conservationist who helped the early development of the science of ecology. He served the Lyndon Johnson presidency as an Assistant Secretary of the Interior Department.

Dr. Cain's academic specialty was botany. Some years ago at a scientific conference in Michigan, he told me that during his teaching at universities in Indiana and Tennessee, he started focusing more on the relationship between people and the environment, coming to believe that industrial and other threats to the land were putting us in increasing peril.

For his first research paper in 1927 on ecological mapping, he took photographs from a biplane in the first use of aerial photography in the biological sciences. Following this episode, he began experiencing problems with loose bowels. He jokingly wondered if it had been due to something he ate or maybe his initial fear of high altitudes. Nothing he took seemed to help him.

"I was getting weaker and weaker, and wondering what else I could try," he stated. "Then an old forester friend of mine told me to eat some blackberries and that would cure my problem. I tried a few cupfuls of them and my problem never returned." During the years since then Dr. Cain has recommended raw blackberries or their juice to friends, relatives and students similarly plagued with diarrhea. He stated that it has always been "the finest remedy I know of for loose bowels."

A Useful Tea

Dr. Cain also told me that the dried leaves of blackberry were useful for blood impurities, sluggish liver, childbirth, mouth and skin sores, and bad breath. He had sometimes made a tea by measuring "an amount of dry leaves pinched by the fingertips of one hand" and put into a 1/2 quart boiling water, and allowed to steep for 20 minutes. He claimed it made a delightful beverage when drunk cold. He recommended about two cups a day for the preceding problems. Or else the skin could be washed or the mouth rinsed out with some of the *warm* tea.

BLACK COHOSH
(CIMICIFUGA RACEMOSA)

Brief Description

Black cohosh is a perennial plant native to North America. It occurs frequently on hillsides and in woods at higher elevations. Its range is from
Maine and Ontario to Wisconsin and down as far as Georgia and Missouri.
The plant has a large, creeping, knotty rootstock that's often scarred with
the remains of old growth. It produces a stem up to 9 feet in height and
has flowers yielding an offensive, stinking smell.

Hypertension in Women

Women in the most common subgroup, Premenstrual Tension Syndrome-
A (PMT-A), were anxious, irritable, moody and nervous 1-2 weeks before
their period. Such women were also inclined to eat five times more dairy
products and three times more refined sugar than women without the disorder.

Because black cohosh is able to reduce hypertension somewhat and
exert a slight sedative action on the nerves, it may be good for such
women. Recommended dosage is about 2 capsules twice daily. Black
cohosh is available from health food stores.

A Medical Testimony for Lung Disorders

In the *Bulletin of The Lloyd Library of Botany, Pharmacy and Materia
Medica* Number 30 (Cincinnati: 1931; p.271) is a testimony given by an
early physician of eclectic medicine in 1823 regarding black cohosh. Dr. J.S.
Gardner recommended this herb in tea form (2 cups daily) for all lung
problems. Speaking of his own experience, he wrote as follows:

> Shortly after commencing the use of this remedy,the hectic paroxysms,
> which had attended me some time previously, were entirely checked.
> The nocturnal evacuations from the surface of the body began to dimin-
> ish. The expectoration of a fluid from the vessels of the lungs and
> bronchia, resembling pus in appearance, was speedily arrested. The
> cough became less troublesome and frequent. My pulse, which for some
> time before was never lower than from 100 to 120 pulsations to the
> minute, was reduced to the minimum standard. The pain in my right
> breast and side left me. My strength and appetite began to improve. I
> speedily abandoned the use of all medicines or other means. A period of

twelve months or more had elapsed, from my primitive ill health to the time of using this medicine. It certainly possesses the power in an eminent degree of loosening arterial action, and at the same time imparting tone and energy to the general system.

BLACK HAW
(VIBURNUM PRUNIFOLIUM)

Brief Description

In some ways black haw resembles the common elder in terms of growth behavior. The deciduous shrub can reach almost 16-1/2 feet in height, with its branches spreading upward. The leaves are dull-colored, finely toothed and nearly 3 inches long. The flowers are quite noticeable, somewhat large, and appear in nearly-topped heads between 3 and 5 inches in width.

In August when the bright red berries ripen into shiny and translucent colors, they make each tree very beautiful in appearance. In Canada, these berries have often been substituted for cranberries in food and medicine preparations.

Possible Preventative for Threatened Miscarriage

The following excerpts were taken from the *Canadian Pharmaceutical Journal* (1882, p.275). Black haw was "first introduced to the profession in 1866 by Dr. E.W. Jenks, of Detroit... But it is particularly valuable in preventing abortion and miscarriage, whether habitual or otherwise, whether threatened from accidental cause, or criminal drugging. It tones up the system, preventing or removing those harassing nervous symptoms that so often torment and wear out the pregnant women... It enables the system to resist the deleterious influence of drugs so often used for the purpose of producing abortions...Black haw was largely employed in slavery times as a preventative of abortion, and to counteract the effects of cotton root [an abortive agent] taken with criminal intent. In dysmenorrhoea [profuse menstrual discharge]... by its sedative and anodyne influences, enables the uterus to bear the burden cast on it with much less suffering..."

A tea was made of the berries by adding a small handful to about a pint of boiling water and steeping for 25 minutes, before straining and drinking. Generally 1-2 cups a day were deemed adequate to prevent miscarriage during the early months of pregnancy. CAUTION: DO NOT EAT THE UNCOOKED FRUIT!

Assistance for Asthma

Stephen LeDeu of Quebec shared a family remedy with me in 1979 when I lectured several times for Nature's Sunshine Products. His mother made a tea of the berries in a manner similar to the previously given recipe. This would be slowly sipped while still rather *warm* in cases of chronic asthma. The tea, he claimed, helped in the evacuation of mucus in the lungs and throat.

Some years later I mentioned this to a friend of mine in Vermont afflicted with asthma and bronchitis. He tried it for a couple of weeks, and reported himself cured of the problem. He said he never felt better or breathed easier after this treatment with black haw berries.

BLACK MUSTARD
(see MUSTARD)

BLACK PEPPER
(PIPER NIGRUM)

Brief Description

Black pepper is such a common commodity and so universally well-known that it needs no physical description. However, not everyone is acquainted with its intriguing history. For a number of centuries, black pepper kept the wheels of world trade turning. Today it is still consumed more than all other spices put together. In fact, it was the pepper trade that primarily brought wealth to Italian, Portuguese and Arab merchants, all of whom made sure that the profits remained sufficiently inflated to please their pocketbooks.

But pepper not only became a way of making money: the spice itself became money. Very few people are aware that during much of the Middle Ages, it served as "hard currency." Some folks stored it under lock and key as a measure of their fortunes, and at one time, a man's liquidity could be judged by his black pepper assets.

Until about 1500, it wasn't understood that black and white pepper came from the same plant; even today, not everyone knows this. In fact, green and black and white pepper are simply three stages of ripeness in the pea-sized berries of this tropical climbing bush. It is native to India and cultivated extensively in other lands such as Indonesia.

An Egyptian Cure for Toothache

Mahoud Faisal, an Egyptian dentist in Cairo, has recommended the following treatment for toothache for those poor people who cannot afford his dental services. "The problem will still be there," he told me, "but at least they will experience some relief from pain."

His cure was simple. People were instructed to make a decoction of the pepper and use it as a mouthwash. To make it just add 1/8 teaspoon (or a generous pinch) of the spice to 1/2 cup boiling water. Stir, cover and simmer on low heat for 7 minutes, then steep, still covered for another 15 minutes. Strain and slowly rinse the mouth with small sips while the decoction is still warm. Retain the liquid in the mouth for a minute or more to ease the aching pain. Repeat as often as needed.

Brings Fever Down

A Philippine folk remedy calls for a generous pinch of black pepper and an equal amount of anise to be combined with one cup of brandy and *gently* warmed over a low heat but not to the boiling point. When it has reached a degree of temperature that is still comfortable to the taste, slowly sip small amounts and retain in the mouth for about 45 seconds before swallowing. It will help reduce an elevated body temperature due to fever by several degrees.

Voodoo Relic

A friend of mine who works for the Miami Police Department has been assigned to what some have euphemistically called "The Voodoo Squad." Their assignment is to canvass the grounds of the Dade County Courthouse early each morning to pick up dead animals, charms, and other objects offered as sacrifices to a variety of Cuban and Haitian gods by relatives of defendants being tried for a variety of crimes. My buddy mentioned some of the food items associated with voodoo rituals that he thought I would be interested in knowing about.

Corn kernels, he said, are supposed to speed up a trial date; eggs are to make a case collapse; cakes are for sweetening a judge's attitude toward the accused in hopes of a lighter sentence; but black pepper is occasionally employed in voodoo practices to keep someone you don't like in jail for a long time. "Put that in your next book!" he dared me. Well, Frank, here it is.

BLACK POPLAR

(see POPLAR)

BLADDERWRACK

(FUCUS VESICULOSUS)

Brief Description

Bladderwrack is common to many New England and Eastern seaboard shorelines that are rocky and have low tide water marks. This sea vegetation is olive-green in color, regularly branched, with branches of spiraling shape and leathery feel. They may occasionally lack air bladders, but usually occur with paired bladders. The midrib is distinct and the stipe unbranched as it comes out of the disc-shaped holdfast.

Senior Citizen Gets Rid of Goiter

Maude Friendly, an octogenarian from Tupelo, Mississippi developed a goiter some years ago. Doctors could do nothing for it and informed her she would just have to "live with it 'til I die," she said.

Angered by their uncaring attitudes, she consulted with a health food store proprietor in another city. He advised her to take some 3 capsules of bladderwrack for one month and then only one capsule every other day thereafter. She did this and "my goiter vanished," she bragged with pride.

Glandular Insufficiency Helped

Bladderwrack should be used to correct an insufficiency of normal glandular performance. The best way to do this is to make a simple clear broth using fresh or dried bladderwrack. The liquid is strained and consumed like soup; it is sweet and delicious and increases glandular activity.

BLAZING STAR
(LIATRIS SPICATA)

Brief Description

Blazing star or liatris was used in colonial times for medicinal purposes, but now is strictly an ornamental. Florists favor it when making cut flower arrangements for some of their customers because of its lovely lavender spikes of feathery flowers. Unlike most other spike flowers, this one is an exception to the rule and flowers from the top of the spike *downward*. The flower spikes may reach 2 feet or longer and can be either lavender or purple.

A Horticultural Approach to Venereal Disease

Who would ever think that a popular outdoor plant used decoratively in wild gardens and borders would have great medicinal use, too? Well, in the case of blazing star this is true when it comes to venereal disease, especially gonorrhea.

A small piece of the root is cleaned, finely chopped and simmered in 3 cups boiling water for 20 minutes. After the liquid has sufficiently cooled, it is then strained and used both as a vaginal douche and wash to get rid of this infection.

Good for Putrid Sore Throat

Sore throats are quite common during cold and flu seasons. But sometimes they can get so bad that the breath develops an offensive smell. To eliminate this problem, just gargle with some tea made from blazing star root every hour, according to the previous instructions.

BLESSED THISTLE
(CNICUS BENEDICTUS)

Brief Description

Blessed thistle was widely used during medieval times. Frequent mention of its uses were made in some of the great herbals of that era (Gerard's *Herbal* in 1597 and Turner's *Herbal* in 1568). This particular herb had religious connotations surrounding it, hence other common names for it like "holy thistle" or "Holy Ghost herb." Blessed thistle apparently helped to relieve pain and inflammation of the heart in the 16th and 17th centuries. William Shakespeare recommends "laying it to your heart" because it "helpeth that doth hurt and annoye the hart," in his play, *Much Ado about Nothing*. The herb is found in moist areas, waste places, meadows and pastures.

Best Thing for Nursing Mothers

Blessed thistle is one of the best medicines for promoting breast milk in nursing mothers. To make a tea for this and also improve the heart, just bring 1 pint of water to a boil. Remove from heat and add 1-1/2 level tablespoons of cut, dried herb. Let steep for 45 minutes. Strain and drink warm, 1 cup at a time about half an hour before nursing an infant. Or for convenience, a mother may wish to take the herb in the powdered form, 2 capsules three times daily during the nursing period. Powdered herb for the tea may be purchased by mail order from Indiana Botanic Gardens in Hammond (see Appendix) or in capsule form under the Nature's Way label from any local health food store. A good blend of this and other herbs for increasing milk flow is available from Old Amish Herbs under the name Thistle Milk (see Appendix).

Liver and Stomach Tonic

Blessed thistle is still very popular in the Black Forest of Bavaria in southern Germany for liver problems and digestive disturbances. There it is taken in 1 teaspoon doses as a fluid extract. A similar dosage can be made easily by combining 1-1/2 tablespoons of powdered blessed thistle in 1-1/2 cups of brandy or vodka. Let stand for two weeks in a pint jar, shaking vigorously each day. Then strain material and put into another jar and store in a cool, dry place. A teaspoon of this extract can be added to 4 fluid ounces of distilled water and taken on an empty stomach.

BLOODROOT
(SANGUINARIA CANADENSIS)

Brief Description

Bloodroot (also called puccoon originally) is an early spring wildflower of eastern North America. Its unmistakable orange-red sap was formerly used by Native Americans as a skin stain for war dances and ceremonial rituals, as well as a fabric dye. It belongs to the poppy family and is allied to the opium poppy from which is obtained important drugs like opium, heroin, morphine, and codeine.

The leaves and flowering stem shoot up from the rhizome in early March or April. In the beginning, the leaves are wrapped around the flower bud, but later on the daisylike flower begins to expand above them as they gradually unfurl. The 8 to 16-inch flowering stems bear a single flower almost 2 inches in diameter, which can have anywhere from as little as six or as many as 12 white petals surrounding the many golden stamens.

Potent Anti-Cancer Remedy

Publishers of health books generally like authors to include information that is safe, simple, and for everyday aches and pains. Few of them venture into areas such as cancer, believing that they are potential minefields of explosive consequences.

However, my publisher is made of sterner stuff and will occasionally manifest the necessary courage it takes to let this author go where other health writers can't. That is possible, I believe, because they have faith in my professional expertise on medicinal plants and the several decades I've been studying folk medicine on an international scope.

Having said all of that, let me now deal with the matter of cancer forthrightly. Those unfortunate enough to get it can choose between orthodox treatments approved by the federal government and national and local medical associations, or unconventional therapies. In either case, a person should expect that whatever is used, be it cobalt radiation and chemotherapy on the one side or botanicals and natural substances on the other, is going to be *potent* and *will* produce some unpleasant side-effects.

So just because I may recommend and explain how to use bloodroot for breast tumors and other cancerous growths is *no* guarantee that the herb is completely safe. Granted that it may not cause hair to fall out or induce violent vomiting as the drugs in conventional medicine so often do. But be advised that *bloodroot is quite caustic and will burn skin tissue* wherever it is applied! However, aside from this serious side-effect, it is quite remarkable for the job it does in helping to treat cancer.

In the 1994 edition of *Folk Medicine Journal,* of which I'm the editor, we featured a lengthy and important article on a variety of anti-cancer salves that are very useful, but certainly very unorthodox when compared to conventional drugs. One of the most famous of these is simply called "The Black Salve" and includes bloodroot as its primary ingredient.

There are different ways to make a salve. I recommend this simple procedure. Take two ounces of fresh bloodroot; grate it or grind it up but be sure you *wear gloves* while doing so. Then add it to 1-1/2 to 2 cups olive oil in a stainless steel pot. Keep the liquid simmering for an hour on very low heat, just enough so that it bubbles but doesn't smoke. Keep a lid on the pot during the cooking process.

In another pot slowly melt about 3/4 ounce of beeswax on low heat. Then add this to the contents of the first pot, stirring the whole time with a wooden spoon to make sure everything is mixed well. Then add a couple of tablespoons of zinc chloride and continue stirring. Put in 1-2 teaspoons of gum benzoin or tincture of benzoin or pine tar to help preserve the salve.

Additional variations to this "Black Salve" formula include the addition of a teaspoon of either powdered goldenseal root or gotu kola herb. If this is done, then decrease the zinc chloride solution by one-quarter. Also, mutton or goose tallow can be substituted for olive oil with good results. Even Crisco, for that matter, may be used if none of the others is readily available.

The salve is poured into clean, empty baby food jars, sealed with their lids and stored in a cool, dry place until needed. A small amount of salve is applied with a gloved hand to the area of the skin where the tumor exists. As mentioned before, it will severely irritate the skin and produce a scab of some sort. The skin should be dry when it is applied. Repeated treatments may sometimes be necessary, but not very often. Generally one application of salve is sufficient and should be left on for a week or longer. When reaction to the salve diminishes or when the affected area grows smaller in size, then that is an indication the therapy has worked.

In the event a scab gets jostled or knocked off prematurely and a small amount of bleeding commences, simply dust the area with a little powdered turmeric or kelp. It is advisable to keep the site of treatment covered at all times with several thin layers of gauze held in place by adhesive tape. The area surrounding it should be frequently cleansed with a moist washcloth, but no water should come in contact with the salve itself.

To prevent permanent scarring once the salve dressing has been removed, rub some aloe vera gel or slippery elm paste on the skin. To make the paste, just mix a little powdered slippery elm bark with a little water and olive oil before applying. Or else bathe the area frequently with any tea made of yarrow, chamomile, or red clover blossoms.

The reader is advised to purchase a copy of the 1994 edition of *Folk Medicine Journal* and read pages 3-51 for more information. To purchase the journal, send a check or money order for $30 to:

John Heinerman
P.O. Box 11471
Salt Lake City UT 84147

I'm not actively encouraging such self-treatment of something so serious as cancer. Yet for those who are determined to do things themselves, I suggest conferring with a nurse or physician's assistant for some fundamental medical directions in the use of this very irritating but highly potent cancer salve to minimize possible injury risk to the skin. **NOTE: Bloodroot is *not* recommended for any kind of internal use!**

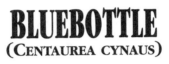

BLUEBOTTLE
(CENTAUREA CYNAUS)

Brief Description

Like a number of other plants, bluebottle also goes by several other common names, depending, of course, on the part of the country in which you live. Gardeners fancy it in their backyards and flower borders. It can also be found growing wild along roadsides and at the edges of pastures and meadows.

It is cultivated in many places for commercial purposes. Various florists with whom I spoke have lauded its striking blue or blue-purple flowers, commenting on how nicely they offset different floral arrangements.

Bluebottle is a slender annual that can reach 2 feet or more in height. Its leaves and stems have a downy exterior. The flower heads get to be an average of an inch in width and are easily recognized by their deep blue hues.

Black Eye and Bruises Easily Treated

A retired professional boxer from Brooklyn Heights, New York shared with me one of his own remedies that he had used for treating black eyes and bruises to his face. He said he made a simple tea from the flowers of bluebottle by adding a handful to two cups of boiling water. He then set the pot aside, covered it, and let the tea steep for 30 minutes. He then soaked a small terry cloth hand towel in the strained liquid, wrung out the excess, and applied it directly over the injured eye or bruise. He left it on until warmed by his own body heat, usually no more than 20 minutes, and then repeated the application with a fresh cool compress. It never failed to ease the swelling and the pain, he confided.

BLUE COHOSH
(Gaulophyllum thalictroides)

Brief Description

This medicinal plant was included in *U.S. Pharmacopoeia* over a century ago and considered then by many doctors worthy of detailed study and use on obstetric and gynecological conditions. Blue cohosh is an erect perennial growing from a rather contorted branched rootstock, which makes it almost appear as if it had been through some agony during its growth period. The flowers are yellowish-green (sometimes of a purple hue), six-petalled, and appear in the late spring, lasting until mid-summer.

A Plant That Is a Woman's Friend

There aren't too many herbs that women can claim as being almost exclusively for them; blue cohosh is the exception. For women suffering from menstrual difficulties and those about to give birth, this little gem of a plant can work wonders.

Lizzie Carver, an herbalist from Reno, Nevada, gave me the following formulas that she routinely prescribes to "all of my PMS patients and expectant moms. I recommend that women suffering from delayed menstruation take 2 capsules twice daily of the powdered root, or else drink 1 cup of tea to correct the problem." To make the tea, just put an ounce of fresh or dried chopped rootstock in 1-1/2 pints of boiling water, simmer on low heat for 7 minutes and then steep, covered, for another 25 minutes. She advises that the tea be taken warm.

If a pregnant woman drinks several cups of the *warm* tea 12 to 24 hours before expected delivery, it will induce labor more easily, she claimed.

BLUE FLAG
(Iris versicolor)

Brief Description

Also called the wild iris, this plant predominates throughout much of the West. In appearance it looks a lot like your common iris—long, smooth spear-shaped leaves and adorned with a light lavender or bluish-purple flower just a tad smaller in size than your garden varieties. Blue flag is a sociable plant, preferring to grow in bunches rather than by itself. Nothing is more beautiful, indeed, than to walk across an entire meadow during late June and early July. What a truly spectacular sight greets the eyes!

Useful for Drug-Resistant Staph Infections

Blue flag roots can be toxic if taken internally, but are very useful for external purposes. I've found them especially helpful to use in cases of staph infection, when all other forms of conventional drug therapy have failed utterly.

Several years ago a 22-year-old student whom I'll call Mike consulted with me about some serious staph sores in his genital area. He had been to several physicians and they had prescribed the usual antibiotics, but nothing seemed to help. He wanted to know if I had something that might work instead.

We went up into the Uinta Mountains to a meadow where a large colony of blue flag was growing. I dug up some of the plants, shook the dirt off, and gave them to him to place in a large plastic bag brought along just for that purpose. We returned to his place and I washed the dirt off some of the roots, dried them in an old towel, and then grated them by hand into a coarse pulp. I spread it out on a piece of cotton cloth folded into a square the size of a washrag and had him apply this to the problem area. He went into his bathroom, closed the door and took several minutes to do this. Because of the location of the sores, he was able to hold this poultice in place simply by pulling his briefs and pants back up again. I told him to keep it in place for several hours and then repeat the process again that night and all the following day with what was left.

He followed my instructions to the letter and happily reported back to me on the third day that the staph sores were "almost gone." "Professor," he said, somewhat humorously, "you sure have a way with plants, don't you?" To which I replied with equal joviality, "And you sure have a way with the women, don't you Mike?" He understood the significance of what I said in relationship to his problem, but took no offense.

BLUE SPRUCE
(PICEA PUNGENS)

Brief Description

Spruce in general can be evergreen trees or shrubs of the pine family and are widely distributed in the Northern Hemisphere. The needles are angular in cross section, rather than flattened as in the related hemlocks and firs. Some species are important timber trees in Europe and America.

Quite a number of spruces are cultivated as ornamentals. The most popular North American garden spruce is the Colorado blue spruce. It is distinguished by its frosty- or silvery-blue needles, but like other spruce has the same strong, light-weight, light-colored, fine-grained, even-textured, long-fibered wood that makes these trees so valuable in the timber industry.

Mouth Sores Eliminated

A retired fur trapper I know who spent years in the Northwest Territories of Canada told me what he did on several occasions when bothered with mouth and lip sores. Being far from the nearest outpost of civilization, he had no access to pharmacies or health food stores, so he learned to improvise from things around him in the outdoors.

He explained how he picked some spruce tree leaves, tore them into smaller pieces to fill 3/4 of an empty cup. These he placed in 1-1/2 pints of boiling water and simmered for 5 minutes, then covered and steeped for 25 minutes. Then he strained the tea through a small piece of clean burlap sack before drinking a small mouthful (about two tablespoons). He swished the tea around with his tongue for several minutes before swallowing. He also soaked a cotton ball in the tea, squeezed out the excess fluid, and then taped it to any external cold sore appearing in the corners of his mouth or on his lip. He said this remedy never failed to work for him.

French Explorer Discovers Cure for Scurvy

In the annals of medical history, some of the greatest cures have been discovered more by happenstance than by painstaking and carefully planned research. The great British bacteriologist, Sir Alexander Fleming (1881-1955) discovered penicillin in 1928 by examining, out of curiosity, some mold that had accumulated on the white bread of his ham sandwich that he was having for lunch one day; he won a Nobel prize in medicine for this in 1945.

A cure for scurvy also came about, partly by accident as well as from necessity. Scurvy is a medical condition due to a nutritional deficiency of vitamin C in the diet and is characterized by weakness, anemia, spongy gums, a tendency for internal hemorrhaging in mucous membrane tissue, and a brawny induration of the muscles of the calves and legs. In the 15th and 16th centuries it was a common malady among European soldiers, sailors and explorers.

The famous French sailor and explorer, Jacques Cartier (1491-1557) made three separate voyages to Canada, exploring the Gulf of St. Lawrence to the site of the present day Montreal. Because his men lacked adequate amounts of ascorbic acid in their bodies, they suffered terribly from scurvy. In a published narrative of his journeys, *La botanique canadienne a l'epoque de Jacques Carter* (Montreal: Contributions du Laboratoire de Botanique de l'Universite de Montreal, 1937; 28:1-77), some 400 years later, an interesting explanation was given of how this malady was eventually cured and the significant role that spruce leaves played in it all. The following excerpts are taken from a faithful English translation made of Cartier's original narrative several centuries ago:

> The captain [Cartier] seeing the aforementioned Dom Agaya healthy and deliberate, was joyous, hoping to learn from him, how he was cured, so that his men could be given aid and help. So when they had arrived near the fort, the captain asked him how he was cured of his sickness [scurvy]. Dom Agaya replied that it was with the juice of the leaves of a tree [spruce] and the water the leaves were boiled in, that he was cured and that this was the special remedy for the sickness. Then the captain asked him if there were any such trees around there, and asked him to show him one so that he could cure his servant, who had caught the aforesaid sickness in the house of seigneur Donnacona [at Quebec] not wanting to let him know the number of his companions who were sick.

> Then Agaya sent two women with our captain, to cure him, they brought nine or ten branches; and showed us how the bark must be pulled off and the leaves of these branches, and all put into water to boil; then the water drunk once in two days. And the juice of the leaves and bark pressed out and the water put on the swollen and sick limbs; and he said that the tree will cure all sickness.

> They call the tree in their [Indian] language, *annedda*. Immediately afterwards, the captain had the drink made, so the sick could drink. Of these however no one wanted to try it, only one or two, who decided to try it. As soon as they had drunk, they felt better, which they found a true and evident miracle. For of all the sicknesses they had suffered from, after having drunk two or three times, they recovered their health and were cured. So that some of the company, who had had syphilis for more than five or six years before getting this sickness [scurvy], by this medicine [spruce leaf tea] were completely cured.

> After having seen this, there was such a demand for this medicine that a tree, as large and as tall as I have ever seen was used in less than eight days, which made such a cure that if all the doctors of Louvain and Montpellier [in France] had tried, with all the drugs of Alexandria [Egypt], they could not have done as much in one year as this tree did in eight days. For it profited us so much, that all those who wanted to try it, recovered health and were cured, by the Grace of God.

BLUE VERVAIN
(VERBENA HASTATA)

Brief Description

There are at least three different basic types of vervains to be found in western and southwestern United States. But the most common one with which most herbalists and folk healers are intimately familiar is the upright, hairy plant with a square stem and sporting widely spaced and toothed leaves similar to mints. The average height is between 24 and 36 inches. This particular kind of blue vervain flowers in midsummer into many long blue or purple spikes; the active blooms form a ring of blossoms that seem to move up the spike as the season progresses, with its seed pods below and flower buds overhead. The toothed leaves get anywhere from 3-1/2 to 4-1/2 inches long in areas boasting better soils.

Wonderful Sedative for Hyperactive Children

For the last 3-1/2 years I have been the editor of *Utah Prime Times*, the Intermountain West's largest monthly newspaper for seniors, which reaches an audience of almost 100,000 people in four states (Utah, Idaho, Arizona, and Nevada). Because of my association with this well-recognized publication, I have been frequently invited to address many senior citizen groups and caregiving associations that cater especially to the elderly.

In April 1995, I spoke to a gathering of elderly residents—all of them women— at the Sarah Daft home in Salt Lake City. It is the oldest continually operating retirement/residential care facility in the Beehive State, established in 1911. After my presentation, one of the octogenarians present took me aside and shared with me some of her own experiences with the use of different herbs.

About 63 years ago, two of her 11 children (a boy and girl, aged 10 and 8 respectively) began showing signs of restlessness at home, in school and in church. She decided to give them each some *warm* blue vervain tea to see what effects it might have on their erratic behavior. She said she made the tea by boiling two pints water and then adding to it two heaping tablespoons dried, crushed flowers and leaves. She covered the pot, simmered only two minutes, set aside and steeped for about 35 minutes. Then she strained a cup for each of them, added a little white sugar ("we used it more in those days than honey") and gave it to them to drink.

"The effect was astonishing," she recalled. "Both of my children calmed down within half-an-hour and stayed relaxed for several hours thereafter. I kept giving this to them several times a day for many months thereafter until they didn't need it anymore." Some of her grown children used it on a few of their hyperactive kids in later years with similar success.

"If today's moms knew just how well blue vervain works," she thoughtfully observed, "they wouldn't be bothered with such cranky and fidgety kids."

Helpful Cold and Flu Medicine

My senior informant also mentioned how well blue vervain had worked for her in treating her children (and in later years, grandchildren) whenever they suffered from a nasty cold or flu, raging fever, or upset stomach. The same tea is taken in between meals and slightly warm, several times daily.

BOG MYRTLE
(see BAYBERRY)

BONESET
(EUPATORIUM PERFOLIATUM)

Brief Description

Boneset is a perennial herb favoring damp places; its range of habitat stretches from Nova Scotia to south of the Carolinas. The plant has an erect, stout, cylindrical hairy stem, that averages between 3 and 4 feet in height, branching at the top. The leaves are large, opposite, united at the base, with their ends climaxing into almost spear points. The lower leaves are between 7 to 8 inches, but the upper ones are only about half this size. The leaf edges are finely toothed with the veins being rather prominent; the bottoms of each leaf appear dotted and have a downy, slightly sticky feel.

The flowers of boneset are terminal and numerous, averaging 10 to 20 white florets. The plant is vaguely aromatic, but with an unmistakable bitter taste that will pucker the mouth immediately if tasted in this fresh state.

How Boneset Got Its Curious Name

Those unfamiliar with herbs would think, at first glance at the herb's popular name, that it is because of its presumed "bone-knitting" properties.

Were this true, of course, then chiropractors and doctors would be clamoring for it all the time. However, such isn't the case. The name was derived from its previous use many decades ago. In the earlier part of this century, it was widely utilized in the treatment of a unique influenza that caused considerable pain in the bones. Doctors began recommending the herb for this break-bone fever (as it was then called) and the name stuck. However, when made into a tea and taken *warm* on an empty stomach (2 cups daily), it can help break a fever very quickly.

Instructions for making a tea are quite simple: add 1 tablespoon boneset herb to 1-1/2 pints boiling water; cover and simmer on low heat for 3 minutes; remove from heat and steep 30 minutes; strain and drink 1 cup twice or thrice daily on an empty stomach.

Knocks the Flu for a Loop

Silena Heron, N.D. of Sedona, Arizona promotes a great "recovery therapy" during cold and flu season. Her standard recommended treatment calls for boneset, equal parts of yarrow, elder flower and lemon balm or peppermint, to be made into a warm tea.

Heron encourages her patients to drink a cup of her special brew, get into a hot bath and then drink a second cup of the "flu brew" while still in the tub. After drying off, the patient should go straight to bed and cover up first with a sheet, then with a heavy wool blanket, followed by plenty of quilts. This will promote heavy sweating for an hour. Then the individual returns to the tub and sponges the body off with apple cider vinegar.

Edward Sieracki of Detroit, Michigan, who followed Dr. Heron's detoxifying regimen, reported that "twenty minutes after drinking this boneset blend tea, I started to sweat profusely. I drank another cup of the tea and went to bed. By the next morning I was fully recovered." Make the tea according to previously given instructions.

To cure a sore throat accompanying a cold or flu, just mix pinches of salt and cayenne pepper with the juice of half a lemon or lime and gargle. It may briefly burn your throat, but the soreness will quickly leave.

BORAGE
(BORAGO OFFICINALIS)

Brief Description

Borage is an annual plant more common to European and Mediterranean countries than it is here, but is cultivated in some places and pretty well known by many North American herbalists. Strangely enough, an herb with such marvelous healing properties grows well in junkyards and waste places, but is much more difficult to grow in tidy gardens and "perfect" nurseries.

To handle the plant, gloves are a requirement because of the white, stiff, prickly hairs covering both leaves and stems. The plant gets about two feet tall and bears blue or purplish, star-shaped flowers during the summer months.

"Herb of Gladness" for the Depressed

The original common name for this herb was "burrage" or "llanwenlys" from the Welsh, which signifies "Herb of Gladness." One ancient Welsh herbalist informs us of "those of our time who do use the flowers in salets to exhilerate and make glad the minde when depressed. There be also many things made of them, used everywhere for the comfort of the harte, for driving away sorrows and increasing the joie of the mind and spirit."

A medical herbalist in the village of Llanybyther in the northern part of Carmarten province informed me some years ago that "a few [two] cups of [warm] borage tea every day, makes those who are very sad, soon very glad." She explained that there is an unidentified component within the plant that responds well to heat and can then enhance the production of beta-endorphins or so-called "feel good" compounds within the brain. For those who frequently suffer from depression, she recommends making a larger amount of the tea. Bring a quart of water to a rolling boil; add 1-1/2 cups coarsely cut borage; cover and simmer 5 minutes; steep 40 minutes away from heat; strain and drink one cup *warm* in between meals.

Fever Reliever

The following remedy comes from a book, *Herbs for Daily Use* by Mary Thorne Quelch, published over half-a-century ago in Great Britain (London: Faber & Faber, Ltd., 1941).

"Sufferers from fever will appreciate a drink made by putting a sliced lemon and half a dozen sprigs of borage into a jug and adding a pint of boiling water. Allow to get cool, then stir and strain. The patient should be allowed to drink freely of this, providing that ordinary lemonade is allowed."

Swellings Reduced

The same reference also suggests: "A poultice of borage leaves is an excellent application for swellings where there is much inflammation, or, indeed, for inflammation of any type."

BOUQUET GARNI

Brief Description

Bouquet garni is the internationally used French name for what domestic cooks or regular recipes might term "an herb bundle." The herbs used usually consist of 5 sprigs of parsley, 2 sprigs of thyme, 1 small bay leaf, 1 piece of dried orange peel, 1 sprig each of sweet marjoram and basil, 2 celery leaves, a small piece of cinnamon stick, a clove of garlic, a small blade of mace, and a pod of red pepper. However, not all of these herbs have to be used to make a good bouquet garni. Since everyone's taste buds are different, the herbs need to be varied to suit individual flavor appeals.

The herbs are usually tied together so that they can be removed at the end of cooking. The same result can also be obtained by arranging the herbs and spices in the center of a square piece of muslin and then drawing the corners together and tying them with a length of thread or string.

Improve Food Flavor and Digestion

The cook who seldom uses some type of bouquet garni should hang up his or her apron, put away the pots and pans, and switch to another vocation. Commercially "mixed herb" preparations or powdered bouquet garni from packets simply won't substitute for the real thing.

One of the benefits of using a bouquet garni when cooking is that it improves the flavor of whatever it is put with. Secondly, and more important, it assists in the digestion of the meal to be consumed. There is less chance of heartburn, intestinal gas, and constipation when it is used in meal preparation.

BOX ELDER
(ACER NEGUNDO)
(also see MAPLE)

Brief Description

The maple group of deciduous trees and shrubs of the Northern Hemisphere are found chiefly in more temperate regions and on tropical mountain slopes. Maples are very popular as shade trees and often have brilliantly colored foliage in the fall.

The box elder or ash-leaved maple is a smaller North American species also frequently planted as a shade tree; its softer wood is used for woodenware, cheap furniture, and paper pulp. It flowers between March and May, during which time many people with hay fever suffer a great deal because of its high pollen count during this time.

Antidote for Mild Burns and Sunburns

It's probably hard for us to conceive of something like box elder being good for anything at all, considering that the tree induces allergic symptoms of itching, watery eyes, draining sinuses and bouts of sneezing in so many people across the country. But this is one of those cases, where something bad for you can also be good.

Boil one quart distilled water. Add 1-1/4 cups coarsely chopped box elder bark, cover and simmer on medium heat for 15 minutes. Remove from the heat, strain, and refrigerate. Use on mild burns and sunburns, both as a wash and cold pack (with a piece of folded, clean cotton cloth). This decoction helps to relieve the itching and inflammation of such burns and expedites the healing process to some degree.

BRACKEN FERN
(PTERIS CRETICA)

Brief Description

Bracken fern is one of the few holdovers from the era of the dinosaurs. Other plants remaining since then include the colossal evergreens and ginkgo biloba. A while back I happened to visit one of the last virgin stands of coastal redwoods in the 560-acre Muir Woods National Monument just north of San Francisco.

In a canyon drenched by winter rain and summer fog, I discovered to my great delight fungi, lichens, mosses, and cloverlike oxalis that thrive in the shade of gigantic redwoods that spire to almost 300 feet or more in height. I also found myself in waist-high bracken ferns, with their rugged, stiff, darkly green fronds. When these plants die in the fall, their wind-rattling brown expanses, if not buried by snow, remain to pinpoint the location of delicious fiddleheads when they arise the following spring. These peculiar entities—each coming into being singly from the usually long, prolific root that extends horizontally underground, where it tends to branch over a sometimes considerable area—curl in such an interesting way that they give the appearance of a violin being tuned before an important concert recital.

Helpful for Lung Problems

The fronds can be made into a useful tea by boiling 1/2 cup of them (cut up, of course) in 1-1/2 pints water for 15 minutes, and then straining. Slowly *sip* 1/2 cup *warm* tea through a straw on an empty stomach for easier breathing. **Caution: Limit the application of this tea to short-term use only due to potential toxicity to the liver.**

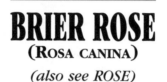

BRIER ROSE
(Rosa canina)
(also see ROSE)

Brief Description

Also called the dog rose, this plant is quite common throughout much of Europe. It is a climbing and trailing prickly perennial shrub growing to about 10 feet in height. The leaves are alternate, ovate to elliptic, average about 1-1/2 inches or more in length, and can be either serrate, acute or acuminate. The flowers of brier rose are aromatic, large, white or pale pink on long pedicels, appearing from mid-to late summer. They are followed by fleshy, scarlet false fruits (called rose hips) that are under an inch long.

Rose Conserve for Illness Recuperation

Often those recovering from serious illness or surgery have a difficult time digesting or holding down the food they eat. One of the simplest foods I know of for such special cases is a conserve made from brier rose petals. It not only tastes good, but also smells good. It has a tonic effect on the system and restores some energy.

To make this conserve, scald a quart of brier rose petals in 1-1/4 cups boiling water for 2-1/2 minutes. Then squeeze through a wire strainer and discard the petals. Boil the rose water with the juice of one lemon and one lime, 8 oz. honey or molasses, 8 oz. brown sugar (with plenty of pectin to help it set up more quickly) and 2-1/4 more cups brier rose petals. Remove from the heat when the setting point is reached. Spoon into jars and cover. Eat a little bit every 2-3 hours.

Rose Leaves for Wounds and Constipation

Gather a handful of brier rose leaves by wearing gloves to protect your hands from plant thorns. Lay them in a small pile between two layers of thin cotton cloth (or two white handkerchiefs) and pound with a hammer until somewhat macerated. Then invert this pulpy mass on to any wound and leave in place for about 20 minutes. The leaves will help to promote healing.

A tea made of the same leaves will help to promote a fair bowel movement in cases of mild constipation. In one pint of boiling water, cook a half-handful of leaves covered for 7 minutes. Remove from the heat and steep for another 30 minutes. Strain and drink two cups of the *warm* tea.

BRIGHAM TEA
(EPHEDRA VIRIDIS)
(also see MAHUANG)

Brief Description

This small- to medium-sized desert shrub doesn't look very promising when you first see it. It tends to remind one of a weather-beaten, long-needled, and stunted pine tree and doesn't exactly inspire confidence as a marvelous medicinal. But looks can certainly be deceiving as we will later learn.

Brigham or Mormon Tea was first used by the great religious leader and colonizer of the American West, Brigham Young, when he relocated his people, the Latter-Day Saints, to the Rocky Mountains. It is said on good authority that he made use of this herb quite frequently because of its purifying properties.

The jointed stems of Brigham Tea have degenerate leaves at the nodes that are reduced to scales, either 2 or 3 depending on the species. The barkless stems range from grayish blue-green with spikelike tips to bright yellow-green or dark green.

Brigham Tea is directly related and very similar in appearance to the Chinese herb mahuang with one notable exception—the latter has ephedrine while the former does not. (Ephedrine is a prescription drug used in modern medicine as a vasobronchial dilator and decongestant in asthma and bronchitis.)

A Frontier Remedy for Sexually Transmitted Diseases

Many are the stories that could be told by colorful characters of the Wild West of how they used Brigham Tea internally or externally as a skin wash for treating various venereal diseases. Grizzled prospectors, cattle drovers and rustlers, buffalo and bounty hunters, fur trappers, freight wagon and stagecoach drivers, Army soldiers and Indian fighters, to name just a few, were continually exposed to syphilis and gonorrhea because of their frequent sexual promiscuity.

During the heydays of mining in different western states, this scraggly and pathetic looking shrub came into favor with many miners and the ladies who frequently catered to their sexual needs. In the bordellos of Nevada, for instance, it was regularly referred to as "whorehouse tea," for obvious reasons.

Even in our current society the same problem continues, but only in greater numbers as more young people every year explore their own sexuality in unsafe ways. The list of sexually transmitted diseases that are possible to contract has grown far beyond the few that existed in the early American frontier areas.

Now, in addition to syphilis and gonorrhea, we have chancroid, lymphogranuloma venereum, and granuloma inguinale, not to mention hepatitis, shigellosis, amebiasis, and giardiasis that can be acquired by nonsexual means.

There are, of course, a limited number of potentially powerful herbs with remarkable antibiotic and antibacterial properties that can arrest the spread of many of these sexual diseases. Herbs such as echinacea, garlic, goldenseal and sarsaparilla are mentioned throughout the text. For overall practical purposes, however, Brigham Tea ranks in the forefront. Not so much for what it may do in killing the viruses or bacteria responsible for these diseases, but more for what it can do in terms of purifying the blood so that the liquid environment in which they thrive is less toxic. A simple analogy may be with chemical pesticides often used to spray for mosquitoes versus draining the swamp in which they breed. Using Brigham Tea on a regular basis can be likened to the latter. For once the body is sufficiently detoxified with a strong blood purifier, then most sexually transmitted diseases either recede considerably in their activity or else clear up of their own accord.

In my years of working with Brigham Tea, I've come to find that, while it works well by itself, it works even better when used in combination with sarsaparilla root and in liquid form better than in capsules or tablets. Bring 1/2 gallon of spring or distilled water to a rolling boil, then add 2 cups each of coarsely chopped Brigham Tea and sarsaparilla root. Cover, reduce to medium heat, and simmer for 15 minutes. Remove from heat and continue steeping, with the lid still on, for another 45 minutes.

Do not strain, but keep the herbs in the tea at all times until entirely used up. Store in the refrigerator and use small amounts as needed. Can be consumed warm or cool, preferably on an empty stomach. Drink 1-2 cups three or four times daily. Also frequently bathe those parts of the body afflicted with one of the previously mentioned sexually transmitted diseases. Continue this therapy for many weeks or several months, if necessary.

Testimony of Allergy Relief

Michael Moore is no stranger to herbs. Since 1968 he has lived and worked among the very plants he writes about. He has picked his own herbs and made them into a variety of useful formulas and products for the health and well-being of others. He has taught the medical lore of herbs at a number of different colleges throughout the American Southwest. He has been the owner or co-owner of at least two separate herb stores in New Mexico for about the last twenty years.

I met him some years ago in Phoenix, Arizona, where we were both speakers before the Arizona Naturopathic Medical Association's annual conference in the Phoenix suburb of Scottsdale. I had concluded my address in a conservative three-piece suit intended for such an august and dignified body of practitioners. Michael followed me in what might charitably have been described as "dressing down" for the occasion. Despite his shaggy and unkempt appearance, there was certainly nothing dishevelled about his knowledge of medicinal plants. The guy really did know his stuff, I quickly concluded, after listening to him for only a few minutes. And the more he spoke, the more impressed I became with his "hands on" expertise. Nothing dissuaded me from my professional respect for him, even when he apologized to the group for looking the way he did "because I slept in my van" to save time and money to get there.

He told of an acquaintance "with a yearly scourge of longstanding pollen allergies," who at some point followed his suggestion to "start drinking [Mormon] Tea as a regular beverage to replace coffee." His unnamed friend began and soon "found that he had taken less than one-tenth his usual amount of little yellow allergy pills for that season." Michael erroneously attributed this decongestant action to an "ephedrine-related alkaloid" he believed was contained within the plant itself. Scientific analysis, however, has shown Brigham Tea to be devoid of such a compound. But it certainly has other wonderful compounds to make it one of the best natural medicines I know of for allergy relief.

Bring 1 quart distilled water to a boil. Add 2-1/2 tablespoonfuls coarsely cut Brigham Tea (fresh or dried). Cover and simmer on low heat for 7 minutes; set aside, still covered, and steep 25 minutes longer. Strain and drink one cup *warm* tea every 4 hours on an empty stomach during allergy season.

BROOKLIME
(VERONICA BECCABUNGA)

Brief Description

Up until about fifty years ago, brooklime was considered a very popular blood purifying herb in much of European and Asian herbal medicines. In fact, many of the old herbal apothecaries throughout Great Britain usually carried a good supply. But in more recent times, it has fallen into disfavor, though still readily gathered because of its widespread abundance.

Brooklime grows in shallow streams, meandering creeks, babbling brooks, and similar waterways. It throws out thick, succulent stems adorned with azure blue flowers, which start unfolding from May to late August. The leaves are opposite, short-petioled, oblong to ovate, and either crenate or serrate. When nibbled on in its fresh form, the herb imparts a taste similar to watercress, but only more bitter. This sharpness probably led to another common name for it, that of "mouth smart."

Complexion Problems, Poor Eyesight, and Persistent Headaches Cleared Up

Over 55 years ago, Mary Thorne Quelch wrote the popular British herbal book entitled *Herbs for Daily Use* (London: Faber and Faber Ltd., 1941) in which she lauded the use of water pimpernel (another name given to brooklime) for skin, eye, and head problems. Here's what she said:

"Our forefathers had great faith in a medicine called Spring Juice, which, taken freely in the early part of the year, was held to be without rival in clearing the blood and improving the digestion. To prepare this, equal parts of freshly gathered brooklime and of scurvy grass [substitute watercress instead] were cut into inch-long pieces and well-beaten with a pestle and mortar [or crush with a rolling pin or gently pound with a hammer on a cutting board]. A small quantity of water [probably no more than

2-3 cups] was added and the herbs left to 'steep' for twelve hours [boiling water is best to pour over them and then cover with a lid]. At the end of that time they were strained, care being taken to extract all the moisture, and juice of Seville oranges [or any orange] to an equal amount was added. A wineglassful [about 4 tablespoonfuls] of this mixture taken fasting each morning for a week was guaranteed to clear the complexion and brighten the eyes, besides curing persistent headaches and healing skin troubles. There is every probability that the draught deserves its high reputation."

To her helpful advice I would only add that a little *more* than her recommended intake could be consumed without any problems. For instance, one could easily take 3/4 cup of this "Spring Juice" every morning, while missing breakfast as she suggested, and not worry about any unpleasant side effects. I would also recommend that the liquid be strained through a coarse cloth and then the herbs themselves squeezed hard to get out all remaining juice.

Wonderful Application for Hemorrhoids and Sores

Several other old British herbals, which I consult from time to time, mention brooklime as very effective for the treatment of hemorrhoids, diabetic leg ulcers, and skin sores. The expressed juice from crushed brooklime may be applied directly inside or to the problem itself for rapid healing. Mixing a small handful of brooklime with 1/2 cup water in a Vita-Mix machine or similar food processor is probably the easiest way to get enough juice to do a sufficient job.

One or two cotton balls or a layered strip of gauze can be saturated with some of the juice and then applied to the problem area and secured with tape.

For an allied plant with similar healing properties, consult the entry WATERCRESS toward the end of this book.

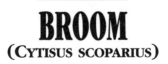

BROOM
(Cytisus scoparius)

Brief Description

The broom, according to Mary Thorne Quelch in her hard-to-find classic *Herbs for Daily Use* (London: Faber and Faber, Ltd., 1941), "reminds us that the small branches [of this shrub], dried and tied together in the familiar besom form, were the first brooms used by housewives of old. Also they were the particular form on which witches rode to their unholy carnivals which accounts for the many legends of spells and witchcraft which cling about the plant."

Broom averages between 8 and 12 feet in height and has very small leaves that are either simply ovate or composed of three little leaflets. Its large, golden yellow flowers open in the early part of summer. It seems to thrive best near the ocean, but may also be found on waste ground and "in coppices all over the country," as Ms. Quelch put it. This is a distinctly British term for a thicket or grove of small trees originating mainly from root suckers rather than seed.

Edema Cure from a Dorset Witch

Some years ago, I had the pleasure of meeting a charming, bespectacled, somewhat rotund older woman with silvery gray hair in the city of Dorchester, England, in the southern province of Dorset, bordering the English Channel. She could have easily passed for different artists' portrayals of the wife of the mythical Santa Claus. She was, in fact, a *witch*. "A *nice* witch, mind ye," she corrected me with a wag of her finger. "I work me charms to bring people good luck," she said. What about those who were bad and maybe in need of a good curse to help them reform their errant ways, I wondered aloud. She simply giggled and said with a shake of her finger again: "Now, now, mustn't be giving away me secrets or telling them things I do in the *dark* now, shall I? Wouldn't want ye to get a bad opinion of me, would I?" I shook my head in agreement and we both enjoyed another hearty laugh together.

She then shared with me one of "me famous cures for dropsy," which is the old medical term for edema or fluid retention. "Put 1/2 ounce of dandyline [dandelion] root into a saucepan with a quart of cold water, which ye bring to a boyle [boil] and simmer until reduced to a pint. Into a jug place 1/2 ounce of broom tops and 1/2 ounce of juniper berries. Over them pour the contents of the saucepan while it is yet boyling. Leave to get cold and then strain. I tell me customers to drink 1/2 pint of this decoction every morning and evening. It works just like me magick does," she said.

In the years since then I've recommended this more than once to different individuals suffering from chronic edema, and they've all reported back, without exception, the marvelous results they got from trying her remedy. In the beginning, I absent-mindedly mentioned its source to one religious extremist, who severely denounced me for recommending to her "a remedy of Satan himself." After that, I learned to be more selective in what I divulged as my true sources for some of the effective remedies I suggested to others.

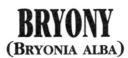

BRYONY
(BRYONIA ALBA)

Brief Description

The common name of bryony hails from the Greek word *bruein*, which means to "grow luxuriantly." In England it is also given the name of "wild vine" to highlight the vigorous growth of the annual stems that rapidly cover hedgerow shrubs. The herb sometimes goes by the name of "English mandrake" because its enormous rootstock is quite similar in appearance to the legendary mandrake mentioned later on in the text. Bryony roots were once carved several centuries ago into human form and often used as shop signs by English herbalists.

The root holds considerable medicinal value, but in large amounts **can be poisonous!** Externally, it is a dirty yellow color, resembling in some ways a parsnip. But it has a horrendous taste and, in former times, when employed as a powerful purgative, could, quite literally, make a person vomit.

Careful Treatment for Whooping Cough and Cardiac Disorders

Bryony is great for a couple of serious health problems, but requires common sense and some skill in using. **It is not to be used indiscriminately. It is not to be used for very long. It is to be used only in very small doses.**

The two most common problems for which I've seen bryony used is in the treatment of whopping cough and cardiac disorders. In both cases, it is administered as a tea, but heavily sweetened with sugar or honey and vanilla to drastically improve its flavor. Several licensed and practicing medical herbalists in London told me that "any lay person with some common sense could safely use it." But good judgment and care are definitely required!

Bring a pint of water to a boil; add 1/4 teaspoon finely chopped bryony root. Cover and let simmer on low heat for 7 minutes; set aside and steep for 20 minutes, then strain. Pour the liquid into another saucepan and reheat until warm but not very hot. Then add some sugar or honey and vanilla flavoring. Cover and steep for 10 minutes, then refrigerate.

Reheat two tablespoonfuls of the liquid at a time and *slowly* swallow when lukewarm to allay spasmodic coughing. Repeat every couple of hours, if necessary. For cardiac disorders, drink 1/2 cup *cold* tea and then eat 1/2 slice bread afterwards to prevent any possible nausea from occurring. Do this only once a day.

In the event of toxicity, evacuate the stomach immediately with syrup of ipecac that you can buy from any drugstore. Follow this with a drink of some kind of herbal demulcent, such as teas made from fenugreek seed, marshmallow root or slippery elm bark, or pearl of barley water. Keep the body temperature stabilized by wrapping in blankets and putting hot water bottles on the feet, abdomen and neck.

Just because I've emphasized some necessary precautions doesn't actually mean that bryony will kill you. It only means that if unwisely and improperly used, it can make a person one very sick individual.

BUCHU
(BAROSMA BETULINA)

Brief Description

Buchu leaves are usually pale green, under an inch in length and less than 1/2 inch in width, leathery and glossy. They have blunt, strongly-curved tips and finely-toothed margins, with round oil glands scattered all over their surface. Quite often the small flowers, with five whitish petals, and the brownish fruits are generally mixed in with the leaves themselves. The leaves are similar to peppermint leaves for strong aroma. Buchu leaves are collected while the plant is flowering and fruiting, and are then dried and exported all over the world.

African Remedy for Gout, Kidney Stones, Urine Retention, Prostate Problems, and Bladder Infection

The Khoikhoi (formerly Hottentots) are a pastoral people, inhabiting the coast of the Cape of Good Hope in South Africa. They are usually much lighter in complexion than their neighbors, the Bantu. The Khoikhoi were the first natives to come into contact (mid-17th century) with the Dutch settlers. In language and physical type the Khoikhoi are related to the San (Bushmen), in that they speak a variation of the Click language and are of short stature.

A scientist named G.R. von Wielligh went among the former Hottentots, gathered up all their healing lore with regard to buchu leaves, and published it in an edition of the *Agricultural Journal of the University of South Africa* (6:80, 1913). The natives once used buchu for successfully treating gout, removing stones, promoting urination, correcting prostate problems, and clearing up bladder infections. They did this by making a tea out of the leaves and drinking it throughout the day. Put an ounce of leaves in one pint boiling water, cover and let simmer for 3 minutes on low heat, then remove and steep for 35 minutes. Strain and drink 2/3 cup 3 or 4 times a day. If buchu leaves are to be taken in the capsule form, it is recommended that 2 capsules twice daily be taken with 8 ounces of liquid.

Local Application for Bruises

The former Hottentots used buchu leaves as a local application to get rid of the swelling and discoloration caused by bruises. They would crush some of the fresh leaves and apply them directly to the site of the injury. You can make a tea with the dried leaves by following the preceding instructions, only double the quantity of leaves to be used. Soak a clean washcloth in the *hot* tea, wring out the excess liquid, and apply to the bruise. Repeat the process when it cools.

BUCKTHORN
(see CASCARA SAGRADA)

BUGLEWEED
(LYCOPUS SPECIES)

Brief Description

Often there are different species of the same plant, as with bugleweed. A couple of species exist in the American southwest and west: L. lucidus is slightly more astringent, while L. americanus is considerably more sedative in its actions.

Bugleweed is a typical member of the mint family, sharing the same square stem and opposing leaf structures as peppermint and spearmint. Bugleweed flowers grow in axillary whorls of tiny pink or white flowers, often only on the leaf-bearing sides of the stems; frequently motherwort, horehound and sage may share this same configuration, provided they don't grow in wet habitats. Bugleweed almost always grows along running water or wet backwashes.

Productive for Nosebleed, Excess Menstruation, Hemorrhoids, Bloody Urine, and Bloody Stool

One of the very best herb formulas that I've ever put together for internal or external hemorrhaging is a combination using bugleweed, shepherd's purse, and stinging nettle. These three herbs make a great hemostatic agent. Bring a quart of water to a boil; add one small handful each of bugleweed, shepherd's purse, and stinging nettle. Cover, simmer 3 minutes on medium heat, set aside and steep 45 minutes. Strain and refrigerate. Works best when used *cold*. Drink one *glass* on empty stomach to stop internal bleeding. Soak cotton balls in cold tea, squeeze out excess liquid and apply inside nostrils with head tilted back to stop nosebleeds. Or apply the same soaked cotton balls inside the rectum to stop bleeding hemorrhoids.

Useful for Mothers Following Labor

A simple tea made from bugleweed is quite helpful for mothers who've just delivered their newborns. It should be taken several days following labor. It helps to tonify their internal organs and circulatory systems. Follow the preceding tea recipe, except eliminate the other two herbs and just use two small handfuls of bugleweed to a quart of water as directed.

BULRUSH
(see CATTAIL)

BUPLEURUM
(BUPLEURUM CHINENSE)

Brief Description

Bupleurum or Chinese thoroughwax is a perennial herb growing wild on the sunny sides of sedge thickets. Its leaves are alternative, and broad linear-lanceolate; its apexes are acuminate; its bases gradually narrowing; the margins are intact and parallel veins 7 to 9 inches. In the autumn, small golden flowers that are either terminal or axillary appear to form compound umbellate inflorescences. The seed capsule is flat and elliptical in shape.

Prolapsed Uterus Mended

Anna Li was formerly a promising student some years ago at Ying Ming University in Taipei, Taiwan. But she suffered from a prolapsed uterus and had to postpone her college education. Regular doctors couldn't help her very much, so she went to see a Chinese herbalist. He was the one with whom I later conferred who told me about her case.

The doctor prescribed for her some bupleuri root. He had her take 20 small BB-size pills daily or drink one cup of the root. He gave her some of the dried, coarsely chopped root wrapped in newspaper and instructed her to put 2 tablespoons of the root in 2 pints boiling water, cover and cook on medium-to-low heat for 20 minutes, then to strain and drink one cup twice a day for two weeks. At the end of this treatment, another examination revealed that Anna's uterus had been restored to its natural position once more.

Headache and Backache Relieved

The doctor also informed me that this same tea brought considerable relief to his patients who suffered from headache or backache. He had them drink it as well as to apply hot/cold packs of the tea to their foreheads or along the top and base of their spines.

BURDOCK
(ARCTIUM LAPPA)

Brief Description

There are basically two kinds of burdock. Common burdock (*A. minus*) is the kind more commonly found intercropped with corn and wheat in the Midwest. Greater burdock is the one primarily harvested for its root as an important source of food in Japan. They use it there as we use carrots here. This variety of burdock has the big, round, brown bristly burrs, hence the common name of cockleburr.

Unsurpassed Blood Purifier

Burdock root is perhaps the most widely used of all blood purifiers, among the best the herbal kingdom has to offer for this, and *the* most important herb for treating chronic skin problems. It's one of the few that can effectively treat eczema, acne, psoriasis, boils, herpes, and syphilitic sores, styes, carbuncles, cankers, and the like.

To make an effective tea, bring 1 quart of water to a boil. Reduce heat to simmer, adding 4 teaspoons cut, dried root. Cover and let simmer for 7 minutes, then remove from heat and let steep for 2 hours longer. Drink a minimum of 2 cups per day on an empty stomach (more if chronic skin problems persist). A larger quantity can be made and used to wash the skin often.

Beating Zits, Naturally

Caroline Vodhanel, of Campbell, Ohio did some self-experimentation with various safe herbs to determine which ones would be the best to take in getting rid of her zits. She wrote: "I discovered that a combination of burdock root, red clover, and dandelion root helped me to relieve my acne vulgaris and blemishes. I took one capsule of each herb in the morning and again in the evening. Now my complexion is beautiful again. You may freely use this testimonial as you see fit."

Eliminating Stones

A great remedy for getting rid of some stubborn kidney and gallstones is to make a burdock-catnip tea. Bring 4 cups of water to a boil and add 2 tablespoons of chopped, fresh or cut dried root. Reduce to simmer for about 10 minutes, covered. Remove from heat and add 3 teaspoons chopped or cut fresh or dried catnip herb.

Let steep for 1-1/2 hours. Then strain and to each cup add 1 teaspoon lemon juice and 1/2 teaspoon pure maple syrup or blackstrap molasses to sweeten. Drink slowly. Exactly 10 minutes later, take orally 1 tablespoon of pure virgin olive oil.

Repeat this regimen 3 times each day. The tea soothes irritated tissues and helps to break up or partially dissolve the stones, while the oil acts as a lubricant to remove them from the body more easily. It's *very important* that *no* greasy, fried foods, soft drinks, refined carbohydrates like white flour or white sugar products or red meat and poultry be consumed during this treatment; otherwise, absolute and complete success cannot be fully guaranteed.

After taking the last cup of tea and spoonful of oil at night just before retiring, be sure to sleep on your right side with a pillow underneath your armpit. This resting posture, some claim, seems to expedite the removal of stones from the body more quickly.

A Wild Vegetable Dessert

Who would ever think that vegetables would serve as delicious desserts in place of more standard fare like pie and ice cream? Well, in the case of burdock root, you have such a tummy pleaser fit for a king.

BURDOCK ROOTS, HAWAIIAN STYLE

Needed: 2 tbsp. sweet butter, 1/4 cup packed brown sugar; 1 tsp. lemon juice; 1 cup canned, drained pineapple chunks (save juice); 1/2 cup pineapple syrup drained from chunks; 2 tbsp. cornstarch; 2 cups burdock roots, cut into rounds and precooked until tender.

Melt butter in skillet over low heat, add brown sugar and lemon juice; stir. Mix pineapple syrup with the cornstarch, stir well and add to the butter and sugar mixture. Stir constantly over low heat and the mixture is a thick sauce, about 20 min. Add the burdock roots and pineapple chunks to the sauce and heat through. Serve warm.

A Nourishing Herb-Fish Soup

An alternative-care medical doctor from Tokyo, Japan told me at a recent conference in Rhode Island what he prescribed to many of his patients recuperating from recent illness or surgery, or who just needed extra vim, vigor and vitality.

First secure a fresh-water fish of some kind from your local fish market or supermarket meat counter. Carp, salmon and trout are the best. About a pound of fish is necessary, along with 1-1/2 lbs. of fresh burdock root, 1 tbsp. of sesame seed oil, 2/3 cup of uncooked barley pearls, 1 tsp. fresh, grated ginger root, several unused green tea bags, 1/2 cup chopped chives, 2 tbsp. lime juice, and some kelp.

Nothing of the fish should be removed; head, fins, scales and bones all kept intact. Chop the entire fish into 1-1/4 inch chunks (approx. a dozen pieces), then cut the head into several more pieces, removing the eyes. Next cut the burdock root into *exceedingly thin* slices. Sautee this herb root for half an hour in sesame seed oil. After this place the pieces of fish on the bed of sauteed burdock. Cover with just enough water to maintain a nearly 3-in. level over the fish.

Next scatter the barley over the fish and roots, along with the chives and kelp. Then place several unused tea bags in opposite corners of the pot *and on top* of the fish. Cover and bring to a boil, then reduce the heat to a lower setting and slowly cook for at least 5-1/2 hours. At the end of this period of time, uncover the pot and remove the tea bags. Then add the grated ginger and lime juice, cover and simmer again for an additional 15-20 minutes. The entire preparation can be consumed over several days' time.

BUTTERCUP
(RANUNCULUS SPECIES)

Brief Description

Buttercup is the common name for the Ranuncualceae, a family of most annual or perennial herbs of cool regions of the Northern Hemisphere. Botanists believe this is one of the most primitive families of dicotyledenous plants. The buttercup family usually has a simple flower structure in which each flower part may be separate rather than fused into a single organ as are most other flowers.

The family includes many familiar wild flowers and a number of cultivated ornamentals. Some of the well-known representatives, a few of which are mentioned in this book, include: aconite, anemone, baneberry, columbine, globeflower, hellebore, marsh marigold (cowslip), and peony.

The largest genus, Ranunculus, comprises the buttercups and crowfoots, names often used interchangeably. Occurring in arctic, north temperate, and alpine regions, with species to be found in the Andes and in subantarctic regions, this genus is characterized by glossy yellow flowers (hence the name "buttercup") and deeply cut leaves (purportedly similar to crows' feet).

Buttercups contain an acrid juice that can inflame and blister the skin. Livestock avoid it for this reason. However, in former times, this root juice was applied to the joints to relieve gout and rheumatism, but since then has fallen out of favor, even with herbalists.

Tincture Cures Shingles and Sciatica

A tincture of the buttercup root can be made for curing shingles very effectively and relieving the excruciating pain accompanying sciatica. Dig up two buttercup root bulbs and wash them under running water to remove any debris. Put on some plastic gloves and chop both roots coarsely with a sharp French knife. (The gloves are to protect the hands from coming in contact with the juice and developing blisters.)

Put the chopped roots in a quart glass fruit jar. Add enough vodka, brandy, gin, or rum to cover. Seal with screw-on lid and set in a dark, cool place. Shake vigorously for one minute every day for 2-1/2 weeks. Then strain the tincture through a fine wire sieve or muslin cloth. For added potency, folk wisdom suggests and scientific investigation confirms that this be done only *during a full moon*. Put the liquid into smaller amber bottles that will keep out sunlight and preserve the tincture longer.

The person suffering from shingles should begin taking this tincture, about 10 drops under the tongue twice or three times daily, just as soon as an outbreak of small pimples appears with its accompanying pains in the rib cage. The treatment is continued until the shingles disappear. The tincture may also be taken internally as well as applied locally to the skin to relieve sciatica.

BUTTERFLY WEED
(see PLEURISY ROOT)

BUTTERNUT
(JUGLANS CINEREA)

Brief Description

Butternut is a member of the walnut family, a group of mostly deciduous, resinous trees marked by large and aromatic compound leaves. Also called the white walnut, the butternut produces a sweet and oily nut that is discussed in one of my other works, *Heinerman's Encyclopedia of Nuts, Berries and Seeds* (Englewood Cliffs, NJ: Prentice Hall, 1995).

Sugar is occasionally obtained from the sap of butternut. And butternut hulls yield a yellow-to-gray dye that gave color to the homespun wear of pioneers and to the "butternut" uniforms of some of the Confederate troops fighting in the American Civil War.

Joseph Smith's Inspired Remedy for Dysentery

Whenever I have occasion to think of butternut bark, my mind instantly harkens back to the time in Nauvoo, Illinois, when the founder of Mormonism, Joseph Smith, Jr., told the people in his usual lively humor to "gnaw down a butternut tree" if they suffered from dysentery. During the time (1839-1846) the Latter-Day Saints (Mormons) resided in their city by the Mississippi River, they had to contend with considerable fever and dysentery due to the brackish drinking water, an abundance of mosquitoes, and excessive heat and humidity.

In 1843, a large company of emigrants, newly arrived from Great Britain and elsewhere, gathered on the hill in Nauvoo, Illinois, near the Mississippi River, beside the half-completed Temple, where the great Mormon leader preached to them for over an hour. A member of the Quorum of the Twelve Apostles of the Church of Jesus Christ of Latter-Day Saints by the name of Elder Willard Richards took notes while Smith spoke. Richards was, by profession a doctor trained in the Thomsonian system of herbal medicine.

Part of his talk focused on matters of health; he explained to the large congregation some of the problems connected with drinking water obtained from the river, springs and shallow wells. "If you feel any inconvenience," he advised, then "take some mild physic two or three times, and follow that up with some good bitters. If you cannot get anything else, take a little salts and cayenne pepper. If you cannot get salts, take ipecacuanha." Then in his typical wit, he added, "Or gnaw down a butternut tree" (as opposed to scraping off the inner bark and making a tea from it). He also recommended "boneset or horehound" as well. (This interesting and helpful information came from *History of the Church of Jesus Christ of Latter-Day Saints* (Salt Lake City: Deseret News, 1909; 5: 354-57.)

For those unfamiliar with dysentery, it can be any of several disorders characterized by inflammation of the intestines, especially of the colon, and attended by pain in the abdomen, painful straining for fecal evacuation, and frequent stools containing blood and mucus. Bacteria, protozoa, or parasitic worms, usually ingested from bad drinking water, are the major causes.

The part of the tree to which Smith referred was the inner bark of the root, usually collected in May or June. It is deep brown in color to the core. Its exterior surface is nearly smooth but a little warty in places, while the inside is smooth and of rather thin, stringy fiber. Powdered butternut bark tends to always be a chocolate brown.

The average intake for the powder is about 3 capsules twice daily in cases of dysentery. Otherwise, a tea made from the root bark is just as effective. Two tablespoons of coarsely chopped bark are added to two pints of boiling water, covered, and simmered for ten minutes on low heat, then set aside and steeped 45 minutes. The tea is strained and one cup twice daily on an empty stomach is consumed.

I might add that I have tried some of Joseph Smith's other suggestions for dysentery when I've been in Third World countries. In every instance his recommendations worked well in stopping watery stool discharges.

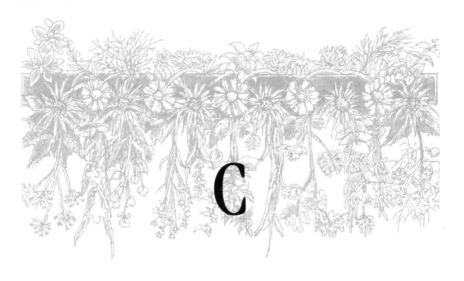

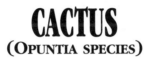

CACTUS
(OPUNTIA SPECIES)

Brief Description

A cactus is any plant recognized for its fleshy green stem, which performs the function of leaves, and for the spines (not always present) of various colors, shapes and arrangements. The flowers of an individual cactus are notably delicate in appearance although often somewhat large and showy. Their colors can vary from species to species, but are usually yellow, white or variations of red and purple. A cactus usually yields edible berries.

The most beautiful place I believe I've ever been to see many different varieties of cactus is in Ajo, Arizona. Some years ago I took a most unusual trip in an open jeep with a guide into the heart of the huge Organ Pipe Cactus National Monument. It is 330,000 stunning acres that showcase the most pristine tract of the great Sonoran Desert of the American Southwest. To this day I can still vividly recall many wonderful moments from that thrilling trip. How could I ever forget those suicidal jackrabbits that flashed across the road and froze in the thin shadows of creosote bushes as our vehicle came within range? Or fail to remember the harsh tenor rasps of the cactus wrens as they screeched madly at each other? Or those Harris' hawks floating overhead in the still blueness like live kites, looking for their next dietary morsel of some scurrying ground rodent? This was cactus country indeed, where the crickets ticked and cicadas droned.

We discovered some 30 different species of cactuses at Organ Pipe. They grew out of rock and sand at whatever crazy angle their footholds required. The organ pipe cactuses are what give the park its name and reputation; they sprout huge vertical arms up to 25 feet high. These cactuses, we carefully noted, had almost reached the northern edge of their range.

Diabetic Potential Validated

The species of cactus known as "prickly pear" has been used by Native American and Hispanic cultures throughout the American Southwest to treat adult and juvenile onset diabetes. The usual method of preparation has been to make a tea from the fruit and pads, but sometimes the powdered cactus is also taken in capsule form. Gloves should be worn when working with these parts and an effort made to remove the spines with pliers and to peel them. Chop up enough to make 2-1/2 cupsful. Then boil them in 1-1/2 quarts water for 25 minutes. After this, the tea is strained and used. Due to the slimy quality of the tea, it may need to be diluted with a little water to improve the taste. Three cups are taken each day with meals.

How effective has the treatment been? Well, apart from individual testimonies from diabetics who've been helped, there is also some validating scientific evidence. A lengthy report entitled, "The hypoglycemic effect of *Opunita streptacantha* studied in different animal experimental models," was published in the *Journal of Ethnopharmacology* (7:175-181, 1983). It stated, in part, that prickly pear cactus "induced hypoglycemic effects when orally administered to intact animals under induced states of moderate increase of blood sugar." What this means in terms of diabetics is that the use of prickly pear cactus fruit and pad is an effective treatment for this disease based on medical folklore and confirmed by scientific fact. Those who use it in the powdered form should take about 5 capsules daily.

Dry, Itchy Scalp Improved

Some Native American tribes of the Southwest have resorted to cactus as a good rinse and conditioner for dry, itchy scalps. The Apache and Pima will take small chunks of the peeled pads, add them to a container of water and shake thoroughly. Then the slimy juice is strained into another vessel, poured over the head slowly and gently massaged in. After leaving it in the hair for about six minutes, it is then rinsed out under cold, running water, leaving the hair silky smooth and the scalp with a clean, tingling feeling.

Indian Remedy Heals Shattered Leg

The following true story happened in the 1870s somewhere along the Utah-Arizona border. It was related many years ago by Albert Lyman, a modern descendant of the principal character injured.

"Jody Lyman was hit by one of the thieves' shots and it shattered the bone in his leg just above the knee. His companions took him to the willows. When darkness came they headed back to Bluff [Utah] more than a hundred miles away. His pain was agonizing with every step of the horse. Six or eight miles out from the river he could bear it no longer. They stopped in the middle of a desert with no water around for seven miles. The wounded man couldn't be moved next morning or the next. It seemed like there was nothing to do but watch the sufferer die.

"His leg, terribly swollen and discolored, had maggots in it. Riding up to the distressed camp was Pah-lilly, a Navajo medicine man. He asked several questions and discerned the gravity of the situation: "What are you doing for him?" he asked in his own language. They made him understand that they were doing nothing. Pah-lilly told them to gather a few prickly pear [cactus] leaves, of which there was plenty nearby, to burn the spines from them and mash them into a poultice to be applied to each side of the leg. His leg was healed [after that]."

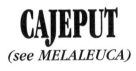

CAJEPUT
(see MELALEUCA)

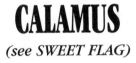

CALAMUS
(see SWEET FLAG)

CALENDULA
(CALENDULA OFFICINALIS)

Brief Description

More popular in Europe than in America, calendula yields bright yellow to orange flowerheads, and is prolific in numerous waste places and gardens as a hardy weed of sorts. An old folk belief says that if its flowerheads should close up after 7:00 a.m., it will rain for sure the next day.

Its greatest value in either salve or dilute tincture form is for any kind of external skin, muscle or blood vessel problems—wounds, sores, varicose veins, pulled muscles, boils, bruises, sprains, athlete's foot, burns, frostbites, etc.

Heals Intestinal Ulcers and Colitis

Two important medical studies published in Vol. 20 of the Soviet journal *Vatreshni Bolesti* for June 1981 confirm the value of calendula in healing duo-denal ulcers, inflammation of both the stomach and duodenum, and intesti-nal colitis. In the first instance, an equal mixture of comfrey root and calen-dula brought healing relief to 19 patients with duodenal ulcers and 19 oth-ers suffering from gastroduodenitis. A tea made of both herbs (1 tbsp. of each herb in 1 quart boiling water, simmered 5 minutes, steeped 40 minutes) was administered to each patient (2 cups daily) with considerable success.

In the second study cited, 24 patients with chronic nonspecific colitis were treated with a combination of herbs consisting of equal parts of dan-delion root, St. Johnswort, lemon balm, calendula and fennel seed, made into a strong tea (1 tsp. of each herb in 1-1/2 qts. boiling water, steeped 1 hour) and given to each of them three times a day, 1 cup at a time. According to the published medical report's brief English abstract: "As a result of the treatment, the spontaneous and palpable pains along the large intestine disappeared in 95.83% of the patients by the 15th day of their admission to the clinic." This is sufficient testimony to demonstrate the clin-ical validity of this wonderful herb for successfully treating all manner of inflammation.

Varicose Veins Disappeared

A West German herbalist, Maria Treben, relates the following episode:

On a visit, the lady of the house showed me her legs covered with varicose veins. I fetched calendula from her garden and prepared the ointment [recipe listed below]. The residue I put immediately on her legs (the residue can be used four to five times). She spread the ointment, the thickness of the back of a knife, on a piece of linen and bandaged her legs with it. You will be surprised when I tell you that four weeks later, when she visited me at home, the varicose veins had disappeared. Both legs had nice, smooth skin.

Making a Healing Salve and Tincture

Finely chop two heaping handfuls of fresh calendula leaves, flowers and stems. Next gently melt enough lard in a heavy frying pan on low heat to equal about 2-1/2 cups. Add the chopped calendula, stir with a wooden ladle for a few minutes, then remove the pan from the stove, cover and let the contents set for an entire day. The next day warm the pan up again, filter contents through cloth and pour into clean jars. Seal tightly and rub liberally on the skin whenever necessary. A ready-made Calendula Dairy Salve from Old Amish Herbs (see Appendix) is unique from all other ointments in one respect—its base consists of pure pork lard, one of the most absorbent materials for the skin. This salve is good for man and beast alike.

To make a tincture soak a handful of flowers in 2 cups of whiskey for 14 days on a window sill in the sun. Shake several times each day. When taking internally for hepatitis, cramps and inflammation, use 12-15 drops at a time.

An Improved Bean Recipe

Calendula flowers tend to impart a more delicate flavor to the creamy smoothness of butter beans, especially when they are complemented by a rich, tasty sauce.

CALENDULA BUTTER BEANS

Needed: 3 cups butter beans, cooked and drained (hold back 2/3 cup of the liquid); 1/4 cup oatmeal; 2 tbsps. butter; 1/2 cup whole wheat flour; 2/3 cup nonfat milk; granulated kelp for flavor; pinch of nutmeg; 1/2 tsp. chopped parsley; bread crumbs; some olive oil; 1 each medium-sized onion, carrot, celery stalk, and tomato, all diced; 1 tbsp. olives; 1-1/2 cups vegetable stock; and 3 tbsps. calendula (or marsh marigold) flower petals.

In a Vita-Mix whole food machine or similar food processor, combine 1 cup beans and oatmeal. In a saucepan, melt the butter, add 1/4 cup flower and cool for 3 minutes. Slowly add milk and reserved bean liquid, stirring constantly, and bring to a gentle simmer. Cook, stirring always until thickened. Add the kelp, nutmeg and parsley; mix with the beans and oatmeal.

Preheat oven to 375° F. Dab a paper towel in some olive oil and lightly rub it over the sides and bottom of a baking dish. Then fill the bottom with bread crumbs. Add the remaining beans and pour the beans/oats mixture over the top. Sprinkle with some more bread crumbs and bake for 40 minutes until nicely browned.

In a saucepan, sautee the diced vegetables in olive oil on medium high heat for 5 minutes, shaking the pan occasionally. Mix the remaining flour with a little stock to form a smooth paste. Remove the vegetables with a slotted spoon and add stock to the pan. Gradually add the flour mixture and bring to a simmer, stirring always. Return the vegetables to the pan and simmer gently for a couple of minutes. Pour this vegetable mixture over the beans and garnish with calendula petals. Serves 4 to 6.

CALIFORNIA LAUREL
(see BAY)

CAMPHOR
(CINNAMOMUM CAMPHORA)

Brief Description

Camphor isn't a plant, but something obtained from one. It is a white crystalline substance obtained from a species of tree known by the Latin binomial cited in the heading. It is a type of evergreen resembling the lime or linden tree (Tilia europa); both reach great heights averaging 120 feet or more and when in full bloom emit very aromatic fragrances that grace the air for some distance around them.

The ancient Chinese highly valued camphor because of its antiseptic and disinfectant properties; they frequently used it to scent soap and for embalming purposes. In other parts of the Orient it has been used for incense burning.

Marco Polo's Medicinal References to Camphor

The famous Italian traveler Marco Polo (1254?-1324) met the famed Mongolian leader Kublai Khan in 1275 A.D., entered the ruler's diplomatic service, and was sent on a variety of missions to all parts of the large Mongolian empire. During these frequent trips, he saw and recorded much in his diaries. Polo mentioned that wherever there was a plague, orders would be sent out for camphor incense to be burned in all the homes of sick and well alike. He noted that this helped to contain the spread of further infection by purifying the air that others would breathe.

He wrote that a little oil of camphor was slightly cold to the touch and used locally on the gumline at the site of an infected tooth to contain the aching pain by numbing the sensory nerves. Based on Polo's observations, I have recommended that a little oil of camphor be rubbed on the lower back to remove backache and on sore muscles to relieve them. It can also be used with good effect locally for sciatica and rheumatism.

Polo spoke of seeing a little camphor rubbed on the temples, foreheads, necks, spines, and abdomens of opium addicts who were in withdrawal from their drug habits. He correctly noted that camphor displayed a very soothing effect upon their highly excited nerves. Again, based on his own historical observations, I have recommended similar treatment for some ex-heroin junkies, trying to kick their drug habit but having a very difficult time. Two reported back to me later just how calming and soothing camphor was to them when nothing else seemed to work.

This great Italian also made references to camphor's wonderful effects in Oriental medicine for treating asthma and bronchitis. Mongolian and Chinese doctors would rub some of the oil of camphor on the chests and backs of their patients suffering from such respiratory disorders. They would also put a few drops in some warm water and have their patients slowly sip this.

The combined therapy, he stated, had the effect of having them cough up considerable mucus and improving their breathing.

Salt Lake Jailer Relies on Camphor

Claustrophobia is what quickly sets in when you take an escorted tour through the 30-year-old Salt Lake County Jail. As I walked the hallways of this basement bastille, I found myself having to hunch my shoulders so they wouldn't brush the walls on either side. The only light was artificial, and in the subterranean gloom the ceiling lowered and the corridors squeezed. It wasn't entirely a trick of my imagination, since the building I was in had settled enough in the last three decades that in the basement the walls bulged six inches inward. The guard showing me through casually joked, "We're just waiting for the rivets to blow."

Now what was I doing in a place like this? Had I forgotten to pay my parking ticket? Hardly! I was there to do a story on the miserable living conditions of the jail for a monthly newspaper (*Utah Prime Times*) of which I am the editor.

Besides the dilapidated state of the jail, there is also another health danger lurking, albeit more minor and subtle. The smell is indescribable. It's as if more than a quarter of a century of dead air, already passed through countless nostrils and mouths and never properly circulated to the outside, had formed fetid knee-deep pools. Stirred up by thousands of passages each day, the scent clung to my hair and suit long after I had returned to the outside. "What happened to you?" asked my secretary Linda Klein when I returned to my research center. "Did a dog urinate on you by chance?"

"That bad, huh?" I asked incredulously.

It was my comment about the dank air to the guard escorting me that led to his short discussion about camphor. He produced a little vial of camphor and said, "I never come to work without this stuff. Every 30 minutes or so I'll take a little whiff of it and it helps clear out the cobwebs from my head. If I didn't do this, the stuffy conditions down here would probably get to me big time, and make me pretty ill. But this way I can put in my eight hours each day without much of a problem. I think the stuff [meaning camphor] probably disinfects my sinuses or something like that. I mean, I don't get anywhere near the colds, coughs, or sore throats that the rest of the jailers or inmates seem to be getting. And let me tell you, when one of the toilets or urinals backs up in a cell, then's about the time you want to die or else go topside for some fresh air. But this stuff here," he noted, while holding up the small glass vial of camphor again, "saves my butt . . . er, I mean my nose every time!"

CAÑAIGRE
(see DESERT GINSENG)

CANNABIS
(see MARIJUANA)

CARAWAY
(Carum carvi)

Brief Description

Caraway is a biennial or perennial cultivated and found wild in the northern and northwestern U.S., Europe and Asia. The hollow, furrowed, angular, branched stem begins to grow in the second year from a white, carrot-shaped root. The leaves are bi- or tri-pinnate and deeply incised, the upper ones on a sheath-like petiole. The small white or yellow flowers make their appearance in the late spring (usually from May to June). The seeds are dark brown, flat and oblong in shape.

Women's Tea for Tardy Menstruation

A nutritious broth or vegetable-herb tea can be made from the following ingredients and taken by women who have delayed periods in order to encourage the onset of their menstrual cycle. Bring 1 quart of water to a boil. Add 1 tsp. caraway seed, 1/2 small chopped carrot, 1/2 of 1 chopped celery stalk and 1/2 tsp. grated ginger root. Cover and simmer on low heat for 25 minutes. Uncover and remove from heat. Add 1 tsp. *each* fresh chopped parsley, fresh cut watercress, dried peppermint and yarrow. Cover again and steep an additional 20 minutes or so. Strain, sweeten and flavor with a few drops and pinches of honey and cinnamon. Drink 3 cups each day on an empty stomach until period commences.

Nature's Anti-Gas Medicine

To prevent heartburn and acid indigestion, simply bring 2 cups of water to a boil, adding 4 tsp. slightly pounded seeds. Simmer on low heat 5 minutes, then steep away from heat an additional 15 minutes. Sweeten to taste with a little honey and drink one cup with each meal for pleasant digestion of food. When taken warm, the tea will also promote the onset of menstruation, help relieve uterine cramps, promote breast milk secretion in nursing mothers, and help clear away mucus from the back of the throat. Small amounts may also be given with good results to infants suffering from intestinal gas.

Culinary Value

Not only do caraway seeds add a certain pungent flavor to cabbage, turnips, potatoes and breads, but they also help to digest the starches in some of these foods. The seeds are indispensable in making rye, pumpernickel and Swedish breads.

Likewise, they find added attraction in many European dishes, especially stews and soups, ranging from Hungarian goulash to Russian borscht. Apple sauce, pickled beets, sauerkraut, squash and pumpkin pies shouldn't be without them either.

CARDAMOM
(ELETTARIA CARDAMOMUM)

Brief Description

Cardamom is a perennial found throughout southern India, but also cultivated quite extensively in the tropics as well. The simple, erect stems reach an average height of 8 feet from a mere thumb-thick, creeping rootstock. The leaves are lanceolate, dark green and glabrous above, lighter and silky-

like beneath. The small, yellowish flowers grow in loose racemes on prostrate flower stems. The fruit is a three-celled capsule holding up to 18
seeds. Cardamom is used in cooking and for flavoring wormwood and
valerian.

Remedy for Celiac Disease

Celiac disease is an intolerance for the gluten in grain commonly occurring
in children, and marked by frequent diarrhea and continual digestive problems. Generally a gluten-free diet is prescribed to help them. But when I
was in mainland China in 1980, I discovered in some city hospitals we visited the use of powdered cardamom sprinkled on cooked cereal to correct
this problem in youngsters. I've recommended it here with relatively good
results. Children who have the same kind of problem are able to handle
grains like cooked oatmeal or whole wheat bread when sufficient cardamom has been previously included.

Spice Improved Digestion of Founder of Gray Panthers

The late Maggie Kuhn, who died in 1995 at the age of 89, was one of the
founders of the Gray Panthers, an activist senior citizens organization with
40,000 members in 32 states and six countries. In an interview with her
several years ago, a reporter with the *Philadelphia Inquirer* learned that
Kuhn sometimes took a little cardamom with a few of her meals because,
she said, it helped to improve the digestion of her food.

The easiest way to take cardamom with a meal is to put a little bit in
a single gelatin capsule before the meal, and swallow with a cup of water.

Culinary Advantages

Because of its mild, pleasant, ginger-like flavor, cardamom can be used in
a number of bean dishes, holiday beverages such as eggnog, or baked
goodies like Danish sweet rolls and fruit cakes. However, as said previously, it's especially valuable in cooked cereals and whole grain breads for
those unable to tolerate the gluten.

CARDAMON COFFECAKE

Needed: 1/4 cup chopped walnuts; 1 tbsp. each white and brown flour; 1
tbsp. white and brown sugar; 1 tsp. ground cinnamon; 1 tbsp. chilled butter,
cut into small bits; 1 cup white flour; 1/4 cup brown sugar; 1/2 tsp. baking

powder; 1/4 tsp. each of baking soda and powdered cardamom; a pinch of salt; 1/2 cup plain yogurt; 1-1/2 tbsps. melted butter; 1 farm egg; some vegetable cooking spray; 2 more tsps. white flour; and 1 medium pear, peeled, cored, and cut into 1/4-inch wedges.

Combine the first four ingredients in a bowl; cut in 1 tbsp. butter with a pastry blender until the mixture resembles coarse meal. Set aside. Next, combine 1 cup flour and the next five ingredients in a large bowl; mix together thoroughly. Combine yogurt and the next two ingredients; stir well. Add this to the flour mixture, stirring just until moistened.

Coat a nine-inch round cakepan with cooking spray; lightly dust with two tsps. flour. Spread the batter into the prepared pan. Arrange the pear wedges on top of the batter like wagon-wheel spokes, around the edge of the pan, overlapping slightly (avoid placing the pears over the center of the batter). Sprinkle the walnut mixture evenly over the top of the coffeecake. Bake at 350°F. for 30-40 minutes. Serves 8.

CARDAMOM COOKIES

Needed: 3/4 cup white flour; 1/2 cup honey; 1/2 tsp. each powdered cardamom and powdered cinnamon; 1/4 tsp. baking soda; 3 tbsps. melted butter; 1 farm egg, lightly beaten; some vegetable cooking spray.

Combine the first five ingredients in a medium bowl and stir well. Add the melted butter and egg; stir thoroughly. Drop the dough by rounded teaspoonfuls 3 inches apart onto baking sheets coated with cooking spray. Bake at 350° F. for 12 minutes. Remove from the pans, and let the cookies cool completely on wire racks. Makes two dozen cookies.

CASCARA SAGRADA
(RHAMNUS PURSHIANA)

Brief Description

The tree from which the valuable reddish-brown bark is obtained is a small- to medium-sized deciduous with hairy twigs, capable of reaching heights near 50 feet in some instances. The tree is native to the Pacific Coast states and provinces of the U.S. and Canada. The bark is removed from trees with trunk diameters of about 4 feet or more. It's then permitted to dry and age for one year before use, as the fresh bark has an emetic principle which is destroyed on prolonged storage or by heating.

Guaranteed Laxative

If your colon isn't functioning like you think it should be, this is the herb for you. The Nov.-Dec. 1982 issue of the Italian medical journal *G. Clin. Medica*, reported that a preparation containing cascara was definitely an effective therapy for clearing up simple constipation in many elderly patients. Up to 3 capsules at a time should do the job nicely. For a more complete "roto rooter" effect on your bowels, try an herbal spice laxative formula from Old Amish Herbs. It is said to be a very "moving" experience. (See the Product Appendix for further details.)

Helps Fight Herpes Simplex

I attended the Second International Herb Symposium held at Wheaton College in Norton, Massachusetts in 1992. Qualified practitioners and scientists gave several interesting workshops covering many aspects of herbal healing.

One of those with whom I spoke told me she had used tea extracts of cascara bark for treating herpes simplex in some of her college-age patients. However, for fear of reprisal from state or federal health authorities for practicing medicine without a license, she asked that I not use her name or even mention where she resided. I agreed to this reasonable request. She described how she made the tea by boiling two tablespoons of the crude bark in one quart of distilled water, covered, for 10 minutes. After letting the tea steep for another 30 minutes, it was strained and refrigerated. She advised her herpes patients to drink three cups a day with meals, as well as to bathe their herpes sores with some of the fluid. She reported that it is about 70% successful in putting the herpes virus back into hibernation. (It is impossible to get rid of the virus, but it can be kept in a dormant state for many years through proper diet, herbal and nutritional supplements, and a relaxed mood.)

CASTOR BEAN
(RICINUS COMMUNIS)

Brief Description

Castor bean responds very well to heat and humidity. The hotter and moister the climate, the taller it becomes, taking on tree-size proportions of 30-40 feet tall. In countries of more moderate warmth and less humidity, it is of more slender growth, averaging only 10 to 15 feet in height. But in colder environments, it is reduced in size to a mere shrub of no more than five feet tall.

It makes a nice cultivated ornamental, however, on account of its beautiful foliage. The handsome leaves are placed alternately on the stem, on long, curved, purplish foot-stalks, with drooping blades, between 6 to 8 inches wide. They are divided palmately about 75% to their depth into 7 to 11 lance-shaped segments which are pointed and coarsely toothed. When they become fully expanded, they are of a blue-green hue.

The flowers are both male and female on the same plant, and are produced on a clustered, oblong, terminal spike. The bean part of the plant contains a very toxic compound.

Medicinal Applications for the Respiratory System

Two Italian medical researchers wrote a paper on the "Various Uses of the Caster Oil Plant," which was published in an issue of the *Journal of Ethnopharmacology* (5:117-37, 1982) some years ago. They noted an old custom practiced in some parts of Italy to splash leaves of the castor bean with vinegar to cure chest inflammation. In Haiti, they use castor oil with an infusion of orange leaves against bronchitis. In the Ivory Coast and Upper Volta on the African continent, natives will rub their chests, backs, throats, and necks with castor bean leaves to recover from pneumonia and similar feverish afflictions.

The foregoing uses can be somewhat justified by scientific observations made in the laboratory that tea extracts of the leaves possess specific activity against *Mycobacterium tuberculosis* and *Aspergillus niger*, both responsible for some respiratory infections.

Infectious Skin Diseases Healed

The lengthy report by these two Italian researchers also indicated that castor oil was very helpful in treating a number of serious skin afflictions from the now-extinct smallpox to leprosy, and from fungal to parasitic infections. In most cases, the afflicted part was massaged with some castor oil, which had previously been lightly cooked on low heat with several unspecified antibiotic herbal drugs.

Some reasonable substitutes here would be to use a little garlic or onion juice (about one tablespoonful) or some goldenseal root powder (approx. 1/2 teaspoonful) in 1/4 cup castor oil, heated for a few minutes and frequently stirred to mix everything well.

CATNIP
(Nepeta cataria)

Brief Description

Catnip is a perennial herb of the mint family. Its erect, square, branching stem is hairy and grows from 3-5 feet high. The oblong or cordate, pointed leaves have scalloped edges and gray or whitish hairs on the lower side. The flowers are white with purple spots and grow in spikes from June to September.

Sure Cure for Insomnia and Hyperactivity

A major constituent in catnip, nepelactone, is quite similar in its chemical structure to the valepotriates, the sedative principles of valerian root. This helps to explain why a "cup of hot catnip tea taken at bedtime insures a good night's sleep." Mice given catnip extract experienced a reduction of overall activity and an increase in their sleeping time. And a hot water extract administered to young (9- and 27-day-old) chicks in a hatchery caused "a significant increase" in their average daily and weekly light sleep time.

To make yourself a truly effective nightcap, simply bring 1-1/2 cups of water to a boil. Remove from heat and add 1 tsp. of preferably the fresh cut herb or else 1 tsp. of the dried material and let steep for about 20 minutes until lukewarm before drinking. Honey may be added if desired. An Old Amish Herbs remedy called Night Nip works pretty well, too, for insomnia (see Product Appendix). Three capsules before retiring is suggested. The tea is also very good for reducing fevers, the miseries of hayfever, and nausea. A small cup of warm catnip tea sweetened with honey is good for calming hyperactive kids.

Relieves Aching Tooth, Gums

Rural residents of the Ozark and Appalachian Mountains employ either mashed fresh catnip leaves or the dried herb powder as a crude poultice application directly to sore gums or aching teeth, to relieve the intense pain and suffering. If the powder is to be used, a piece of cotton is moistened with water and then some of the powder applied on the surfaces, after which the cotton is put into the mouth and held firmly against the aching tooth or just rubbed on the gums for quick relief. The fresh leaves seem to bring nearly instant relief, while the dried powder takes a little longer to work.

Remarkable Eyewash

A strong catnip tea can be used as an effective eyewash to relieve inflammation and swelling due to certain airborne allergies, cold and flu, and excess alcoholic intake ("bloodshot eye" syndrome). Bring 3 cups of water to a boil and add 5 tsp. of cut fresh leaves. Reduce to low heat and let simmer for only 3 minutes. Remove from heat and let steep an additional 50 minutes. Strain and refrigerate in a clean fruit jar. Use as an eyewash with an eye cup several times each day. Or soak a clean terry-cloth towel in a warm solution of the tea and apply over the eyes for half an hour. Used catnip tea bags, while still warm and wrung out, can also be put on the eyelids for some relief.

Marijuana Substitute

In my occasional campus lectures before college students or high school kids on the subject of herbs in general, I am often asked the familiar question, "What herbs are there that you can legally smoke to get you high?" My answer, based upon solid clinical evidence, has invariably been catnip, even though I believe young people shouldn't be using them as such.

In a past issue of *JAMA* (*J. of the Am. Med. Assoc.* 236:473,1976), UCLA psychologist Dr. Ronald K. Siegel has also mentioned catnip in this regard. But the most compelling evidence for catnip's psychedelic effects comes from the Feb. 17, 1969 issue of *JAMA*. Several cases were reported, of which one is excerpted here for the benefit of readers who may personally know young people who might benefit from a safer and more legal herbal hallucinogen, than those which are harmful to the health and definitely illegal.

> A 17-year-old white female high school student has been undergoing psychotherapy for two years for relatively mild behavior disorders. The patient has smoked marijuana for approximately one year, usually twice a month. She has used cataria for 3 months, approximately once a week. She describes the effects of catnip as being similar to marijuana, i.e., relieving depression, elevating mood and producing euphoria...The subject can voluntarily reactivate this experience for up to 3 days after having smoked cataria and often does so to escape the boredom she experiences in school.

Catnip cigarettes and tea are also very good for overcoming any kind of dizziness.

'Frisco SPCA Loves Their Cats and Catnip, Too

Some time ago I paid a visit to the San Francisco Society for the Prevention of Cruelty to Animals (SPCA). A staff member showed me around its facilities and offered me a warm cup of catnip tea. I mentioned the irony of them having catnip on hand, considering that their organization deals in cats (as well as dogs and other domestic animals). My hostess, Eileen, was quite forthright as to why they kept plenty around. "We find that when things get pretty stressful around here, nothing seems to quite relax us like a warm cup of this tea. Catnip is so soothing to the nerves, you know." I chimed in with good humor: "I gather it's the pu-r-r-r-fect herb for the occasion."

Eileen then told me that a person can learn a lot about a cat's disposition by reading it's tail signals. "The tail is a handy guide to a feline's heart," she said. "A swishing tail indicates anger. A straight-up tail expresses pride or happiness. A tail curled tightly around the body may express fear or insecurity." I thanked her for this timely advice and will, hereafter, pay closer attention to the tail messages my own office cat, Jake, routinely sends out to me and the rest of my staff.

CATTAIL
(TYPHA LATIFOLIA)

Brief Description

Cattail is easy enough to recognize by any lake, marsh or swamp: on each separate, substantial and round stalk with its long, tapering, pointed, ribbonlike green leaves there grows at the end a plump, brown weiner. At the start of the growing season each of these hot-dog-shaped protuberances is crowded with initially green feminine flowers. Above these later are shriveling, microspore-crammed tops which, when maturing, drop their male cells of their own free will to fertilize their sisters; this eventually produces golden pollen and hoardes of tiny, white-tufted seeds that the winds disperse across the landscape for considerable distance.

Just about every part of the cattail, from its large starchy roots to its cornlike buds and later the flourlike pollen, is quite edible and very good for your health.

An experienced tracker and backwoods survivalist, Tom Brown recounted some of his own childhood experiences with the common cattail in his book, *Tom Brown's Guide to Wild Edible and Medicinal Plants* (New York: Berkley Books, 1985; pp.87-88). A portion of that narrative has been included here with the kind permission of the publisher.

"As time passed and we learned more of what the cattail could be used for, we began to experiment and come up with our own ideas. We certainly used the cattail head (punk) soaked in tallow, to burn as a torch and as a smudge to rid the area of mosquitoes, and as an addition to our tinder bundles [for making campfires]. We soon discovered what a great insulation the cattail down was, and began to incorporate it into our clothing. One of my favorite things was to get two old blankets and sew them together with an opening at the top. Into the opening we would stuff cattail down until it made a huge pillowlike affair. These we used as sleeping bags through the winter, and they kept us warm and snug in all types of weather. At the end of the season, we would shake out the cattail down, thus reseeding the swamps, and wash our makeshift bags."

Flour for Medicinal and Nutritive Purposes

A handy flour can be obtained from the rootstock of cattails. I thank James E. Churchill for letting me copy from an old issue of the now-defunct *Mother Earth News* (May 1970, pp.59-60) his technique for extracting the starch.

"Fill a large container with cold clean water. Dump in peeled [cattail] roots and mash with a potato masher or large stick. When the roots are crushed, reach down and get a bundle and begin tearing them apart. Wring and tear until you have nothing left but what looks like a string. Tear until every bit of pulp is gone from the fibers and remove the fibers from the water. Strain the water through a cloth until a lump of pulp and starch is left. Strain with fresh water three times or until the pulp is nice and clean. Dry it [spread out on a cookie sheet in the sun] and run it through a grinder until all pieces are reduced to powder. Then store in an empty coffee can with a plastic lid as you would regular flour."

Diarrhea: Make a tea by adding a small handful of cattail flour to 1 1/2 cups of hot water. Stir thoroughly before drinking. Two to three cups daily is advisable until problem ceases.

Poison Ivy Rash/Burns: Make a medium-thick paste by adding just enough water to a small handful of cattail flour. Mix thoroughly with a wooden spoon to get out the lumps. Then spread a thin layer on the injured skin using a cake spatula. Leave for several hours before changing the dressing.

Insect Bites/Stings: Mix 1 teaspoon of water with 1 tablespoon cattail flour. Mix until an even paste forms; then spread this rather thickly on the injured site.

Tooth Problems: Believe it or not, nature has provided *both* a toothbrush as well as the toothpaste in the same plant! Remove all of the down from a cattail stalk, which then becomes a handy toothbrush. Wet a little dab of cattail flour and rub the paste on your teeth with one forefinger. Then brush with the fuzzy stalk.

At the base of each green leaf may be found a sticky substance. Tom Brown claimed he had "used this sticky juice for deadening the pain of toothaches with good results."

Cuts/Abrasions: Apply some of this same sticky juice to a cut or a scrape; it makes a wonderful antiseptic and coagulant agent.

Hair/Scalp Problems: An equal mixture of cattail flour and pure lard or Crisco shortening makes a temporary but effective hair conditioner when you're out in the wilderness where your hair can suffer some potential damage from wind, rain, or sun.

Nervousness/Stress: Some Hopis, who formerly lived in the ancient Indian village of Old Oraibi in northeast Arizona, made a chewing gum by mixing some of the brown fuzz scraped from a few cattail stalks with a little mutton tallow. This they would then chew on for hours to alleviate stress and nervousness.

Physical Weakness/Fatigue: Cattail flour adds beautiful color, flavor, nutrition, body and thickening to any soup for which it is used. It also gives appetite to someone who doesn't feel like eating much. Try adding a handful to a beef or chicken broth and notice the difference it makes.

The following recipe makes very delicious muffins that are easily digested by those with weak stomachs and poor appetites.

CATTAIL MUFFINS

Needed: 1 cup each of cattail flour and whole wheat flour; 2 tsps. baking powder; 1/2 tsp. salt; 1 egg beaten; 1/4 cup each of sunflower oil and honey; 1-1/2 cups milk.

Combine the dry ingredients first before adding the wet ones. Stir only minimally, probably no more than 15 seconds. Ignore whatever lumps there may be in the batter. Grease or paper a muffin tin, then fill two-thirds with batter. Bake for 20 minutes in a preheated 400°F. oven. Makes about two dozen delicious muffins.

Serve some muffins with a bowl of soup which has had a little cattail flour added to it. Not only will the person eat heartily, but will also gain much strength from both.

CAYENNE PEPPER
(CAPSICUM FRUTESCENS, C. ANNUUM)

Brief Description

Cayenne pepper is a perennial in its native tropical America, but is an annual when cultivated outside of the tropical zones. Growing to a height of three feet or more, its glabrous stem is woody at the bottom and branched near the top. The leaves are ovate to lanceolate, entire and petioled. The drooping, white-to-yellow flowers grow alone or in pairs of three between April and September.

The ripe fruit, or pepper, is a many-seeded pod with a leathery outside in various shades of red or yellow. There is a host of hot chili varieties; serrano, yellow wax and jalapeno are the most common California chilies around. Capsaicin is the particular compound which accounts for the fiery properties in all chilies.

A pharmacist, Wilbur Scoville, devised a way early in this century of scoring capsaicinoid content; hence, they are called Scoville Units. Most peppers fall into a range from 0 to 300,000 Scoville Units. Green bell peppers rate zero because they lack the necessary capsaicinoids. Jalapenos measure 2,500 to 5,000, while the Tabasco peppers and Cayennes rank between 30,000 and 50,000. At the upper end of the scale are the Scotch Bonnet from the Caribbean and the Habanero from the Mexican Yucatan—both are a definite 300,000 each.

These days, however, many chile writers use a new system, the Official Chili Heat Scale, with a rating of 0 to 10. Bell peppers still fall to the bottom, with zero; Jalapenos come in at 5, Tabascos and Cayennes at 8, and the Scotch Bonnet and Habanero at 10.

Keeping Cool with Hot Chilies

The active ingredient in cayenne and other chili peppers, capsaicin, delivers the fiery kick to Mexican food, turns plain pickle juice into Tabasco sauce, makes ginger ale a real thirst quencher, lets the good times roll in Cajun cuisine, and makes curry powder a more interesting spice all around.

Capsaicin, in fact, is able to first stimulate and then to desensitize the warmth detectors in the hypothalamus gland, so that a drop in body temperature is evident. This enables natives in hot southern climates like Central and South America and Africa, for instance, to tolerate the heat a lot better than we would. That's one of the reasons why they consume so much capsicum and other chili peppers, to keep themselves cool, believe it or not!

Burn Away Body Fat by Eating Red-Hot Chili Peppers

The chemical capsaicin has a molecular structure very similar to vanilla, but a thermal rating equal to the molten hinges on the gates of hell! Some recent European studies have suggested that adding cayenne pepper to your meals not only boosts your vitamin C levels, but can also rev up your body's metabolism. It seems the capsaicin somehow "resets" the individual "fat thermostats" (called "brown fat"), which enables the body to burn off more fat through chemical combustion, rather than storing it in muscle tissue.

The next time you go to one of those big chili festivals held periodically in different parts of the American Southwest, take the time to look around and observe those in attendance. You'll find that among *true* chili enthusiasts, there is very little obesity.

Halts Bleeding Quickly

For any sudden gash, nick or serious cut, just apply enough cayenne pepper or powdered kelp or both to the injury until the bleeding stops. Several years ago I cut my hand while dining in a restaurant. I drew a small crowd around my table when I requested some capsicum to dress the injury; there were more than a few comments on the success of my treatment when all bleeding ceased within a matter of minutes.

How Capsaicin Can Relieve Rheumatoid Arthritis

More and more doctors these days are recommending new creams whose pain-fighting ability is drawn from the source that gives chilies their incredible punch. The hotter the pepper, the more capsaicin it contains. And the more capsaicin, the greater the body's response.

For as little as $13.95, you can get arthritis relief from an over-the-counter tube that contains capsaicin. Topical creams like Zostrix and Capzasin-P are very effective on arthritic shoulders, elbows, wrists and other painful parts.

Dr. Roy Altman, a rheumatologist at the University of Miami's medical school, participated in a demonstration of the effectiveness of such capsaicin-based creams in a controlled study. Some of his team's arthritis subjects got capsaicin; others received a placebo. Those who spread the pepper-powered cream on achy joints reported the most relief.

When I spoke with him some time ago, he seemed really enthusiastic about capsaicin. But how can a substance that *induces* pain also stop it, I wondered aloud. Capsaicin fights pain, he told me, by entering nerves and depleting them of the substance that transmits pain signals to the brain.

"Over the past several years we've gotten a better understanding of nerves and how they work," the doctor explained. "There are certain nerves that transmit pain signals and those that do not." Capsaicin, he noted, zeroes in on those that release "substance P," a neurotransmitter that sends pain signals to the brain.

To understand better how substance P works, consider this simple analogy. You're hanging a picture on the wall and accidentally bang the end of your thumb with the hammer. Or maybe you burn your fingers by touching a hot pot on the stove. In each of these episodes, substance P has just been released into the system.

Blended in an inert cream, capsaicin permeates the skin, enters the nerve and eliminates substance P—at least temporarily. If pain relief is to continue, Altman said, the cream has to be used faithfully. Capsaicin is by no means a cure. The salve offers a way to manage arthritis, Altman concluded, while reducing the amount of oral medicine that can cause stomach problems.

Topical creams containing capsaicin are intended for the temporary relief of minor aches and pains of muscles and joints associated with arthritis, simple backache, strains and sprains. Adults and children two years of age and above may safely use them. They should be applied to affected areas not more than four times daily. Transient burning may occur upon application, but usually disappears in several days. For optimum relief, the treatment should be continued every day, 3 to 4 times daily.

CAUTION: Be sure to wash your hands with soap and water after applying. Do not apply on broken skin or pre-existing rashes. Do not use with a heating pad. Keep it away from your eyes.

Prevents Blood Clots and Strokes

The New England Journal of Medicine reported that residents of Thailand have virtually no blood clot problems because of their frequent consumption of red pepper. If you use capsicum on a regular basis, you won't ever have to worry about getting blood clots! About 2 capsules a day is good for general health maintenance and eating more Mexican, Indian and other spicy foods laced with red pepper will virtually guarantee keeping your blood pretty thin. It also means you have a reduced risk of ever suffering a stroke.

An Ulcer Healer

How can something so hot help something so painfully raw and sensitive as a stomach ulcer heal up quite nicely in the course of time? The internal consumption of capsicum stimulates the gut's mucosal cells which release more slimy mucous that neatly coats the walls of the intestines, including sore, bleeding ulcers. If you've ever watched a dog lick its wounds or held a burnt finger in your mouth, you'll know about the kind of relief I'm talking about which comes to stomach ulcers covered by lots of mucous. That then is about how cayenne pepper helps to heal ulcers. Suggested intake is one capsule twice to three times daily with meals.

Knocks Out Cold and Flu Miseries

Some Jewish grandmothers in Brooklyn, New York have relied upon a pinch of cayenne pepper and a finely chopped garlic clove in a bowl of hot chicken soup as the best way to fight the aches, pains and fever accompanying colds and flus. Called "Jewish penicillin" by many, it's often recommended by medical doctors in place of antibiotics.

Cayenne also seems to work quite well with vitamin C. In fact, vitamin C doesn't perform as well unless cayenne accompanies it. An Old Amish Herbs remedy called Super C has cayenne, ginger and vitamin A in with vitamin C to make it more potent (see Product Appendix in back of book for more information).

Brings Down Blood Sugar Levels

A report in the *West Indian Medical Journal* (31:194-97) mentioned how a pack of mongrel dogs picked up off the streets in Kingston, Jamaica were given powdered cayenne pepper. The result was a dramatic plunging of their blood sugar levels for up to several hours at a time.

If you're diabetic an average of 3 capsules of Nature's Way or any health food store brand of capsicum will help bring down high blood sugar levels very nicely. If you're just the opposite and hypoglycemic, you'd better avoid cayenne altogether, both in food and in herbal formulas as well.

Lowers Cholesterol and Reduces Risk of Heart Disease

Rodents were fed high fat diets but given some cayenne pepper as well. There was an increased excretion of cholesterol in their feces and no rise in their liver cholesterol to speak of. So when you're consuming any kind of greasy food, be sure to drink an 8 oz. glass of tomato juice with it that has a pinch of cayenne pepper and a squeeze of lemon juice. This also should help lower your risk of heart disease.

Getting Rid of Cluster Headaches

Cluster headaches usually last between 30 minutes and two hours and occur several times each day for months on end. They are generally characterized by excruciating, throbbing pain in and around the eye. The pain can be so intense at times that it seems as if a hypodermic needle is being jabbed into the eyeball.

But thanks to pioneering research done in Italy, cluster headaches can almost become a thing of the past for nearly two million suffering Americans. Dr. Bruno Fusco, a professor of internal medicine at the University of Rome, tested the effects of one capsaicin-based cream (Zostrix) on 45 patients for up to a week. His team of researchers applied a little of the cream with cotton swabs about an inch inside the nostrils on the side of the head where the pain was felt. After the swabs were removed, those sides of the nose were gently massaged for about 15 seconds to make sure the cream had been evenly distributed and to help it penetrate the mucous membranes.

The results were incredible: cluster headaches vanished in 34 patients and they remained pain-free for a year or more. Five others reported a 50% reduction in their headaches, and just six got no benefits at all. The only reported side effect was a burning sensation in the nostril when some of the cream was applied, but after 4-5 applications, the burning ceased.

Keeping Your Toes Warm in Winter

Cayenne pepper sprinkled in your socks keeps your feet warm in winter. I know an old duck hunter from Idaho who always put some cayenne in the bottoms of his woolen socks and also into the fingertips of his gloves when staying out in the cold for long periods of time.

Increases Color Brilliance of Body's Own Electromagnetic Energy Aura

Capsicum and paprika are known to increase energy levels within the body to a certain extent. Capsicum especially is included in some herbal energy products currently found on the market, such as Nature's Way Herbal Up sold in most health food stores nationwide. When I was in the Soviet Union in 1979, Dr. Venyamene Ponomaiyov, professor of chemistry and pharmacology at the Pyatigorsk Pharmaceutical Institute in Georgia informed me that he and some of his colleagues had discovered that cayenne pepper dramatically increased the intensity of electrical energy auras around the volunteers who used capsicum frequently in their diets. This finding indicates just how strength-promoting cayenne can be.

Antidotes for Reducing Pepper's Hotness

Capsaicin, which gives hot peppers their fiery properties, dissolves in either fat or alcohol. That's why either milk or beer is so popular for helping to quench the flames when any of these species are ingested for dietary or medicinal purposes.

Salve for Sprains and Bruises

An ointment used in mainland China and Taiwan for treating athletic and work-related injuries such as sprains, bruises, and swollen painful joints is made with one part ground hot pepper and five parts Vaseline. Prepare by adding the ground hot pepper to the melted Vaseline, which is then mixed well and cooled until it congeals. This ointment is applied once daily, or once every two days, directly to the injured area.

In a 1965 report from a journal of traditional medicine from Zhejiang, 7 of 12 patients thus treated were cured and 3 improved, while 2 did not respond to this treatment. In the effective cases, 4-9 applications were usually used.

Naturopathic Remedies for Sore Throat

According to naturopathic physician Jane Guiltinan, "cayenne pepper will literally 'knock the socks' off the worst sore throat pain imaginable." Relief will last for up to four hours, she claimed. Dr. Guiltinan is the chief medical officer at the John Bastyr University Natural Health Clinic in Seattle, Washington. She noted that the cayenne hastens the depletion of substance P in throat nerve endings. This provides relief until the nerves can replenish their supply of this pain-inducing chemical.

Dr. Guiltinan recommends a mixture of lemon juice, cayenne pepper and salt to be used as a gargle. Her simple formula not only relieves sore throat pain, but also fights viral infection. The addition of a sour citrus juice like lemon or lime adds an astringent element to the remedy, which shrinks swollen membranes and helps to eliminate mucus deposits. The salt discharges further bacterial growth in warm, moist places such as the throat.

Instructions for making her searing gargle are quite simple: Combine the juice of one-half lemon or lime with one full tablespoon of salt. Stir both into one-half cup of lukewarm distilled water. Next stir in one-quarter teaspoon of cayenne pepper. Gargle small amounts of this potent medicine for as long as you are able, but DON'T SWALLOW!

Variations of this basic remedy may include the addition of honey, blackstrap molasses or pure maple syrup and pure vanilla extract to add some flavor and improve the horrible taste. Gargle with some of this mixture about every four hours or as often as needed until the sore throat goes away.

Decreasing Pain Associated with Shingles, Trigeminal Neuralgia, and Diabetic Neuropathy

Some time ago medical investigators at the pain clinic at Toronto General Hospital in Canada discovered a new way to treat prolonged cases of shingles. In about 15% of cases, the disease includes a chronic phase of severe ongoing pain called post-herpetic neuralgia. Even the touch of a bedsheet can hurt so much that it is nearly impossible for the sufferer to rest comfortably. But when these researchers applied a capsaicinoid-based cream to their patients' shingles-sensitized skin, 78% experienced a modest decrease in pain, while another 56% reported a substantial decline in their pain thresholds.

Lung Diseases Possibly Prevented

Although scientific evidence is still somewhat scant, a few medical studies have already suggested that including cayenne pepper and other chilies in your diet regularly should help reduce your risks of ever contracting viral pneumonia and other diseases of the respiratory system. In some ways not yet fully known to scientists, capsaicin is able to strengthen the lungs through improved immune defenses, so that infections can't set in so easily.

Perhaps this phenomenon may be due to the high amount of vitamin C present in chili peppers. The late Hungarian scientist Dr. Albert Szent-Gyorgyi was studying cayenne pepper (especially paprika) in the early 1930s when he discovered and isolated this important nutrient; this eventually earned him a Nobel Prize in medicine. Overall, chilies contain considerably more vitamin C per unit weight than do oranges or grapefruits. This probably explains why Spanish sailors from the 16th century on preferred taking on board with them as many pickled peppers as they could pack. The chilies prevented scurvy, a vitamin C deficiency disease that was once very common among sailors.

Famous Radio/TV Commentator's Bad Home Experience with Chilies

Cokie Roberts is pretty well known in the corridors of power within the nation's capitol. She is a political analyst for National Public Radio during the week and is a regular on ABC Television's *This Week with David Brinkley*. I'm indebted to Porter Anderson, a managing editor of *The Islander* (the newspaper of the sea islands of South Carolina) for this story.

Ms. Roberts told of a recent episode when her husband brought into their kitchen "this basket of purple, red, green, and yellow peppers . . . Beautiful, I mean, these are the peppers that are $1.89 a pound." She disolved into that trademark laughter of hers, for a moment, one gutsy giggle and a half.

"But Steven tried to kill us . . . and he came close [to doing it]. He decided that instead of hanging all his little red peppers in the window to dry over the winter like he usually does, that he'd dry them in the microwave.

"Don't try it. Toxic fumes. It was like tear gas. I had to get the animals out. We were coughing uncontrollably. It was awful. Everybody's all right, but no thanks to Steven. Fortunately, there are lots of windows and doors in the kitchen, so we could blow the fumes out.

"Well, about seven at night, Steven decides to take a nap before dinner, goes upstairs, and he can't breathe on the *second* floor. All the fumes had moved upstairs. We had to blow it out completely. Thank [goodness] it wasn't the dead of winter. But I think we gassed the whole neighborhood."

CEDAR BERRY

(see JUNIPER)

CELANDINE
(CHELIDONIUM MAJUS)

Brief Description

The name for this plant comes from the Greek word *chelidon* for "swallow." The ancient Greeks believed that the plant flourished with the spring arrival of these birds and withered in the autumn when they departed for warmer climates. Another old wives' tale claimed that swallows used celandine juice to improve the eyesight of their fledglings. Based on this folk notion, celandine juice was once used in the form of eyedrops for treating cataracts, but the practice has long since been abandoned.

Celandine is a perennial herb with branching stems that reach almost a yard high and swell at the nodes. Its smooth leaves are deeply divided with lobed leaflets spread alternately along the lower stem. The plant yields golden yellow flowers. When any part of the herb is broken, it exudes an acrid, sticky orange juice with an unpleasant odor.

Foot Calluses Come Off Quickly

Dr. Ernest Tavel is a successful podiatrist who, for some time now, has been experimenting with a few natural remedies in portions of his medical practice. Consenting patients have small dabs of fresh celandine juice smeared on their corns and calluses with wooden popsicle sticks.

Dr. Tavel said that the sticky juice somehow manages to soften even the toughest ones sufficiently so that they can be easily removed with very little discomfort. He prefers using celandine juice over conventional chemical drops. He claims it also works well for plantar's warts, blisters and pimples.

CELERY
(APIUM GRAVEOLENS)

Brief Description

Celery is one of the oldest vegetables ever used in recorded history. The ancient Egyptians were known to gather wild celery from marshy seaside areas for food. It is a plant of many uses and little waste; the leaves and dried seeds make good seasoning; the outer ribs are best cooked and the inner ribs may be consumed raw because they are good for the heart.

The variety most commonly available is the light-green to medium-green Pascal celery. Stalks are firm and solid with a maximum of green leaves. They usually have a glossy surface and snap easily. As a member of the distinguished parsley family, it enjoys some of the same reputable medical claims often attributed to the former herb. The ancient Greeks on the Isthmus of Corinth around 450 B.C. regularly crowned their winning athletes with crowns of celery stems and leaves.

In 1982, the average American ate 7.8 lbs. of celery, 11% more than 5 years earlier. In l983, it was a $235 million crop in America, compared with $184.5 million for carrots and only $152 million for broccoli. California supplies the nation with more than 60% of all celery production.

Calm Frayed Nerves

The seeds and the stalks of celery both contain a sedative compound called "phthalide" (the "ph" is silent). In mainland China, celery juice was useful in reducing hypertension in 14 out of 16 patients. The juice was mixed with equal amounts of honey and about 8 tsps. were taken orally three times each day for up to a week. Make your own celery juice at home with a juicer or buy it fresh from a health food store. Mix equal parts of it and carrot juice together and drink an 8 oz. glass once a day to help strengthen frayed nerves.

Quick Relief for Hornet Stings

Several years ago a barefoot participant in our plant identification hike in Provo Canyon accidentally stepped on a black hornet. Intense pain and swelling commenced within minutes.

There was no plantain or yarrow available. Another participant had some celery sticks in a plastic bag; I started chewing one vigorously until I had ground it to a pulp with my back molars. I then applied this wad of celery and saliva directly to the wound and held it there for about 15 minutes. The throbbing ceased and she felt more comfortable thereafter. A crudely-made mud pack with more chewed celery inside brought added relief for some hours later.

Helps Keep Weight Off

Robin W. Yeaton, Ph.D., who worked for the UCLA Program Development Symposia in 1985 told me that she lost over 30 lbs. in 2 1/2 months, by nibbling on a lot of celery sticks whenever the urge to snack came over her. The sodium seemed to have a positive effect in helping her to shed additional pounds, too.

Using Celery in Recipes

Be sure that the celery you use is always as fresh and crisp as possible. Avoid any kinds that are wilted, brown or diseased-looking. Above all, *do not* store celery in your refrigerator for longer than three weeks. According to the Nov.-Dec. 1985 *Journal of Agricultural Food Chemistry*, the furocoumarins present in very small amounts in fresh celery can increase 25 times or more after about 3 weeks' storage. Old celery has caused cancer in animals.

For a simple dish on the stir-fry principle, add sliced celery to bite-size pieces of chicken and allow to simmer covered for 20-30 minutes. Or use lamb with celery in much the same manner. Creamed celery, popular in the '30s and '40s, can be adapted to today's cooking styles by spicing it up with either cheese or nut meats. Toasted almonds add the crunch to this interesting version.

CREAMED CELERY WITH ALMONDS

Needed: 8-10 celery branches with leafy tops intact; 1 tbsp. diced shallots (an onionlike plant); 3 tbsp. butter; 1/4 tsp. sea salt; 1 tbsp. whole wheat flour; 1/2 cup cream; 1/2 cup chicken broth; 1 cup toasted almonds.

Slice the celery on the diagonal, melt the butter in a heavy pan with a tight-fitting lid. Add the shallots first, then the celery. Cover the pan; cook until celery is tender, about 8 minutes. You should not have to add liquid. Shake the pan every now and then to prevent scorching. When the celery is tender, add the sea salt and sprinkle in the flour. Toss celery with a mixing spoon to distribute flour.

Place the pan over a double boiler; add cream and chicken broth. Cook until the raw flour taste is gone, and mixture thickens slightly, about 5 minutes. Add 3/4 cup of the toasted almonds and toss. Place the celery mixture in a serving dish; top with the remaining almonds. Sprinkle paprika over the top and serve. Serves 3-4.

CENTAURY

(see AMERICAN CENTAURY)

CHAGA

(see BIRCH)

THE CHAMOMILES

GERMAN CHAMOMILE
(MATRICARIA CHAMOMILLA OR RECUTITA)

ROMAN CHAMOMILE
(ANTHEMIS NOBILIS OR CHAMAEMULUM NOBILE)

Brief Description

German chamomile is a fragrant, low annual herb, with lovely flower heads and can reach a height of 16 inches. The leaves are pale green and sharply incised. Roman chamomile is a strongly fragrant, hairy, half-spreading and much branched perennial with white ray-like flowerheads and can grow to a foot in height. Both chamomiles are extensively cultivated throughout Europe and the Mediterranean countries, as well as found growing in the U.S., Canada and Argentina.

Calms Headaches and Hyperactivity

If you've ever suffered from an occasional migraine headache or have hyperactive children or grandkids, then you should consider the success that the famous French herbalist, Maurice Messegue, had with chamomile. After just 14 days of intensive treatment with chamomile, a man who had debilitating migraines was cured. To make a relaxing tea, simply steep 2 tbsps. of fresh or dried flowers in 1 pint of boiling water for 40 minutes. Strain, sweeten with pure maple syrup and drink 1-2 cups at a time.

Fantastic Beauty Aid

European herbalists rave about the great cosmetic benefits to be derived from the use of chamomile. When the face is washed with the tea of the herb several times a week, it will show a healthier and softer glow. The same tea also makes a wonderful hair conditioner, especially for blond hair, making it more manageable and shinier.

To make a tea, simply bring 1 pint of water to a boil, then remove from heat and add 2 tsp. of dried flowers. Cover and let steep for 45 minutes. Strain and use when lukewarm to cool.

Wonderful for Skin Problems

Chamomile is especially useful on the skin for a number of problems from flaky scaliness and inflammation to wrinkles and stretch marks. A remarkable chamomile cream preparation imported from Europe has been receiving rave reviews from skin care specialists and consumers here in America. Called CamoCare, it is now available at most health food stores nationwide or from Abkit, Inc. (see Appendix).

I have received a number of testimonies concerning people's success with this wonderful chamomile cream made in Frankfurt. John Sinnette, 78 years old, of Tustin, California is one of these.

> I was frankly a bit skeptical that it would do any good for the rash on my belly and legs, since it had been of long duration and the anti-fungal cream that a doctor had given me had done very little good. Much to my surprise, the red rash almost completely disappeared within about four days of application twice a day!

Reduces Inflammation and Swelling

Chamomile may be used as a compress and wash for all external conditions of inflammation and as an oil rub for muscular stiffness and temporary limb paralysis. To make an effective tea to be drunk and also as a wash, just bring 1-2 pints of water to a boil, adding 2 heaping tsp. of dried or fresh flowers. Immediately remove from heat and steep for 20 minutes or so. Drink a cup at a time 2-3 times daily and wash inflamed areas of skin with the same several times each day as well.

To make a good massage oil for limb stiffness and paralysis, including lower backaches, simply fill a small bottle loosely with some fresh chamomile and then add some olive oil until it covers the flowers. Put a tight lid on the bottle and keep it in the sun for two weeks, thereafter storing in the refrigerator and using as needed. Warm whatever oil is going to be used before massaging well into the skin.

And to help soothe tired, irritated eyes, just soak some chamomile tea bags in a little ice water and then apply to the eyelids for incredible relief This is especially good to do during allergy season.

Great Relief for Allergies

One of the chief components in both chamomiles, especially in the German variety, is azulene. This compound has helped in the prevention of allergic seizures, even in guinea pigs, for up to an hour after administration. Azulene might also possibly cure hayfever. Chamomile is good for relieving asthmatic attacks in kids and adults. An effective chamomile throat spray is marketed to most health food stores under the CamoCare label, and has been used for this purpose. An asthmatic can spray some of this chamomile concentrate in the mouth toward the back of the throat to relieve choking sensations and to better facilitate breathing.

Besides drinking 3-4 cups of warm chamomile tea on a daily basis during allergy season for adults, and 1-2 cups per day for young children, it's also advisable to inhale the warm vapors by covering the head with a heavy bath towel and holding the face about 8-10 inches above a pan containing freshly-made tea for about 12-15 minutes at a time.

Regenerates the Liver

Only a few herbs in the plant kingdom are capable of regeneration or producing brand-new liver tissue. Tomato juice is one of these and German chamomile tea is another. Two compounds, azulene and guaiazulene, initiated new growth of tissue in rats which had had a portion of their livers surgically removed, according to Vol. 15 of *Food & Cosmetics Toxicology* for 1977. For encouraging the formation of new liver tissue, it's recommended that up to 6 cups of chamomile tea be consumed every *other* day or an average of 3-4 cups per day. In this particular instance, the tea seems to work much better than powdered capsules would. This treatment would probably be especially good for those suffering from degenerative liver diseases such as infectious hepatitis or the more deadly AIDS virus.

CHAPARRAL
(LARREA DIVERICATA)

Brief Description

Chaparral is one of the most amazing herbs ever found in the plant kingdom. It thrives on nutritionally bankrupt soil and settles in where even the hardiest of cacti fear to tread. Chaparral secretes a powerful anti-growth substance that keeps all other vegetative intruders away. *Nothing* grows around the immediate perimeter of this shrub—not even other chaparral!

This incredible plant survives in the hottest of desert hells on as little as a few tablespoons of water per year, yet somehow manages to still retain its distinctive bronze to mustard-green hue.

Naturalist Douglas Rigby described this hardy plant (which he called "the creosote bush") in his charming book about the wonders of the great American Southwest. Entitled *Desert Happy* (New York: J.B. Lippincott Co., 1957; pp.108-109), it tells about one man's love affair with the desert. I'm grateful to Mr. Rigby for the permission he granted to quote selected excerpts regarding chaparral.

We met the creosote bush after a rain one afternoon. Walking northwest...we ran that day into an odor strange and pungent, not noticed on any previous stroll. Sniffing our way... we came upon a stand of conventional-looking shrubs in symmetrical goblet form, slim-twigged and airy-branched. The shiny leaves, quite small, were split half-way up the middle like a tiny pair of Dutchboy breeches...In summer these leaves would change to mustard green, but now the green was overlaid with a varnished bronze, a brooding desert tone, rather sinister; and indeed a dark alliance may be suspected that such a Simple Simon plant should prosper here unarmed and in full leaf the year round.

Yet creosote bush is far from sinister. In truth, the bush is a plant genius. With unparalleled ingenuity it has surmounted, point by point, the challenges of a fiercely challenging environment. Against animal assailants, including most insects, its repellant odor and taste serve as armament and cause its avoidance by all except now and then a starving jackrabbit or a nest-building packrat. As for the supreme desert enemy, this pliant plant can outride aridity. Not only are its small-surfaced leaves thrifty of transpiration by virtues of their form, but they are covered also with a lifetime protective varnish to ensure a double-tight grip on moisture. If the plant's superstructure appears lightheaded, its root system is profound. The taproot may delve to a depth of 5-1/2 feet, and in some localities its root-laterals have been measured embracing a territory of 55 square yards. And with good reason, since unlike the night-blooming cereus or the narrow-leaved yuccas with their redoubtable tuberous reservoirs, creosote bush has no underground safe-deposits to tide it over hard times.

It settles by preference on bankrupt land and lives tranquil in meanest clay or sand above a caliche hardpan that would blanch and curl brown its stiletto-bearing competitors. Besides thrifty leaf and resourceful root, creosote bush, so it is claimed, employs a shrewd system whereby it poisons most of its own seeds so that they cannot germinate; thus it prevents suicide by overpopulation in a land of scarcity. Count in finally the secret of the bear, the bacillus, and the bedbug—the ability of the organism (in this case, the seed above all) to sleep on [or hibernate] when energy must be conserved. For that matter, in bad years the entire plant is privy to the allied secret of 'drought dormancy.' This is the decisive factor in the survival of many eminent desert plants, and in times of direst emergency even the usually bland creosote bush employs it.

Ideal Dandruff Remover

In times spent with Mexican American residents in New Mexico and with the Pima Indians in Arizona, I've learned that chaparral is a most effective remedy for helping to get rid of dandruff. In fact, it works even better than the popular shampoos that are advertised nationally.

Here's how to use it. Bring 1 quart of *cheap whiskey* or some *cheap* brand of *wine* to a boil. Add up to 6 tbsp. of dried chaparral, which you can get from any health food store or by mail-order from Indiana Botanic Gardens (see Appendix). Reduce heat and simmer for 20 minutes, then remove and steep for up to 8 hours. DO NOT use any aluminum cookware, only enamel, silverstone or stainless steel.

Strain into a fruit jar and keep in bathroom. Every time you shower and wash your hair with soap, first be sure to rinse it well before using this chaparral-alcohol mixture. Pour a cup of the stuff into your scalp and work in well with your fingertips. After this DO NOT RINSE with water. In less than a week, dandruff problems should be virtually eliminated. After that, use it several times a week to keep dandruff from ever recurring.

The same mixture can be used on cats and dogs suffering from lice or fleas. After bathing them, just apply it as you would to your hair for the same wonderful results.

Candida Disappears

The same solution used either as a douche or taken internally every day, 1 cup at a time, but with the tea made from water instead of liquor this time, will help to combat yeast infection and cause any *Candida* present to virtually disappear. The feet may also be soaked in the same strong *alcoholic solution* to fight athlete's foot.

Longevity Factor

The world's oldest living organism is *not* a bristlecone pine tree in the White Mountains north of Bishop, California. Rather it is a ring of creosote bushes in the Mojave Desert 150 miles northeast of L.A. The age scientists have assigned to these chaparral bushes after careful anaiysis—11,700 years old! This is due to their NDGA content.

The second most important content in chaparral is called nordihy-roguaiaretic acid or NDGA for short. It is a very strong anti-oxidant, meaning it's been used in numerous food products in the past, especially in fats and oils, to prevent rancidity. The authors of *Life Extension—A Practical, Scientific Approach* say that if you want to live a long time, you need to be taking some kind of anti-oxidants to hold your "free radicals" in check.

"The tiniest killer in your body," they say, "isn't a virus at all"—it's a type of recklessly delinquent molecular fragment with considerable irregular behavior that can cause blood clots, arthritis, senility, and greatly hasten the aging process in all of us. They say that "when you cook with food containing fats and oils, it's wise to include anti-oxidants if you plan to store any leftovers."

But food like ground hamburger, they point out, "is a particularly rich source of these dangerous free radicals." With this in mind, it seems like a good idea to take one chaparral capsule after consuming a Big Mac and french fries in order to offset some of the damage all of those free radicals you've ingested are capable of doing. And while chaparral may not hold quite the same promises expected of ginseng for longevity, it can certainly help to slow down the aging process quite a bit from the foods we eat on a daily basis.

Holds Cancer in Check

The medical doctor most involved with the limited success that chaparral has achieved with some kinds of cancer, is Charles R. Smart, M.D., an internationally known cancer specialist, who was Chief of Surgery at LDS Hospital in Salt Lake City until 1985. In an interview published in the June 1978 *Herbalist* magazine, he was quoted as saying "that chaparral tea produced regression of tumors but *not* necessarily cures" with "the possibility of reacquiring the cancer continuing to exist." Therefore, it's in this context as a control mechanism rather than as a purported cure that chaparral is being offered for the reader's serious consideration.

Dr. Smart's initial experience with this wonderful desert shrub began in 1967 when an 85-year-old Caucasian man was evaluated at the University of Utah Medical Center for a rapidly growing malignant melanoma of the right cheek associated with a large tender mass just adjacent to it. The sore on his cheek was surgically removed, examined, and pronounced malignant. Dr. Smart's medical report, which was subsequently published in the April 1969 issue of *Cancer Chemotherapy Reports*, mentioned that this gentleman returned several more times for further lesion excisions and finally a wedge biopsy of the facial area and a needle biopsy of the growing neck tumor.

By this time his physical appearance looked terrible. He had lost considerable weight and had become pale, weak and fairly inactive. Major surgery was suggested, "but the patient decided to return home without treatment, feeling that his age and condition precluded surgical treatment."

According to Dr. Smart's report, the patient "began taking 'chaparral tea' by steeping the dried leaves and stems in hot water—about 7-8 grams (approximately 1 tbsp.) of leaves per quart of water—and drank 2-3 cups of tea, only rarely missing a dose, and taking *no other* medications." Smart's patient began this home treatment for his cancer sometime in November 1967 and by February 1968 had experienced a substantial decrease in his facial lesion, with the neck tumor completely disappearing. "He looked better and had begun to gain weight and strength," Dr. Smart reported.

The patient returned to the University of Utah Medical Center in September 1968 "and was re-examined. Doctors were quite astonished to say the least—the cancer was virtually gone, their patient had gained about 25 lbs. and looked greatly improved in color and general health."

The unidentified patient was a Mormon temple worker named Ernest Farr, who then resided in Mesa, Arizona. He lived for another 9 years, passing away at the remarkable age of 96 of, believe it or not, the very same cancer which his chaparral had held in check all this time! The irony here was that some of his children and grandchildren wouldn't permit him access to any more chaparral, believing the success he had attributed to it to be merely a figment of his tired imagination.

The medical community never completely rejected chaparral, nor its main anti-cancer component, that lightweight, yellowish-white crystal powder known as NDGA. Based on the limited success which Dr. Smart and his medical team had had with chaparral on several other cancer cases besides Mr. Farr's, Dr. Meny Bergel and a medical team in Rochester, N.Y. began a lengthy series of experiments using NDGA from chaparral on a group of 32 cancer patients with inoperable tumors or where surgery and radiation had been unsuccessful.

In an unpublished paper entitled "The Use of NDGA in Therapeutics," Dr. Bergel recounts the success his team had in being able to at least substantially reduce the excruciating pains which many of the group experienced with their various tumors, although nothing was said about the cancers themselves regressing.

Chaparral is also useful for holding leukemia in check, according to one medical publication. And several other impressive successes have been recorded with this desert shrub in *Unproven Methods of Cancer Management* published by the American Cancer Society in 1970. Four patients responded well to treatment with tea—two with advanced melanomas, one with metastatic choriocarcinoma and with widespread lymphosarcoma. After just 2 days of treatment, the patient with lymphosarcoma experienced a 75% disappearance of his disease. The choriocarcinoma patient who hadn't responded well to other therapies, responded well to chaparral tea for several months. And of the two melanoma patients, one experienced a 95% regression and the remaining disease was excised, while the other remained in remission for up to 4 months before another lesion developed.

A final historical footnote to Dr. Smart's report on chaparral would provide a fitting climax to one of nature's most superb immune system strengtheners. About the time that his study was made public, another Arizona couple by the name of Murdock was facing a bout with cancer similar to Ernest Farr's. Tom Murdock's wife suffered an incurable tumor which several previous operations and radiation treatment had failed to correct.

Hearing of Dr. Smart's cautious but positive optimism expressed in regard to chaparral, they decided to try the herb for themselves. Mrs. Murdock began drinking as much as 2 quarts of the tea a day. As reported in the Sunday, October 16, 1983 issue of the Salt Lake City newspaper, *Desert News*, "After drinking the chaparral tea Mrs. Murdock started getting better."

This started Tom Murdock on the road to selling herbs. His first product choice was obviously chaparral capsules. "What started out as a last-ditch effort to save Mrs. Murdock's life worked and resulted in the formation of the largest health food company in the country," the newspaper account related. That company is Nature's Way, now managed by one of the Murdock's sons in Springville, Utah.

CHERVIL
(ANTHRICUS CEREFOLIUM)

Brief Description

Chervil comes from a Greek word meaning "leaf of rejoicing" or "cheer-leaf." The 16th century English herbalist Gerarê confirmed this original meaning when he wrote: "It is good for old people—it rejoiceth and comforteth the heart and increaseth their strength."

Chervil is of East European origin and is found growing wild in southeast Russia and most of Iran. It found its way to England thanks to the ancient Romans. Today, however, the leaves and stems are principally used in France for seasonings, salads, soups and as a pot-herb.

This annual plant has a round, finely grooved, branched stem which grows 12 to 26 inches high from a thin, whitish root. The leaves are opposite, light green and bipinnate, the lower leaves petioled, the upper sessile on stem sheaths. The small, white flowers grow in compound umbels from May to July. The elongated, segmented seeds ripen in August and September.

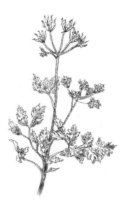

Excellent for Eye Disorders

Chervil has an outstanding track record in parts of Europe (especially France) for successfully treating a variety of eye disorders, among them severe inflammation of the deeper structures of the eye (ophthalmitis), separation of the retina from the choroid (detached retina) and loss of eye lens transparency (cataract). When used in conjunction with other eye herb remedies, such as eyebright, the results are nothing short of simply amazing.

A distinguished oculist in Paris in the last century used chervil locally in ophthalmia. He proposed applying chervil poultices to the affected eye and also washing the eye with a decoction of the same plant. This treatment has been recommended due to the good results obtained by other specialists.

The medicinal virtues of this herb are very much linked with its smell and this is quickly destroyed by heat. So it's a plant that should not be cooked, not even broiled. "The ancients used it for eye troubles," notes Maurice Messegue, a famous french folk healer, "and I have been able to confirm for myself its value in such cases. I myself like to use parsley and chervil against conjunctivitis and other eye inflammations. Steep the chopped leaves in boiling water, cool to body temperature and apply the solution with an eye cup. It soothes the burning sensation and acts as a disinfectant."

Remedy for Cataracts, Detached Retina, and Glaucoma

One of the most successful formulas for many eye disorders to ever come out of France has been attributed to professor Leon Binet, a prolific author of medical books and a former Dean of the Faculty of Medicine in Paris.

His remedy calls for equal parts (or 1 tsp. each) of freshly cut chervil, parsley, Roman chamomile (*Anthemis nobilis*, NOT German chamomile) and lavender flowers, all to be added to 1 pint boiling water and permitted to steep away from any heat for about 20-30 minutes. I recommend that an equal amount (1 tbsp.) of fresh or dried eyebright herb also be added to the solution, which is later strained and applied to both eyes with an eye cup three times a day. This is good for cataracts, detached retinas and occasionally glaucoma.

CHICKWEED
(STELLARIA MEDIA)

Brief Description

This apparently feeble member of the pink group is actually a lusty annual with matted to upright green stems that take over many areas. Commencing its growth in the fall, it vigorously thrives through the sleet and snowstorms of winter, even in the far north, survives most weed killers, beginning to bloom while the snow is often still on the ground, and many times it finishes its seed production in the springtime. It's so abundantly fruitful, however, that it flowers throughout most of the country every month of the year.

Growing to a foot high in matted to upright trailing stems, it has egg-shaped lower and median leaves and stemless and highly variable upper leaves. In the star or great chickweed (*S. pubera*), the characteristic blooms, brightly white and about 1/2 inch across, have such deeply notched petals that their 5 appear more like 10—the number of stamens. Usually gathering themselves together at night and on cloudy or foggy days, they unfurl under the brilliant sun.

Antidote for Blood Poisoning

Chickweed ranks beside herbs such as burdock root as being terrific blood cleansers. Where there exists a threat of blood poisoning or tetanus due to chemical dye or dirt getting into the bloodstream, here's what you should do. First make a poultice and apply it directly to the affected area in order to draw out as much of the poison as possible. To make the poultice, simply blend together 1 tbsp. each of the powdered ginger root, capsicum and kelp, adding just enough honey/wheat germ oil (equal parts) to form a smooth paste of even consistency. Spread this on clean surgical gauze and apply to the area. Cover and leave for up to 7 hours before changing again, if necessary.

At the same time administer internally capsules of chickweed (6 at a time) or a tea (2 cups at a time) made by adding 1 tbsp. dried herb to 2 cups boiling water and steeped for 20 minutes before straining and drinking. The same steps can also be followed with great success in treating carbuncles, boils, venereal disease, herpes sores, swollen testicles and breasts.

Nice Salve Relief for Itching, Rashes

Chickweed brings great comfort to the miseries of chronic itching and severe rashes. Just make a salve using fresh chickweed, if possible; otherwise the dried powder will have to be used instead.

Needed: 1-1/2cups coarsely cut fresh chickweed (or 1/2 cup liquid chlorophyll with 1 cup powdered chickweed); 2 cups pure virgin olive oil; 6 tbsp. beeswax. Warm up the oil and beeswax in a pan on top of the stove on medium heat. Then combine all the ingredients in a heavy cast iron skillet or small heavy roast pan and place in the oven for about two hours on just the "warm" setting. Then strain through a fine wire strainer while mixture is still hot, pour into small clean jars and seal tightly.

Herbal Weight-Reducing Program

Most of the herbal literature, past and present, recommends using chickweed in treating obesity. My friend, Mike Tierra, a licensed, practicing herbalist in Santa Cruz, California, mentioned in his *Way of Herbs* that "chickweed is particularly useful for reducing excess fat, having both mild diuretic and laxative properties."

Mike here gives his own weight-reducing program which has helped many of his heavier patients shed unwanted pounds.

Needed: The following powdered herbs: kelp (5 parts), cascara sagrada (1 part), senna leaf (1 part), cinnamon (1 part), and licorice root (1 part). (I've omitted Mike's 1 part of poke root because I don't consider it that safe to use.) Fill some "00" gelatin capsules purchased from any drugstore with the above herb mixture and take 1-2 capsules three times daily, *before* meals, with a cup of herbal tea.

To make the herbal tea, combine equal parts of these cut, dried herbs: chickweed, cleavers or bedstraw and fennel seed—or approx. 2 1/2 tbsp. of the same in 1 pint of boiling water. Let steep for half an hour before drinking. Both methods should have the scales soon dropping in your favor.

Naturalist's Recipe

The late great nature lover and herb forager, Euell Gibbons, devised several recipes using fresh chickweed.

GIBBONS' CHICKWEED AND GREENS

"Chickweed is so tender that it cooks almost instantly," he wrote, "and it should always be short-cooked to preserve the maximum amount of its health-giving nutrients. To make Chickweed and Greens, I always use about 2 parts chickweed and 1 part stronger greens. The stronger greens are put on first, covered with boiling water, and cooked about 10 minutes; then the chickweed is added, and after the water has regained a boil it's cooked about 2 minutes more. Drain, but don't throw away that cooking water. Chop the greens right in the cooking pot, using kitchen shears; season with salt, butter, a little pepper and some finely chopped raw onion. Sprinkle each serving with some crumbled crisp bacon. This makes a hearty and palatable dish that requires no apologies.

I've made the above omitting the fried bacon because I so intensely dislike pork, believing it's bad for your health, and have substituted kelp for the salt and capsicum for the black pepper. Also, I've squirted the juice of halves of lemon and lime over the cooked greens and stirred just before serving. They give the dish an extra lip-smacking goodness. He suggests that the chickweed/other green cooking water be drunk for obesity problems.

CHICORY
(CICHORIUM INTYBUS)

Brief Description

Chicory is a scruffy, weedy perennial that is usually cultivated but also found wild in the U.S. and Europe. The plant has many 2- or 3-foot, stick-like stems, open, widely space foliage and milky sap. The striking thing about chicory, however, is its bright, almost iridescent blue flowers that bloom incongruously on the stems as if stapled to the wrong plant. The rootstock is light yellow outside, white inside and contains a bitter milky juice.

In the U.S. the name "endive" usually refers to the small, pale, cigar-shaped plant, while escarole refers to the broad, bushy head with waxy leaves. Endives have slightly bitter taste. All three salad plants in this family—endive, chicory and escarole—were believed to have been some of the bitter herbs consumed by the Children of Israel during the Passover before their exodus from Egypt. Chicory root is frequently used in natural coffee substitutes and added to regular coffee to give it a richer flavor and reduce its caffeine content somewhat.

Chicory Coffee for Male Birth Control

There is some clinical evidence that chicory root might be helpful in rendering male sperm temporarily infertile. Scientists in India administered brewed water extracts of dried powdered chicory roots to 30 male adult Swiss mice, while a corresponding group received no chicory at all, only water to drink instead. In a week and a half, the mice were autopsied. Those which had been on the chicory root brew registered considerable infertile sperm counts as well as decreased weight in their testicles. This information may prove helpful for men not desiring to use condoms.

Good-quality roasted chicory root, either cut or powdered, may be obtained from better health food stores or through mail-order from Indiana Botanic Gardens in Hammond (see Appendix). Brewing the roasted root with the drip method of coffee making works best to give you a very flavorful and rich blend. Making the chicory coffee extra strong and drinking up to 6 cups per day should be enough to render the average adult male's sperm infertile for at least a week without having to resort to other means of birth control.

Effective Liver Cleanser

The same above brewing method makes an excellent drink for cleansing the liver and spleen as well as treating jaundice. An average of 2 cups per day for these purposes seems sufficient.

Combats Fat in the System

Lab rodents that were deliberately fed a very high fat diet containing chicory roots experienced a remarkable decrease in their blood cholesterol levels later on. This suggests that whenever deep-fried foods or fatty meats are to be consumed, a cup or two of chicory root brew be consumed with the meal for protection against eventual hardening of the arteries.

Lowers Rapid Heartbeat

Over a dozen years ago a group of Egyptian scientists investigated the potential use of chicory root in treating tachycardia or rapid heartbeat. Their study showed the presence of a digitalis-like principle in both the dried and roasted root which actually decreased the rate and volume of the heartbeat. Its effects were demonstrated in the toad heart, for instance.

While further research obviously still remains to be done before determining its full impact on human health, it would seem that a cup or two of the root brew by the drip method might just help alleviate this condition somewhat, whenever it occurs.

Neutralizes Acid Indigestion

A cup of the *cold* root brew is excellent for settling an upset stomach or correcting acid indigestion and heartburn.

Dissolves Gallstones

Chicory root and endive tea are very good for getting rid of gallstones. To 1 quart of boiling water, add 3 tbsps. of cut root, reduce heat and simmer for 20 minutes, then remove from the heat and add half a cup of finely cut, raw endive; cover and steep for 45 minutes. Drink several cups at a time twice a day in between meals, but especially so about 2 hours before retiring for the night.

A Complete Chicory Snack

To enjoy something different and slightly off the beaten path that's both healthy and exhilarating, try a snack using all three kinds of chicory species. Accompany the following "wild" salad idea with a cup of instant Country Beverage containing chicory from Old Amish herbs (see Appendix).

WILTED CHICORY GREENS SALAD

Needed: 1 medium-sized onion, sliced and separated into rings; 1 cup sliced, fresh mushrooms; 1 minced clove garlic; 2 tsps. butter; 1/2 tsp. dried, crushed basil; 1/2 cup loosely packed raisins and 2 cups each of endive and escarole snipped into pieces with kitchen shears or scissors.

In a large saucepan cook the onion, mushrooms and garlic in butter on low heat until tender, but don't brown. Stir in the dry basil and a dash of kelp if you like. Then add both kinds of chicory greens and 2 tbsp. of apple cider vinegar. Cook and toss mixture occasionally for 2-1/2 minutes or until the greens begin to turn limp or wilty-looking. Just before removing from the pan, add the raisins and give everything a final stir.

Transfer right away to serving dish. Should be eaten relatively soon while still warm. Two pieces of lightly buttered pumpernickel toast and warm chicory coffee also make a great addition to the salad.

CHINESE CUCUMBER
(TRICHOSANTHES KIRILOWII)

Brief Description

One of the "hottest" herbs in the market place today is Chinese cucumber. For almost a half-century, this perennial and herbaceous vine with the withered-looking melon fruit has been the source of an important drug classified as GLQ223, or simply "compound Q." But more about that later.

Chinese cucumber grows wild along hillsides, in weed patches, and along the edges of forests in mainland China and elsewhere in the Orient. The climbing plant has a thick root, climbing stem, alternate leaves, axillary white flowers, and a gourd-type fruit. In some ways, the plant resembles bryony (Bryonia dioica).

Wonderful Folk Remedy

Nearly all parts of the plant are used for medicine of some sort. In herb shops and open market places throughout Hong Kong and Taiwan, the brownish-yellow dried skin of Chinese cucumber is sold as a natural drug for treating conditions of dehydration, glandular inflammation, and poor urination in cases of elevated fever. About two tablespoons of the broken rind are boiled in two pints of water and a cup of the strained tea drunk every couple of hours through the day.

Oriental herb doctors also strive to relieve asthma, bronchitis, measles, mumps, chickenpox, laryngitis, abscesses and breast inflammations with strong teas made from the dried roots. These roots are usually in irregular pieces, between 2-3 inches in length, and often the size of my thumbs. Worms seems to like them, because I have yet to find any dried roots devoid of worm-nibbling.

Some of the Oriental doctors whom I've observed preferred to boil the root in some type of alcohol (usually rice wine), believing that such improved its medicinal benefits greatly. Generally, a small handful of the broken root was tossed into a pint of boiling wine and gently cooked for about 20 minutes. The resulting tea always tended to be a little on the starchy side, because the older roots were often employed in the belief that they nourished sick people better than young roots did.

"Compound Q" for AIDS

Some years ago in the early stages of AIDS research, a few particularly daring and adventuresome medical doctors decided to experiment with some natural substances outside the realm of accepted drug therapy. One such brave soul was Michael McGrath, M.D., who first tested "Compound Q" from Chinese cucumber on willing AIDS patients under his care at San Francisco General Hospital. To his astonishment, this radical treatment proved worth the risk, since he found that "Compound Q" killed *only* those T-cells which had been infected by the AIDS virus, but left alone healthy macrophages (scavenger cells which are a part of our immune systems). Remember, however, that this protein compound is *rather hazardous without strict and expert medical supervision!*

For those who have AIDS and want something other than AZT (the conventional drug currently used for this disease), Chinese cucumber root in capsule (6 daily) or tea (1-1/2 cups daily) may offer some hope; and "Compound Q," *when properly administered by a trained physician,* may help more than expected.

CHIVES
(ALLIUM SCHOENOPRASUM)

Brief Description

Chives is common to many countries, both in its cultivated as well as wild states. This perennial plant grows to around a foot tall from a small, elongated-shaped bulb. The leaves are hollow and cylindrical, closed at the top and dilated to surround the stem at the base.

Anorexia Nervosa and Similar Eating Disorders Helped

A Philadelphia gastroenterologist has come up with a pretty simple remedy for eating disorders like anorexia nervosa, an abnormal fear of becoming fat which causes a cessation of eating.

His own adolescent daughter went through a period when she suffered from this. What his wife found by accident, he told me, was the daughter's sudden interest in the *smell* of chives. "My wife was cooking for some guests we were having over for dinner that night," he said. "A few minutes before our daughter came home from school, my wife chopped some chives and had sprinkled them into whatever she was then cooking. Our daughter passed through the kitchen soon thereafter, and the aroma caught her off guard. She told her mother how good that smelled and lingered long enough to savor the aroma of the chives.

"This set us to thinking," the doctor continued, "that if the *smell* of this herb inclined her to pause momentarily to consider what was being cooked, then *a tea* made of the same might just give her enough of a renewed interest in food to get her eating again. My wife chopped up about two heaping tablespoons of chives and simmered them in a pint of boiling water, covered, for about twelve minutes. She added a tiny dab of butter and pinches of salt and white pepper. This she then strained and poured into a cup and set before our daughter, encouraging her to drink it. She told her it was only liquid, not food, and therefore wouldn't interfere with her determined fasting.

"The aroma of the warm tea, of course, hooked her, and she slowly started sipping it, while doing her homework. Pretty soon, she started looking around for things to nibble on. And before long, she was rejoining us at the dinner table for normal helpings of food." This doctor credits chives for removing her weight obsession and renewing her interest in food.

CHRYSANTHEMUM
(CHRYSANTHEMUM SPECIES)

Brief Description

It is conservatively estimated by horticulturists that about 165 species of chrysanthemum are native to the Old World. There are, however, a lot of hybrids currently being sold by florists all over the country as cut flowers that have their origins in *chrysanthemum indicum*. One hybrid, *C. x morifoliun*, is forced into bloom by commercial growers and sold in pots by florists and nurseries for both indoor and outdoor display purposes. Still other cultivars of this particular hybrid are sold as cut flowers; the spider mum is an example of this. *C. frutescens*, also commonly known as the Boston or Marguerite Daisy, is sold as a potted plant.

'Mums the Word with Hypertension

A number of related studies appearing in the scientific literature within the last several decades from China and Japan report positive benefits for high blood pressure using chrysanthemum flowers. For example, a 1972 report mentioned the clinical use of 'mum tea in treating hypertension and its associated symptoms of headache, dizziness and insomnia. A mixture of close to an ounce each of 'mum flowers and Japanese honeysuckle flowers was divided into four portions. Boiling water was added to one portion and permitted to steep 15 minutes, and the resulting tea was consumed. A second steeping of the flower heads was made and the tea was also drunk. The same procedure was followed three more times that day. All four portions of the mixture were used each day for up to a month. Of 46 patients thus treated, 35 showed improvement in their symptoms, with blood pressure returning to normal in three days to one week. The remaining patients also showed varying degrees of symptom relief and lowering of blood pressure after 10 days to one month of consistent treatment.

A more recent report from a team of scientists working in Okinawa and Ibaraki, Japan underscored the findings in the 1972 study and reconfirmed the significance of 'mum flowers in treating hypertension. This second report was entitled "Effects of *Chrysanthemum indicum Linn.* on Coronary, Vertebral, Renal and Aortic Blood Flows of the Anesthetized Dog" and appeared in the scientific journal *Archives of Internal Pharmacodynamic Therapeutics* (288-300, 1987).

Experiments were carried out using six male and female mongrel dogs, which had their chests surgically opened in order to carefully observe the continuous changes induced by a tea extract of chrysanthemum flowers which was then freeze-dried and the resulting powder dissolved in a compatible saline solution and administered to each animal intravenously.

These tests showed that the 'mum flower extracts "produced decreases in aortic blood pressure" of each dog, thereby confirming this herb as valid and very useful as a tea for treating high blood pressure.

'Mums for Angina Pain

Angina attacks create a horrible pain and a spasmodic choking which feels akin to suffocation. It is "almost like dying," one sufferer vividly remembered. It frequently occurs following extreme exercise, emotional stress, or considerable excitement. Such attacks can occur without any advance notice and may even happen during rest or sleep.

An interesting study published in 1973 in an obscure Chinese medical journal mentioned the clinical use of 'mum flower tea in treating 61 angina pectoris patients. Doctors made a tea by steeping 3-6 flower heads in one cup of boiling water per patient, for about 15 minutes, before having each of them drink it. This procedure was repeated 2 or 3 times daily, as needed. The response overall was 80% positive.

'Mums for Dry Mouth, Coated Tongue, Bad Breath, Bitter Taste, and Bloodshot Eyes

During one of my several trips to mainland China, I spent some time in Guangzhou (formerly Canton), a major deepwater port city on the Pearl River, when one of the great national trade expositions was in full swing. Thousands of businessmen from all over the world were in attendance.

A prominent local business figure explained that in this part of China, people frequently suffered from what is popularly called "feverish air." Symptoms, which are both real and imagined, include headache, dryness in the mouth, a metallic taste on the tongue, bad breath, dry throat, and sometimes bloodshot eyes.

To remedy this unpleasant situation, the local Cantonese frequently resort to taking a tea made from 'mum flowers. The tea is made according to the instructions given previously. Anywhere from three to five cups are taken each day for up to several days or until the symptoms of this "feverish air" *evaporate* into thin air!

CICELY

(see SWEET CICELY)

CILANTRO

(CORIANDRUM SATIVUM)

Brief Description

Cilantro is the leafy part of coriander, which is best known for its orange-scented seeds (see CORIANDER). Cilantro bears a close resemblance to Italian parsley and adds a characteristic cool snap to salsa, salads, curry and Chinese stir-fry dishes.

Former School Superintendent Finds Relief from Accidental Food Poisoning

For almost three decades, Dr. M. Lynn Bennion was a highly respected education official in Utah. Beginning in 1946, he took on the challenging job of Superintendent of Salt Lake City schools. In one of his first public speeches, as reported in the Sunday edition of *The Salt Lake Tribune*, he censured the "horror-packed, fear-provoking" serial programs that were very popular on radio in those days, as being "detrimental to the emotional life of our children." Condemning the use of "over-exciting sound effects" and a "predominance of crime" existing in many "adventure" serials, he said such programs "lacked constructive and applicable patterns of good conduct and good citizenship. He warned parents that "bad dreams," nervousness, "irritable dispositions and neurotic tendencies," would develop in their children if they permitted them to reglarly listen to such mayhem and violence over the airwaves. With what is being shown on television and movie screens these days in the way of graphic gore and raw sex, it is, indeed, interesting to ponder what he might have to say regarding all of this *visual* programming so readily available to young people, not to mention the filthy vulgarity spouted over the radio by such talk show "shock jocks" as Howard Stern.

I met him once many years ago. We chatted amiably and he casually related something that had happened to him a long time ago at a large banquet on the East Coast. He said that a number of people who ate in this particular restaurant, including himself, came down with ptomaine poisoning, which was eventually traced to a bad salad.

He doesn't remember exactly how he was introduced to some cilantro, which the restaurant had on hand, but it was probably by a waiter. Anyhow, he remembers being offered a small bowl of these dark green, pungent baby leaves of coriander and munching on them while eating the rest of his dinner.

While many others became "sicker than dogs," his worst discomfort was a slight gut ache and considerable gas. He attributes the mildness of this ptomaine attack to the amount of cilantro that he had consumed.

Terrific Salsa

MILD FLAVORED SALSA

Needed: 2 large ripe tomatoes, diced; 1 small onion, minced; 6 cloves garlic, minced; 2 green onions, sliced; 4 small tomatillos or 2 large tomatoes, minced; and 3/4 cup cilantro, finely minced.

In a small bowl, mix all ingredients. Refrigerate for at least an hour to allow the flavors to blend and the juices to come out. Serve with your favorite tortilla chips. This is one salsa you'll definitely enjoy, because there are *no* chili peppers in it to bite you back.

CINCHONA
(CINCHONA LEDGERIANA)

Brief Description

Originally called "Peruvian bark" by the Europeans because of its introduction by Peru to the Old World in 1640, it also went by the name of "Jesuits' powder" due to its frequent use by priests of this Catholic order to cure many fevers. It received the name "cinchona" after the Countess of Chinchon helped to popularize its fine medicinal qualities throughout more of Europe.

Although cinchona has been principally exported from South America in past centuries, it now enjoys much wider cultivation in places like India, Sri Lanka, and Indonesia. Of some forty species in this genus, close to a dozen have served as commercial sources for this important drug.

The shrubs or trees can reach 100 feet in height. They possess a bark which has a corky appearance and vertical or horizontal cracks when older. The bark is bitter, astringent, and slightly aromatic and contains the important medicine quinine, which was liberally used by physicians on numerous workers during the construction of the Panama Canal (from 1906 to 1914) to prevent or treat malaria fever.

Still the Best Fever Medicine Known to Man

Until World War II and the introduction of synthetic drugs, quinine from cinchona bark was still held in high esteem by the world medical community as the most valuable and *natural* malaria remedy available. In some Third World countries, such as Sri Lanka, it is still preferred over modern conventional antibiotics. The thinking among some European and American doctors also has been that cinchona deserves a second look, considering how more and more bacteria and viruses are becoming well adapted to the antibiotic drugs in current use. They believe that quinine is still an old, reliable standby for some of the infectious diseases that are now getting much tougher to treat.

The usual therapeutic oral dose for adults has generally ranged from 167 to 333 mg. three times per day (following meals) for two days, followed by 600 mg. three times per day for four days. Quinine sulfate, containing approximately 83% quinine, is the most common salt of quinine given orally. For those who are unable to tolerate the horrendous taste, there are quinine-containing capsules or even syrups.

You cannot obtain these in health food stores or nutrition centers, but must do so with a doctor's prescription from any local pharmacy or drugstore. Still, quinine in these forms is certainly much more preferable to synthetic antibiotics.

An Appetite Stimulant, Flu Medicine, and Remedy for Neuralgia, Headache, and Sore Throat

Cinchona bark makes an ideal medicine for suppressed appetites, influenza and the common cold, sore throat, headache, and neuralgia. In 1-1/2 pints of boiling water, simmer for 12 minutes one level tablespoonful dried and broken cinchona bark pieces. Drink two cups of tea daily *after meals.* Gargle the throat with some warm tea and apply hot packs of the same for external discomforts.

CINNAMON
(CINNAMOMUM ZEYLANICUM)

Brief Description

Cassia or Chinese cinnamon comes from Burma, while true cinnamon is a native of Ceylon. Cassia is more pungent, while true cinnamon is more light and delicate; it's also more expensive than cassia. Cassia nips the tongue and is more suited to spiced meats, pilaus (rice or cracked wheat with boiled meat and spices) and curries, while true cinnamon is more desirable in sweet dishes, pastries, breads, and cakes. Cinnamon was included as a major ingredient in a "holy annointing oil" that Moses used.

Fantastic Mouthwash

In place of Listerine try another antiseptic mouthwash that really does "kill germs on contact." Half a teaspoonful of tincture of cinnamon added to half a tumbler of warm water makes an excellent mouthwwash when the breath is unpleasant and the teeth decayed.

To make a tincture, combine 10-1/2 tbsp. powdered cinnamon in 1-1/4 cups of vodka. Add enough water to make a 50% alcohol solution. Put in a bottle and let set somewhere for two weeks, shaking once in the morning and again in the evening. Then strain and pour the liquid into a bottle suitable for storage. This tincture will last a long time.

Settles Upset Stomach

One of the most delicious, if not helpful, remedies for acid indigestion, heartburn and cramps is to sprinkle a little cinnamon and cardamon on hot, buttered raisin toast and slowly eat, chewing thoroughly before swallowing.

Cold and Flu Fighter

To make an effective French folk remedy for colds and flus, combine 2 cups of water, a small stick of cinnamon and a few cloves together in a saucepan and bring to a slow boil for about 3 minutes. Remove and add 2 tsp. lemon juice, 1-1/2 tbsp. dark honey or blackstrap molasses, and 2 tbsp. good quality whiskey. Stir well, cover, and let steep for 20 minutes or so.

Drink 1/2 cup at a time every 3-4 hours. It's pleasant tasting and really breaks up the fever and congestion accompanying either the common cold or influenza.

Reduced Yeast and Fungal Infections

An incredible experiment in the *Journal of Food Science* for 1974 demonstrates the power of cinnamon over most yeasts and fungi. Slices of white, raisin, rye and whole wheat breads, manufactured without the usual mold inhibitors, were subjected to various aflatoxins, a group of toxic molds so dangerous that they can cause liver cancer and kill humans and animals alike. These toxins often occur in food.

The toxic molds grew like crazy on all of the other breads, except for the raisin bread where growth was described as being "scant or not visible at all." In trying to identify whether it was the raisins or cinnamon responsible for this, food scientists discovered that as little as 2% or 20 mg. of the spice per milliliter of a yeast-extract and sucrose broth inhibited 97-99% of these molds.

What this tells us is that cinnamon is a super remedy for reducing the incidence of *Candida albicans*, a widespread yeast infection, and for clearing up athlete's foot. Use either a strong vaginal douche or footbath for these problems. To make a solution, bring 4 cups of water to a boil and add 8-10 broken cinnamon sticks. Reduce heat to low setting and let simmer for about 5 minutes or less. Remove and let steep, covered, for 45 more minutes. Use while still lukewarm for either problem.

Can Help Prevent Cancer

Two cancer specialists with the British Columbia Cancer Research Centre in Vancouver reported that the cinnamic acid in cinnamon helps to prevent cancer induced by chemicals in many of the foods we eat. They suggest cinnamon be used more often in food preparations as a preventative measure.

Old Fashioned Recipe

CINNAMON-MOLASSES COOKIES

Needed: 1/2 tsp. baking soda; 1/2 tsp. sea salt; 2 1/4 tsp.ground cinnamon; 1 cup (2 sticks) soft butter; 1 cup blackstrap molasses;1/4 cup dark honey; 1/4 cup brown sugar; 2 large eggs; 1/2 cup plain yogurt; 4 cups sifted all-purpose flour. Blend the first four ingredients together. Gradually add the molasses, honey and sugar. Beat in the eggs. Stir in the yogurt and flour next. Mix all ingredients thoroughly. Drop rounded-teaspoon portions of dough, 2 inches apart, onto cookie sheets covered with lecithin from your local health food store. Bake in a preheated hot oven at 400°F. for 12 min. or until lightly browned around the edges. Store in an airtight container. Makes 48 large cookies as a rule.

CINQUEFOIL
(POTENTILLA CANADENSIS)

Brief Description

Cinquefoil is a creeping perennial with stem runners that are capable of reaching up to five feet in length. Leaves with toothed edges, hairy veins and divided into five or seven leaflets grow on long stalks. The bright yellow flowers appear from the late spring to late summer and are born singly on leafless stalks.

Cinquefoil was an ingredient in different spells in the Middle Ages, cast by those who worked in the black magic arts. In one centuries'- old recipe called "Witches Ointment," for instance, the juice of the herbs cinquefoil, smallage, and wolfsbane was recommended to be mixed with the fat of children dug up from their graves and added to fine wheat flour.

Good for Sore Throat, Tonsillitis, and Gum Inflammation

Years ago when I spent a great deal of time in the Canadian provinces, I got to know some of the people there quite well, like Mark Fowler, who not only showed me how he used cinquefoil, but also gave me a new appreciation for seals and caribou in a way I had never expected.

Whenever someone he knew experienced a sore throat, tonsillitis or gum inflammation, he would show them where some cinquefoil was growing and how to make a strong tea from it. He would pick enough of the fresh plant, which when cut into small (one-inch long) pieces with scissors or a knife would equal about half a cup. This would then be added to two pints of boiling water and gently simmered, covered, for about fifteen minutes and then permitted to steep for another thirty minutes. This made a strong tea which the individual could use to rinse the mouth in cases of gum inflammation. The tea, he noted, should be held in the mouth for a minute or two before expectorating. A similar amount of half a cup is gargled in small sips for throat problems with good results.

Now about that different perspective on wild game that I got while visiting Mark in the city of St. John's in Newfoundland Province. Residents there looked beyond the cute cuddliness of seals, and saw something else that tasted quite good with a dash of Worcestershire sauce. I'm speaking, of course, about the tasty seal flipper pie, which routinely appeared on many restaurant menus during the Spring I was there. It is a dish that is guaranteed to stick in the throat of any self-respecting animal rights campaigner; but, oh is it *ever s-o-o-o good!*

Mark and I visited the Stone House, a restaurant located in one of the oldest buildings in St. John's. There we supped not only on flipper pie, but also on more exotic fare that included—are you ready for this, animal rights lovers?—seal, caribou, and cod tongues, served lightly seasoned and pan fried. Hmmm! Hmmm! Hmmm! Did it ever taste great! I remember telling Mark in between bitey morsels, "Things don't get any better than this, do they?"

I'm almost tempted to share with readers a delicious recipe I brought back with me from St. John's on how to prepare *baby* seal casserole, spiced with sage and sherry, but shall resist doing so for fear of raising the blood pressure and ire of some of my readers who are animal activists.

CITRIN
(COMMERCIAL EXTRACT OF GARCINIA CAMBOGIA)

Brief Description

One of the newest and hottest things to hit the American natural products industry is an extract from the rind of Malabar tamarind (*Garcinia cambogia*).This fruit has been utilized in India, Pakistan, and Sri Lanka for centuries as both a food and medicine. For instance, *Chopra's Indigenous Drugs of India* (Calcutta: U.N. Dhur & Sons Private Ltd., 1958; pp.508-09), a standard reference work on Indian botanicals for many years, states that this fruit is used for conditions of edema, delayed menstruation, obstinate constipation, and intestinal parasites or worms.

The tamarind rind is rich in the substance hydroxy citric acid (HCA). The Sabinsa Corporation was the first American company to import Malabar tamarind, beginning in 1991, for the purpose of extracting HCA, which is very similar to the citric acid found in grapefruits, oranges, lemons and limes. At Sabinsa, the extracted HCA became neutralized with calcium, and was soon marketed to natural food and food supplement manufacturers under the trademarked name of citrin. Soon cheaper imitations appeared utilizing slightly varied forms of HCA, such as (-)hydroxycitric acid (hydroxycitrate), also known as HCA. But the genuine HCA extracted from Malabar tamarind by the unique methods developed at Sabinsa has always been considered to be the most effective.

Miracle Weight Loss Cure for Obesity?

In the last couple of years Citrin HCA has periodically been in the news, because of its remarkable weight loss-inducing properties. Citrin slows down the enzyme process that produces fat in our body cells. When less fat is produced, then there is obviously less fat and cholesterol or, ideally, none at all available for storage in body muscle tissue. And apart from producing fat, our body cells also tend to chemically "burn" it up. When citrin slows down fat production, the chemical combustion or "burning" dramatically accelerates. The correct name for this process is *thermogenesis*, or the burning of calories.

Some alternative-minded doctors began using citrin in preparations such as CitriMax with many of their obese patients, who were only too willing to try something new in hopes of alleviating some of the emotional and physical baggage of overweight. These doctors found that citrin helped to control appetite and food intake in most of their volunteer subjects. However, they advised pregnant women or lactating mothers and young children against taking or being given citrin.

CitriMax, the product utilizing HCA from Malabar tamarind, was clinically tested on 50 heavy people. They were divided into two groups of 25 each. One group was given CitriMax and the other a placebo lookalike every day for two months. The study was conducted using the standard "double-blind" method, meaning that neither the test subjects nor those conducting the experiment knew who was getting what. All the volunteers were encouraged to eat low-fat meals, and were advised to drink a minimum of five large glasses of water every day.

At the end of the two-month test period, the average weight loss for each group was measured. The group taking the Malabar tamarind-derived HCA (with chromium added) lost an average of 11.1 pounds per person. In the group that received the placebo, the weight loss was only 4.2 pounds. The CitriMax group experienced a weight loss that was *2-1/2 times greater!* They also reported having more energy and less inclination to always nibble and snack on foods that were high in fat and sugar.

The company which revolutionized the process for extracting citrin from Malabar tamarind has a book available entitled *Citrin: A Revolutionary Herbal Approach to Weight Management.* It is a compilation of the research writings of three Ph.Ds and one M.D. It retails for $5.95 and may be obtained by sending that amount to:

Sabinsa Corp.

121 Ethel Road West, #6

Piscataway, NJ 08854

Or call: 1-800-CITRIN4/ (908)-777-1111

Those desiring to pursue a deeper investigation into this Malabar tamarind HCA extract may consult the following scientific literature, some of which I have used in this entry:

MEDICAL HYPOTHESES (27:39-40): "A natural food, the Malabar tamarind, may be effective in the treatment of obesity."

RECENT ADVANCES IN OBESITY RESEARCH: II, PROCEEDINGS OF THE 2ND INTERNATIONAL CONGRESS ON OBESITY (Westport, CT: Technomic Publishing Co., Inc., 1977): (Chapter 46), "Novel pharmacological approaches to the treatment of obesity."

THE BARIATRICIAN (Summer 1993, pp. 17-19): "A non-prescription alternative in weight reduction therapy."

CLARY SAGE
(SALVIA SPECIES)

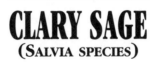

Brief Description

Clary sage is somewhat similar in appearance to common sage, although its blue or white flowers are slightly smaller. The flower buds grow out of large, pinky mauve bracts. Branches of these bracts radiate out in pairs from a spectacular central stem that reaches a height of five feet. Both the broad, wrinkled leaves and pointed bracts are highly aromatic.

Ideal Aphrodisiac for Crippled Sexuality (Frigidity, Impotency) in the Senior Years

In Germany clary sage is known as "muskateller salbei" because the powerful aroma strongly resembles that of cheap muscatel wine. In his classic work *The Art of Aromatherapy* (Rochester,VT: Destiny Books,1977; p.211), author Robert B. Tisserand described his own surprising experience with this rather arousing smell.

"The first time I used clary sage oil was when giving a massage, and both myself and the patient became rather intoxicated. At first I was not sure if it was the clary oil, but every time I have taken it, or inhaled it for a time, it has had a similar effect. It slows one down, brings on a feeling of euphoria, and makes concentration difficult. It is much more like the effect of cannabis than alcohol."

Further along, he noted that "the aphrodisiac quality of clary is intimately related to its euphoria-producing property." Only a little is necessary; too much can 'result [in possible] poisoning and a severe headache," he warned. The essential oil is clear and its sweet, nutty scent helps to relax a person when used either in very warm bath water, as an inhalant, or as a wonderful massage oil when combined with equal parts of sandalwood or lavender oil. **It is not recommended for internal consumption without strict medical supervision from an experienced aromatherapist or herbalist.**

An elderly couple that I know have reported to me their own unique discoveries regarding this singular herb. The husband, a retired banker, mentioned to me that "the sexuality we had enjoyed in previous years seemed to have gone" out of their lives. "We still cared for each other in a psychological sort of way," he remembered, "but nothing much was happening between us beneath the bed sheets at night. My wife decided to consult an herbalist in the neighborhood to see what could be done for our 'crippled sexuality.'"

The result was several imaginative and delightful ways of using clary sage oil. The herbalist recommended that each one of them soak in a warm bath of clary sage, advising them to add no more than 10 drops to half a tub full of *warm* water (not hot since heat will quickly dissipate the strength of this essential oil). They were each to remain in the water no more than 25 minutes.

After drying themselves off, they were to give each other a short but relaxing massage lasting no more than fifteen minutes and using 3/4 teaspoonful of clary oil on the spine, upper shoulder blades, lower back, and on the abdomen in front. She showed them how to keep their fingers spread apart, using the whole palms of each hand, and give long, smooth, gliding strokes (called effluerage).

Following this relaxing treatment, she recommended a simple form of aromatherapy for each, to "put us in the proper mood and right frame of mind," the husband noted. The herbalist had each one sprinkle a blend (1/4 teaspoon each) of clary sage and sandalwood oils on a clean handkerchief, press it gently to their nostrils, and inhale deeply four times.

"By then," my informant concluded, "we were both calmed down and in enough of a euphoric state, that we actually started feeling sensual emotions towards one another, just like we had done when we first got married some 45 years ago. We soon discovered that these two essential plant oils created a physical attraction in us for each other. We spent the rest of the evening in, how shall I say, rather intimate terms that gave us both much physical pleasure and emotional happiness. In some ways, clary sage may have helped save our marriage."

Relieves Sore Throat, Laryngitis, and Hoarseness

Clary sage oil has a very calming and soothing effect on any type of inflammation of the mucous membranes lining the mouth and throat. A simple mouthwash and gargle will help to relieve sore throat, laryngitis and hoarseness. Just add three drops of clary oil to three-fourths glass of distilled *warm* water and stir thoroughly with a spoon before taking each mouthful. Rinse out your mouth, or gargle with the liquid, before expectorating it. Works well for mouth sores, too.

CLEAVERS
(Galium aparine, G.verum)

Brief Description

Cleavers is an annual plant found in moist or grassy places and along river banks and fences in Canada, the eastern half of the U.S., and the Pacific Coast. A slender taproot produces the weak, square, procumbent or climbing, prickly stem that grows 2-6 feet in length. The rough, oblong-lanceolate-to-almost-linear leaves occur in whorls of six to eight around the stem. The small, white or greenish-white flowers appear from May to September. The plant exudes a strong, honey-like odor and is best gathered in July.

Helps Tighten Loose Skin

Cleavers makes an excellent facial wash as it tightens the skin. For those with the customary wrinkles and sags that come with age, this might be an herb to consider.

Bring one quart of water to a boil. Remove from heat and add 3-1/2 tbsp. of dried herb. Cover and steep for 40 min. Wash the face and neck often. Packs consisting of a wash cloth or small terrycloth hand towel soaked in the tea, lightly wrung out and then applied to the entire facial area for up to 10 minutes several times a day should help to tighten up loose skin folds. Gradual results should become evident within 2 weeks. One of the first things to look for is a new kind of life feeling in formerly tired, worn-out skin.

Calms Epileptic Seizures

The late naturopathic physician, John Lust, recommended cleavers for epileptic seizures. A tincture probably is the most effective. Use 10-15 drops once a day as a rule or twice a day if seizures are too frequent and close together. A tincture is available from Eclectic Institute of Portland, Oregon (see Appendix). And the cut, dried herb for tea is available from health food stores or Indiana Botanic (see Appendix).

CLEMATIS
(see BUTTERCUP)

CLOVER
(see RED CLOVER)

CLOVES
(CARYOPHYLLUS AROMATICUS OR SYZYGIUM AROMATICUM)

Brief Description

Cloves are one of the most famous of all spices. The 30-foot trees stand like evergreen sentinels with their clusters of crimson flowers and seem to flourish best near the sea. That's probably why the island of Zanzibar today is the most renowned clove-growing country of all. "On a hot, muggy evening when the light breezes filter through the trees," describes Tom Stobart in his *Herbs, Spices and Flavorings*, "if one approaches the island from downwind, one can smell cloves even before the land comes in sight."

Stops Toothache and Bad Breath

Rubbing oil of cloves on sore gums or generously applied on a cotton wad, then placed on an aching tooth, will, in both instances, bring rapid relief for several hours. Clove is a powerful, penetrating antiseptic which makes it ideal for an effective mouthwash. In 2 cups of hot water, put 3 whole cloves or 1/4 teaspoon ground cloves, and steep for 20 minutes, stirring occasionally. Then pour through a fine strainer and use as a mouth rinse and gargle twice a day for bad breath.

Curbs Cravings for Alcohol

Reformed alcoholics who continue to get the yen every now and then for a taste of hard liquor, should just put 2 whole cloves into the mouth for a while, slowly sucking on them but being careful not to chew or swallow them. By doing this their cravings are temporarily but effectively curbed.

Food Flavor Improved

Because of their fragrant odor and sharp taste, cloves are frequently used in cooking meat and vegetable dishes. Or a person can lightly crush four or five buds, add them to boiling water, and make a spicy tea that stimulates even the most sluggish appetite. Red wine can be turned into a refreshing beverage by heating it and adding 3 or 4 cloves.

As I observed in one of my earlier books, *The Complete Book of Spices* (New Canaan, CT: Keats Publishing, Inc., 1983), cloves are handy to use with beans, some desserts like cake and cookies, pork, venison and other wild game, sweet potatoes (yams), some soups, and some vegetables (especially those which are yellow or orange in color).

CLUB MOSS
(LYCOPODIUM CLAVATUM)

Brief Description

Rare in America, this species is found throughout Europe and much of Asia. The spores of club moss are collected principally in Germany, Switzerland, Russia, and some of the former republics of the old Soviet Union; this is generally done in the mid-summer months. The tops of the plants are cut as the spikes approach maturity and the powder shaken out and separated by a sieve.

The part of the plant collected is the minute spores which, as a yellow powder, are shaken out of the kidney-shaped capsules growing on the inner side of the bracts covering the fruit spike. Originally, several centuries ago the entire plant was used, but then just the spores began to be used alone in the 17th century.

Medical Treatment for Skin Problems

Dame Edith Wiggins is a middle-aged lady of the upper class in Great Britain. I was introduced to her through a Lord Kingsbury at a special Medical Herbalists' Symposia in London several years ago. Both had come by special invitation of their personal doctor, who was a licensed, practicing Medical Herbalist. (A unique charter drawn up by King Henry VIII a couple of centuries ago permits herbalists to practice their wonderful craft without interference from the regular medical profession.)

After one of the morning sessions had concluded, Dame Wiggins, Lord Kingsbury, their doctor and I went off in one corner and had a pleasant little conference of our own. This very prim and proper lady with the regal bearing, insisted that I "pay *close* attention" to what she wanted to tell me. So, I readily complied, always being eager to learn something new.

Dame Wiggins asked me to look at her bare arms and hands, which I did. She wondered if I could detect any traces of eczema or erysipelas. I said that I couldn't. She then declared that she had previously suffered from bad cases of both skin afflictions, but had been "totally healed by wonderful club moss," which her herbal doctor had prescribed. Lord Kingsbury and the doctor (whose name, unfortunately, I never learned) seconded and confirmed what she had just told me.

The method of application was very simple. The doctor had her fill a glass pepper shaker with some of the club moss powder. He then showed her how to liberally "dust" her afflicted skin with this every morning and evening. She stayed with this treatment faithfully for several months, never daring to appear in public for fear of what might be said about the color of her arms and hands. But soon everything cleared up and she was "quite satisfied with the outcome of the whole affair."

My "Million Dollar" Formula for Energy and Stamina

In my nearly 2-1/2 decades of working with herbs, I've been sought out by some of the biggest food supplement and herb companies in America to create special formulas for them. In doing so, I always find out exactly what they have in mind, and what they hope to achieve with whatever is given them. Of course, my services never come cheap, and such clients often end up paying me thousands of dollars for the marketing rights to one of my formulas. I've always had a policy to *never* take royalties of any kind on each bottle of whatever formula is made by me and sold by them. By wisely adhering to this, I've been able to avoid entanglements with the Food and Drug Administration and have continued merrily along my own way of writing more health books that give *real* solutions to *complex* problems.

Now one of the fastest growing areas in the gigantic health food business is energy products. This market has experienced sales increases of *300 to 500%* within the last 7 to 10 years. The growth rate has been nothing short of phenomenal and doesn't appear to be slowing down anytime soon. At one point I was requested to make some kind of energy product that was different from all the others in the market place.

I bought up samples of every energy formula I could get my hands on. My staff and I studied the ingredients of each product. We found that all of them shared one or two things in common, namely kola nut and/or ephedra (mahuang). The first contains caffeine and the second ephedrine; both dramatically stimulate the central nervous system and can, with long-term use, injure the body by creating a druglike dependency on them.

Naturally I refused to go this route and opted for something else instead as the "kicker" to making an herbal energy formula work. My studies led me to look at club moss very carefully. Here was an interesting herb with compounds capable of penetrating the blood-brain barrier and doing some wonderful things to the limbic area (pleasure center) of the brain. Yet the activity I desired to be created within the body was done *without* causing any addictions.

Next, I looked at ginger root, because of what it can do to *increase* blood circulation. This was very important for the *rapid* delivery of an herbal formula throughout the body for the creation of energy. But not just any old ginger would do; I wanted the *good* stuff from Jamaica.

My third key ingredient was gotu kola, a common weed equivalent to crab grass that is pervasive throughout all of Southeast Asia. It, too, affects circulation in a very positive way, but also does some wonderful things to certain "master glands" of the body. This, I realized, would also be important to an *effective* energy compound.

Now I had my *base* from which to work. Whatever else I piled on top would, more or less, be what I have always termed "label herbs." That is, plants that *look* good on the label and impress the consumer, but actually have little or nothing to do with the performance of the formula itself. So I threw in "pinches" of this and that, a little ginseng here and a little damiana there. But the real "heart" of my energy formula rested in this trio of herbs: club moss, *Jamaican* ginger root, and gotu kola.

The company made up about a hundred bottles of 60 capsules each and passed them out to their employees, family members, relatives, friends, and neighbors. Our research center directed the sampling of some volunteers. Just about everyone who took *two* capsules on an *empty* stomach (very, very important) with a full 8 fl.oz. glass of water, reported feeling "sensations of energy and stamina" within about ten minutes. And these feelings of physical exuberance were sustained for up to *five hours* in many cases. But, best of all, when the effects wore off, there were no sudden "let downs" or recurring bouts with fatigue. And *no one* who took the formula for weeks or months at a time ever reported an addiction to it, once they ceased using it.

This, dear friends, is how my famous "Instant Energy" came into existence. The company started marketing the formula right away, and soon health food stores were ordering more than could be properly turned out at any given time. People started clamoring for more, once they heard the excellent results by word-of-mouth. Company officials were ecstatic beyond belief, and paid me some B-I-G D-O-L-L-A-R-S for the rights to my little invention.

Ultimately, though, greed and mismanagement overtook the partners in this venture and their business eventally became unravelled like a ball of yarn does after a kitten gets through playing with it on the floor for awhile. I had to take back the rights to my own formula, because company owners failed to pay me the rest of what they still owed me. So, until now, this remarkable energy formula has sat in the back room of our research center, gathering dust and doing no one any good.

But it's time now to bring it out of moth balls once and for all, and share it with *you* the reader and the rest of the American public, who may eventually buy this book. I'm going to give you the *precise* amounts of each of these three *key* ingredients. Once that is done, the formula will no longer be a company "secret" and the proprietary information no longer "confidential." By doing this, I'm giving away the proverbial key to the bank. But, as I see it, ordinary people like yourself are more deserving of it than some greedy businessmen connected with a high-powered supplement company.

Here's what you do to make my "million dollar" herbal energy formula. First, consult the Products Appendix to learn where to purchase club moss, Jamaican ginger root, and gotu kola. Personally I recommend Great American Natural Products, Inc. of St. Petersburg, Florida (813-521-4372).

Once you get the *powdered* ingredients and some double size capsules to fill, make up a small mixture as follows:

4 parts (teaspoons or tablespoons) club moss

3 parts (teaspoons or tablespoons) *Jamaican* ginger root

2 parts (teaspoons or tablespoons) gotu kola

Mix them thoroughly together by hand in a large bowl or dry mix in the plastic container that comes with a Vita-Mix whole food machine or similar processor.

After this, spread out a clean piece of cotton cloth on a flat surface. Fill each gelatin capsule by pushing the larger open end into the powder, lifting it up, and then pushing the small end of the other part together with the filled portion. Lay it down on one half of the cloth; after you've filled about ten capsules this way, then pull some of the cloth over the top of them and gently roll the capsules back and forth to remove any unpleasant herbal powders.

When feeling weak and fatigued, take two capsules with a *full* 8 fl.oz. glass of water. By all means, remember to do this on an *empty* stomach morning and evening. And now that you know the "secret" to my "million dollar" energy formula, you should soon be feeling like a "million dollars." The only thing that remains unresolved is putting a million dollars in your pocketbook. But you'll probably have to take your chances with the lottery or travel to Atlantic City or Las Vegas in the hopes of ever winning that!

An Important Homeopathic Drug

Homeopathy is a philosophy of health and a formal system of drug therapeutics generally credited to Samuel Hahnemann (1755-1843). In 1810 he published the first edition of his book *Organon of Rational Healing* (later retitled the *Organon of the Healing Art*) in which he systematically spelled out the principles of the homeopathic doctrine.

In this book he mentioned that a large number of substances were biologically inert in their crude forms, but when subjected to his serial dilution and succession process (or trituration) they acquired remarkable medicinal powers. One of the examples he used to illustrate this was club moss. The spores in their crude state were believed by many herbalists in Hahnemann's day to be utterly worthless as a medicine. But when he ground them up into a fine powder with mortar and pestle (trituration) and administered them that way, results were incredible. Consequently, club moss has become one of the most important and powerful drugs of the homeopath's armamentarium of medicines.

COCA
(ERYTHROXYLON COCA)

Brief Description

Coca is native to the highlands of Colombia, Ecuador, Peru, Bolivia and western Brazil. It is thought that the ancient Incas were the first ones to discover its use for medicinal and well as pleasurable purposes.

Coca is a small, bushy tree that grows to about 18 feet tall at higher altitudes, but quickly descends to the rank of a common shrub no higher than about six feet at lower altitudes. The branches are slender, with red-brown bark roughened by leaf scars. The leaves are evergreen, alternate, mostly near the ends of the branches, oval to elliptic, pointed at both ends or occasionally rounded at the apex. The fragrant flowers are wide, five-petaled, ten-stamened, appearing in groups of 6 to 20 in axils of absent leaves from the previous season, and can be either white or yellow in color.

How Cocaine Is Extracted

The principal alkaloid of coca is cocaine. Plant leaves picked when fully ripened in Bolivia and Peru often contain the highest amounts of cocaine (75% of total alkaloids).

In the processing of the leaves to cocaine, many farmers will themselves engage in the first few steps by turning the leaves into coca paste, which is easier to transport to a cocaine processing laboratory hidden deep in some jungle to avoid detection. More than 100 kilograms of dried leaves are required to make a single kilogram of the paste. The leaves are collected from twigs that are cut off in the spring, pruned again in June, and pruned for a final time in early fall. The dried, crushed leaves are then mixed with water and calcium carbonate or lime to produce an alkaline reaction. The mixture is next crushed, with kerosene or gasoline added, while everything is thoroughly stirred with wooden paddles. After the leaf pulp is discarded, the kerosene is mixed with acidified water, and the aqueous layer is separated and made alkaline with ammonia or baking soda. This precipitates a thick, aromatic paste containing not only cocaine, but also several other alkaloids. The smoking of coca paste has become a drug abuse problem in peru, Bolivia, Colombia, and Ecuador.

Another method is used stateside for extraction purposes about which most people are unaware. I, too, was totally ignorant of this until recently tipped off by a friend of mine in the eastern United States. Coca leaves are imported from Peru and Bolivia by ship and unloaded in New Jersey, where they are immediately transported under heavy security to a particular chemical factory at a location I'm not at liberty to disclose right now. There the cocaine is extracted for medical use, and from what is left of the leaves comes a flavoring agent that, in small amounts, goes into soft drinks enjoyed by hundreds of millions of drinkers in 155 countries worldwide.

A number of very potent chemical solvents are used to soak the leaves so that all cocaine is effectively removed. These powerful agents include separate solutions or mixtures of the following: acetone, alcohol, carbon disulfide, chloroform, ethyl acetate, hydrochloric acid, petroleum, turpentine, and water. My friend said that in spite of the best precautions taken, tiny residues of many of these chemicals still turn up in the cocaine and soft drink flavoring agent. Since he began working at this facility some years ago, he has entirely sworn off drinking cola beverages and has managed to persuade hundreds of his friends and relatives to do the same.

Wonderful Anesthetic

The medical profession depends heavily on cocaine for its legal use as a local anesthetic. Cocaine blocks nerve conduction, causing numbness. It also constricts blood vessels; that's why each year surgeons in the U.S. and Canada prefer it for some 225,000 nasal operations, in order to shut down the nose's mass of capillaries. In many hospital emergency rooms, nurses routinely swab areas of skin on patients requiring stitches with a colorless liquid containing cocaine. This way there is less blood and virtually no pain upon sewing.

Doctors also rely upon cocaine for other types of surgeries. When limbs require amputation, then a cocaine solution is injected at the site of amputation in order to lessen the pain which the amputee will be experiencing upon awakening. Back operations sometimes require a hypodermic injection of liquid cocaine into the spine to greatly reduce the severity of the pain which the patient would otherwise be feeling some hours afterwards.

An old-time dentist once told me that his profession routinely used liquid cocaine a number of years ago when pulling teeth, especially wisdom teeth. He noted, "They were tough buggers to get out and caused a helluva lot of pain, I remember that cocaine made it easier on the patients and us, too."

Some Bolivian Folk Uses for Coca Leaf

Almost a decade ago I made a trip to El Alto, Bolivia. There I met Jorge Baton, an Aymara Indian, who took me to one of a number of Indian sorcerers in the city, regularly consulted by many of the inhabitants for a variety of problems, both real and imagined.

Now Jorge had been suffering from a terrible headache for some time and couldn't get rid of it. The sorcerer wet a couple of coca leaves, beat them a few times with a flat rock, and then applied them across Jorge's forehead. Within ten minutes, Jorge felt a lot better, paid his fee, and walked away with me, obviously a very happy man.

Jorge said that another time his young son cut his leg on a sharp object. Jorge took him to the same sorcerer who bruised some coca leaves, laid them on the open would, and bound them in place with some strips of gauze. The child ceased moaning in about thirty minutes, all pain having entirely disappeared.

On yet another occasion, Jorge's wife paid a call on this same *yatiris* (sorcerer), who gave her some fresh coca leaves to chew while delivering her child. She then went to the local hospital and gave birth, all the while chewing some of the coca leaf, which helped to deaden most of her labor pains. Afterwards, she offered the rest to visiting friends and relatives to help celebrate a successful delivery.

The Addiction Factor

For an estimated 5,000 years, the people of the Andean highlands in South America have been chewing coca leaves for pleasure and stimulation. In the Museum of the Bank of the Pacific in Guayaquil, Ecuador, there is a three-inch ceramic head in a glass case of a man with the characteristic chewer's bulge in his left cheek; the artifact is dated around 1500 B.C. and assigned to the Valdiva culture.

By 1862 German chemists had taken coca leaves brought by an Austrian scientific expedition from Peru and had isolated from them the alkaloid which they called *cocain* (later anglicized to "cocaine"). Today more than ten million Americans keep buying it—to sniff, smoke, or inject. This brings them indescribable pleasure, unbounded energy, but more often misery and sometimes death.

Cocaine creates a "fire in the brain" of electrical and chemical excitation. Current research suggests that this action occurs in the forebrain, where cocaine prolongs the action of the neurotransmitter dopamine, thus firing reward and euphoria circuits in the brain. Cocaine also appears to increase the effects of the neurotransmitter norepinephrine, thereby stimulating the sympathetic nervous system. The combined effect seems to have worked well enough to make it in constant demand by millions of American users from all walks of life. This enormous market of the illicit buying and selling of cocaine generates stupendous quantities of cash. Enough, in fact, some economists claim, to wipe away the national debts of a number of Third World countries! But wherever cocaine is being used illegally, there will be money to be made, pleasure and exhiliaration to be found, and death—either from long-term addiction or murder most gruesome.

"The Pause That Refreshes"

No discussion of coca leaf would be complete without including its previous use by The Coca Cola Company of Atlanta, Georgia. Did you know that once upon a time, a tiny amount of *pure* cocaine was added to one of the world's favorite beverages? In my research center here in Salt Lake City, I have some memorabilia from the turn of the century which proves this. An old 1901 letterhead from the "Office of The Coca Cola Company" bears a familiar trademark logo with these descriptive phrases on either side of it: "Delicious • Refreshing • Exhilarating • Invigorating." And then directly beneath these words and the centerpiece logo are the following lines: "The New & Popular Fountain Drink, containing the tonic properties of the wonderful COCA PLANT, and the famous COLA NUT. ON DRAUGHT AT ALL POPULAR SODA FOUNTAINS AT 5¢ PER GLASS." And a full-color 1903 advetisement depicted actress Hilda Clark holding a paper cup clearly marked "Coca Cola" and a piece of paper on which was written in cursive these words along with her signature: "Coca-cola makes flow of thought more easy and reasoning power more vigorous. —/s/ Hilda Clark."

In 1904, however, the federal government insisted that the Coca-Cola Company remove all the cocaine and caffeine from its highly addictive beverage. The company retaliated with threat of a major lawsuit, and the government came back with its own implied threats of arrest of key company officials, seizure of its existing properties, and forfeiture of all assets. Eventually a compromise was reached between both parties that was agreeable to everyone concerned: the government would back off its intended use of force, and, in return, Coca-Cola would remove the cocaine but be allowed to retain the caffeine.

Quite a remarkable history, wouldn't you say, for a beverage that began as a doctor's prescription for lethargy and forgetfullness in some of his patients? Today, an estimated 72,000,000 bottles are consumed on a daily basis in the United States alone.

Call 1-800-COCAINE and Get the Cops

Apparently Kevin Bibby isn't very good with numbers, especially phone numbers. When he allegedly tried to page his dope dealer on the weekend of May 12-14, 1995 for another batch of cocaine, he misdialed one number and beeped a Uintah County (Utah) sheriff's deputy instead.

Narcotics detective Steve Hatzidakis became suspicious and returned Bibby's call. He got Bibby to talk by pretending to be a buddy of the drug dealer. The suspect, who lives near Vernal, Utah, ordered several ounces of pure cocaine, Hatzidakis said.

But when he was busted, Bibby, 26, didn't have any cash. He said he was trying to introduce the narc cop to a man who wanted some methamphetamine. That bumped up the charge from a third-degree felony to a second-degree felony.

It kept getting worse for Bibby, though. He lives within 1,000 feet of a Mormon Church meetinghouse. That also enhanced the charge, making his alleged crime a first-degree felony, punishable by 5 years to life in prison.

Detective Hatzidakis, from whom I got this story, said in conclusion: "We're gonna put a dictionary together and under the word 'dope' we're gonna put his [Bibby's] mug shot."

COFFEE
(COFFEE ARABICA, C. CANEPHORA)

Brief Description

Different types of coffee are preferred in various parts of the world. Arabica coffee is produced mostly in South and Central America, particularly Brazil, Colombia, Mexico and Guatemala, while robusta coffee is produced mainly by African counties such as the Ivory Coast, Uganda, Angola and so forth. In the U.S., Colombian and Central American coffees are preferred over Brazilian and African coffees. The March 1981 *National Geographic* concluded that the world's annual bean production could make 3,644,000,000 cubic feet of liquid coffee, a volume equal to the Mississippi's outflow for an hour and a half. And although internal consumption can possibly cause a variety of health problems, ranging from pancreatic cancer and genetic birth defects to elevated serum cholesterol levels and hypoglycemia, it does have several therapeutic benefits.

Grounds Make a Brisk Body Rub

Some health authorities have recommended rubbing the skin with a dry luffa brush in order to enliven the skin more. But in Japan, people are buried up to their necks in roasted coffee grounds and rub the grounds all over their bodies to shed old dead skin and stimulate circulation. You may try the same thing on a more limited scale with the warm grounds rubbed on your face and neck in a rotating fashion. You'll find your skin will feel like new in a short time!

Coffee Enema for Really Good Clean-Out

Robert Downs, D.C., an Albuquerque chiropractor, claims that an occasional coffee enema several times a year is good for getting rid of hidden toxins that might lurk somewhere in the colon. And the *J. of the Am. Med. Assoc.* for Oct. 3, 1980 mentioned that coffee enemas, in particular, have become very popular throughout the country for treating chronic, degenerative diseases.

Fill a hot water bottle two-thirds full of lukewarm, *freshly brewed* coffee. The coffee should be as strong as possible. Next add one-third lukewarm water to which has been added 2 tbsp. of olive oil. Insert the syringe, and then bring your upraised knees and legs together a little and release the control stem just above the syringe on the hose. Water will commence to flow into your bowels, but you should keep your fingers on top of the control stem in case the water needs to be quickly shut off for some reason. It's a good idea to permit the water to enter in short spurts, rather than in longer moments, by pressing down and then releasing the control stem every 10 seconds or so.

This way more water can safely enter the colon without causing undue discomfort. *Only take in that amount of water which your bowels can adequately handle with minimum pain!* To attempt more than what can be contained is only asking for trouble—not only in the mess created, but also the potential damage that could be done internally as well if one doesn't use good judgment. Neither the coffee nor the olive oil is going to hurt you. In fact, they are probably the best combination of enema ingredients I know of to really tackle impacted fecal material in a quick and direct way. Unfortunately, some overzealous health enthusiasts and cancer quacks working in substandard Mexican border town clinics tend to overdo a good thing and administer several such coffee enemas in a single 24-hour period, day after day, and sometimes week after week. Common sense says this is excessive and harmful, to say the least. Soap suds enemas ought to be avoided, says Volume 83 of *Postgraduate Medicine,* because they may be harmful to the delicate membrane linings in the colon and rectum.

Colon Cancer Possibly Prevented

The following information appeared in the April 20, 1995 issue of *Food & Drink Daily.* Medical research conducted in Stockholm, Sweden under the auspices of Karolinska Hospital noted that those who drink an average of six or more cups of coffee or two cups of black or green tea every day reduced their incidence of colo-rectal cancers. The data was contained in a report entitled "Coffee, Tea, Tobacco, and Cancer of the Large Bowel." NOTE: Excess coffee consumption can aggravate some existing nervous conditions and compound the impact of stress upon the body.

Hot Coffee Helps an Asthma or Bronchial Congestion

Based on several personal experiences, I now routinely recommend that a cup of *hot*, black coffee (no cream or sugar, please) slowly sipped through (preferably) a plastic straw works magic in helping those with mucous congestion in their lungs to breathe better.

A while back I drove to Reno in the middle of a dry winter to give a lecture at a local health convention being held, in all places, in part of a shopping mall! I'll have to admit I wasn't the best example of good health since I was recovering from a nasty cold at the time. On the way there I stopped several times for hot, black coffee which I sipped through a straw. I remember how good it felt to my lungs going down. By the time I reached my destination, nearly all of my wheezing and chest congestion had cleared up. I felt like a million bucks! The only downside to this wonderful remedy was that I couldn't sleep a wink that night, but was forced to stay up and watch the late, *late, late* show.

Another time, when working on our family ranch in southern Utah, I became choked up with dust and had a rough time breathing at night. I got up, heated some water, stirred into a glass of it two tablespoons of instant coffee, and drank it hot and black. After that, I returned to bed without further problems and slept like a baby!

COHOSH
(see BLACK, BLUE COHOSH)

COLTSFOOT
(Tussilago Farfara)

Brief Description

Coltsfoot is one of those quirky creations of nature which involves putting the cart before the horse. Or, in this instance, "the son before the father" as its old Latin name of *Filius ante patrem* implies. Very early in the spring, coltsfoot develops flat orange flower heads, but only after they eventually wither do the broad, hoof-shaped, sea-green leaves develop. Coltsfoot is fairly common and isn't picky about the soil it grows in.

Relieves Respiratory Congestion

In the Soviet city of Donetsk, 151 men and 60 women metal construction workers exposed to fumes from welding and metal varnish and paints were given herbal inhalation therapy to improve their breathing capacities. Factory workers were given a tea consisting of equal parts of coltsfoot, yarrow, and plantain leaves and flowers to inhale as well as drink afterwards.

Bring 4-1/4 cups of water to a boil. Remove from the heat and add the above three herbs. Steep them for 1 hour. Then lean over the pot, covering your head with a heavy bath towel, holding your face about 5 inches above it. Remove the lid and slowly begin inhaling. Do this for 5 minutes, then strain the tea and drink 1-1/2 cups. Repeat the routine several times each day, always making a fresh brew the next day. Follow this treatment for two weeks in severe cases of congestion like bronchitis and hay fever.

A Good Chew for Inflammation

A new kind of smokeless product, containing absolutely no tobacco whatsoever but strictly natural herbs, has been developed by Coltsfoot, Inc. of Grants Pass, Oregon (see Appendix). Two of the main constituents are coltsfoot herb and cinnamon, along with orange peel, angelica, hawthorn, tang kuei and bee pollen. A pinch of this can be placed in the mouth, mixed with a little saliva by the tongue and then removed and applied directly on any burn, bee sting, mosquito bite or general sore for immediate relief.

Sure "Cure" for Asthma

My father Jacob Heinerman turned 82 on January 5, 1996. For almost half a century he has been periodically bothered with asthma. He experimented with different herbs, always in tea form, to determine what would work best for him. Eventually, after a couple of decades of trial and error, he came up with a winning combination of herbs that has proven to be a salvation for his health. He describes it as a "sure cure" for asthma because the tea tends to loosen accumulated phlegm in the bronchial tubes, which can then be easily expectorated with very little difficulty.

The tea formula consists of the following herbs: 1 heaping tbsp. coltsfoot, 1 tsp. each yarrow herb and mullein leaves, and 1/2 tsp. wild cherry bark. He brings 1-1/2 pints water to a rolling boil before adding the wild cherry bark; then the sauce pan is covered with a lid and the tea simmered on low heat for no more than 15 minutes (longer than this will make the tea too strong, resulting in possible nausea). The heat is then turned back up, the lid removed and when the liquid starts boiling again, the remaining herbs are stirred in. The lid is replaced, the heat turned off, and the tea allowed to steep 1-2 hours. He drinks 1/2 cup of this strained, *warm* tea morning and evening on an empty stomach.

COMFREY
(SYMPHYTUM OFFICINALE)

Brief Description

Comfrey is a perennial plant common in moist places in the U.S. and Europe. The rootstock is black outside, fleshy and whitish inside and contains a glutinous juice. The angular, hairy stem bears bristly, oblong lanceolate leaves, some petioled, some sessile. There are also tongue-shaped basal leaves that generally lie on the ground. The whitish or pale purple flowers have a tubular corolla resembling the finger of a glove and grow in forked racemes that look scorpionlike.

Comfrey Rapidly Heals Wounds and Ulcers

The Soviet medical journal *Vutreshi Bolesti* for June 1981 contained a report of 170 patients hospitalized for severe gastrointestinal ulcers, and of 90% of them being healed with a combination of comfrey root and calendula (equal parts) made into a warm tea and taken (2 cups) twice a day.

Comfrey, the article noted, is also an effective antacid. A brief testimony from Christine Hays of Culver City, California published in the Nov. 1977 *Prevention* magazine related how her own stomach ulcers disappeared by her drinking comfrey tea for a while. Comfrey's success with this, as well as with external wounds and sores may be attributed in part to the silicon, potassium, phosphorus and nitrogen found in the allantoin.

Allantoin is a very healing substance because it promotes cell regeneration, particularly important for deep wounds and open sores. And, interestingly enough, the reason some surgeons have used live maggots inside of open wounds to promote more rapid healing is because they secrete the same allantoin found in comfrey root.

Comfrey for Cancer

At least three major medical journals in the past have given positive support for comfrey's remarkable ability to reduce certain types of tumors. These include *The British Medical Journal* for Jan. 6, 1912, Vol. 114 of the *Proceedings of the Society for Experimental Biology & Medicine* for 1963, and Vol. 16 of *Chemical & Pharmaceutical Bulletin* for 1968. An incredible recovery from jaw bone cancer with the use of comfrey by a retired American Air Force colonel was recorded in the Feb. 1979 issue of *Let's Live* health magazine.

In my article entitled "Comfrey, the herb of herbs," I mentioned how this military officer was cured of cancer of the lip and lower jaw (caused by excessive pipe smoking) by drinking 3-5 cups of comfrey leaf tea each day for nearly three months. He was skeptical of my recommended treatment, but finally started the program at his wife's insistence; however, once cured, he became an ardent fan of comfrey for life.

This astonishing success with various forms of cancer may be attributed in part to germanium and cobalt present in root and leaf alike.

By the same token, unfortunately, some species of comfrey, especially the closely related Russian comfrey (*S. x uplanicum*) contain a group of compounds called pyrrolizidine alkaloids which, in large amounts, can have a deleterious effect on the liver over a lengthy period of time. The herb may be used with relative safety provided one doesn't overdue a good thing.

Heals Bumps and Bruises

A contributor to Rodale's *Natural Home Remedies* book related how her young son, who fell from a grocery cart and sustained severe bruises to his face, was cured the next morning by her application of ice packs first, followed by a cloth soaked in comfrey root tea. This also works well for getting rid of black-and-blue marks and taking some of the dark blue or purple out of varicose veins, including reducing their size substantially if applied frequently enough.

To make a tea for this and all of the other preceding uses, just bring 1 quart of water to a boil. Reduce heat and add 2 tbsp. dried, cut leaves and steep for 1 hour. Use tea internally and externally as needed. And for a terrific paste for burns, sprains and setting fractures, combine 3 parts of powdered comfrey root or leaves and 1 part powdered lobelia herb with 1/2 part of wheat germ oil and 1/2 part of honey. Store in a cool place until needed. Works great for the above problems.

CORIANDER
(CORIANDRUM SATIVUM)

Brief Description

Coriander is a small annual plant that has been cultivated for several millenniums and is still grown in North and South America, Europe and the Mediterranean countries. The round, finely grooved stem grows almost 2 feet tall from a thin, spindly-shaped root. The leaves are pinnately decompound while the flowers appear in flat, compound umbels that may be either white or red in appearance. The brownish, globose seeds have a disagreeable smell until they ripen, at which time they acquire a distinctly spicy aroma.

Eliminates Genital Odors and Bad Breath

In the southeastern mainland China city of Canton, coriander leaves and seeds are used to help remove unpleasant odors occurring in the genital areas of men and women, as well as of halitosis or bad breath. Bring 2 quarts of water to a rolling boil. Reduce heat and add 3-1/2 tbsp. of seed. Simmer for 1 1/2 hours until the amount has been reduced to slightly less than a quart of liquid. At this point add 2 tsp. fresh, finely grated orange peel and one pitted, finely chopped date. Simmer for an additional 15 minutes, at which time remove from heat entirely. Add 1 tsp. each of dried coriander leaf (if available) and finely chopped fresh parsley, with a drop or two of peppermint oil or wintergreen oil (if available, but not necessary).

Steep mixture for about half an hour, stirring occasionally. Strain through a fine sieve or filter paper and store in a pint fruit jar with a good

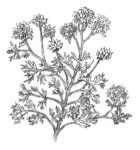

lid to seal it. Store in refrigerator until needed. When using for genital problems, warm up whatever is needed and rub all around genital area. Let the air dry it. Or gargle and rinse mouth with 1/2 cup while cool, but not heated. Also very good to hold in the mouth or soak cotton with and insert to relieve toothache.

Culinary Favorite

Toasting intensifies the flavor of coriander seeds. Toast them in a small skillet over high heat, shaking the pan until the seeds brown slightly. Then crack them between sheets of wax paper with a rolling pin or wooden mallet.

YOGURT AND CORIANDER BREAD ROUNDS

Needed: 1 tbsp. coriander seeds. toasted and cracked (as previously described); 1 cup warm water; 1 tbsp. brown sugar; 1 package Fleischmann's dry yeast; 1 tbsp. salt; 4-1/2 cups unbleached white flour; and 1-1/4 cups nonfat yogurt *warmed* to room temperature.

In a small bowl, combine the water, sugar and yeast. Set aside until foamy for about 12 minutes. In an electric mixer fitted with a dough hook, combine the yeast mixture, one cup yogurt and salt. With the machine at medium speed, add flour and knead until smooth and elastic, for about 10 minutes. (NOTE: A Vita-Mix whole food machine can be used in place of the other, if a dough hook isn't readily available. Consult the Product Appendix for information on how to obtain one of these units; instruction and recipe books accompany every unit sold.)

Alternately, mix ingredients in a large bowl, then transfer to a floured surface and knead by hand for 10 minutes. Coat a large bowl with oil. Transfer the dough to this bowl, cover with plastic wrap or a dish towel, and let it rise in a warm corner for about 45 minutes. Punch the dough back down with your fists and divide it into 16 equal pieces. Knead each piece by hand to form a roll and place on 2 lightly oiled baking sheets. Cover with plastic wrap or dish towels and let rise until doubled in size for about 20 minutes. Preheat your oven to 545°F. With the palm of your hand, flatten each ball to form a 4-inch round. Let rise 5 minutes. Spread a scant teaspoon of yogurt in the center of each and sprinkle with coriander. Bake for about 12 minutes, until golden. Makes 16 individual loaves.

CORNFLOWER

(see BLUE BOTTLE)

CORNSILK

(ZEA MAYS)

Brief Description

Corn is so easily recognizable by most people that it doesn't beg for much of a description. The corn plant has a pithy noded stalk supported by prop roots. The staminate (male) flowers form the tassel at the top of the plant. The pistillate (female) flowers are the kernels on the cob, which is enclosed by a leafy husk. Beyond this extend threadlike styles and stigmas or cornsilk which catch the pollen. The entire plant with its ornamental tassel and ears has been a motif of American art since colonial times.

Urologist Claims Healing Miracles from Cornsilk

Dr. Alexander Fischbein, a recently retired urologist in Texas, got in touch with me after receiving one of my other national health best sellers, *Heinerman's Encyclopedia of Fruits, Vegetables and Herbs* (Englewood Cliffs, NJ: Prentice Hall, 1988). He was intrigued with the many diverse applications for a large number of foods and herbs cited in the text, particularly for cornsilk. He gently chided me for being so skimpy with the information on cornsilk. My reply was that a previous manuscript editor with a very large pair of scissors had, quite literally, cut and trimmed the book down to its present size. We both enjoyed a hearty laugh over this.

He said that when I recommended cornsilk for kidney problems and kidney stones, I hadn't gone far enough. To repeat the data I had included in the former book: "Steep 2 tsps. of cornsilk in 1 cup of boiling water for 20 minutes, strain, sweeten with honey and then drink 1/2 cup luke-warm every 3-4 hours. It is ideal to curb bedwetting habits when used with equal parts of catnip....and valerian root." Dr. Fischbein pointed out that I had neglected to give instructions for preparing the latter combination. So now here it is: in one pint of boiling water gently simmer 1/2 tbsp. coarse-ly cut, dried valerian root, uncovered for about 7 minutes. Then add 1/2 tbsp. finely cut, dried catnip leaves, cover, remove from the heat and let steep for almost an hour. Strain and reheat one cup of the tea until luke-warm; add a little honey or pure maple syrup for flavor and drink. Do this about an hour before retiring.

Dr. Fischbein then shared different examples of how he used cornsilk and goldenseal root together for treating various types of cystitis, which is caused by a bacterial infection of the bladder resulting in severe inflam-mation. He mentioned that two forms of chronic cystitis (interstitial cystitis and cystitis senilis feminarum), which are very common in women ages 30 to 65, were always helped with both of these herbs. He would instruct his female patients to drink two or more cups of cornsilk tea every day and with each cup take one capsule powdered goldenseal root. He said that "this winning combination worked health miracles every time, where con-ventional antibiotics failed to."

He also praised this pair of herbs for successfully treating pyelitis, which is an inflammation of the pelvis of the kidney and is attended by pain and tenderness in the loins, agitation of the bladder, remittent fever, bloody or purulent urine, diarrhea, vomiting, and a peculiar pain on flex-ion of the thigh. It is more common in women than in men, and can occur in women after their first sexual intercourse as a result of infection follow-ing rupture of the hymen. The only change he made in his "natural pre-scription" was to increase the dosage of goldenseal/root to two capsules daily instead of one.

He also mentioned that cornsilk tea by itself "does some amazing things for oliguria and edema." The first is a diminished excretion of urine in relation to the amount of fluid intake and the second is any abnormally large amounts of fluid in the intercellular tissue spaces of the body. He noted that the edema can be localized, say in the abdomen, or it can be systemic due to congestive heart failure or kidney disease. In either case, five cups of cornsilk tea every day "moves fluid out of the body like you wouldn't believe."

To make a larger amount of cornsilk tea, just add 3 heaping table-spoonfuls of the threadlike material to 1-1/2 pints boiling water; cover, remove from heat and steep for an hour. Strain and drink one cup every few hours, or as often as needed.

Cornsilk is a major ingredient in two wonderful herbal formulas. The first is a Kidney formula made by Great American Herbs, and the second is an H_2O diuretic formula made by Old Amish Herbs. Both companies are in St. Petersburg, Florida (see Product Appendix for more information).

Downhome Cooking

I would be somewhat remiss if I neglected a recipe calling for the use of corn. The one I've chosen is a dish that has been served to me every time I've visited friends in the deep South. While one of the ingredients may not be too healthy, it sure tastes lip-smacking good when served hot.

GENUINE SOUTHERN SUCCOTASH

Needed: 2 cups shelled green peas or black-eye peas; 6 cobs of sweet corn, cut from cob; 2 medium onions, chopped; 2 green peppers, chopped; 1 jalapeno pepper, seeds removed, chopped (this is optional); 1/2 lb. slab bacon, cut in 1/2-inch chunks; some salt and pepper for flavor.

The way my friends do it in the South is to just cook everything together at once, instead of the more conventional 1-2-3 step way called for in most recipe books. The succotash is served with hot cornbread, creamery butter, honey, and mint julep or iced tea (with a slice of lemon and a sprig of mint included). Yields: Don't know, nor did the folks who gave me this recipe. "It makes 'nuff fer someone hungry and then again," so they told me.

CORYDALIS
(CORYDALIS CAVA)

Brief Description

Corydalis is a perennial herb common to the forests of France and Germany and to the tickets and hedges of the British Isles. It grows anywhere from half-a-foot to a foot in height and bears soft, bluish-green, pinnately decompound and incised leaves. In the spring it is adorned with flowers that may be white, purple-red or rose-colored in appearance.

Effective for Parkinson's, Palsy and General Trembling

An alcoholic tincture is sometimes made of the rootstock and employed by licensed medical herbalists in Great Britain to treat conditions of trembling, palsy, and Parkinson's disease. Two tablespoons of cleaned and finely chopped corydalis rootstock are put in 1 1/2 pints of a strong, dark ale, mead or beer and set aside for two weeks. The contents of the container are shaken every evening, preferably around the time of a full moon, so I'm reliably informed, in order for the full potency of the medicine to be realized. After this, the herbal liquor is strained and 14 drops are taken beneath the tongue in between meals twice daily, or in 5 tablespoons water.

Depression Helped with Herb Combination

The following placebo-controlled, randomized, double-blind study appeared in *Complementary Therapeutic Medicine* (2:5-13, 1994) and is briefly summarized here.

Sixty patients, aged 40 to 75 and suffering from mild to moderate depression, were given a specific herbal formula or a lookalike placebo for two months. The herbal formula consisted of 40 milligrams each of corydalis, California poppy (Eschscholzia california), passion flower, and valerian, as well as 80 milligrams of St. Johnswort. The medicine was taken in the form of tablets (two a day).

Within 8 weeks of treatment, the Depression Status Inventory or DSI (an index commonly used to score the severity of depression) had improved from a pretreatment score of 55.71 (considered to be borderline severe depression) to 38.42 (for a normal population). In the placebo group the DSI improved from 56.83 to 43.8 The herbal combination significantly improved mild-to-moderate depressive symptoms in this group of patients when compared with the placebo group.

Those unable to secure the exact milligrams of each herb may substitute as follows: 1 capsule each of corydalis, California poppy, passion flower and valerian, and 2 capsules of St. Johnswort once or twice daily as needed, with meals. In the event your local health food or herb shop doesn't have some of these ingredients, consult the Product Appendix for companies that can supply you with all your herbal needs by mail-order. Great American Herb Products in St. Petersburg, Florida is one of these.

COTTON
(GOSSYPIUM HIRSUTUM)

Brief Description

The cotton plant belongs to the genus Gossypium of the Mallow (Malvaceae) family. It is generally a shrubby plant having broad three-lobed leaves and seeds in capsules, or bolls; each seed is surrounded with downy fiber, white or creamy in color and easily spun. The fibers flatten and twist naturally as they dry.

Innumerable products are made from cotton. From the lint (that is, the fiber separated from the seed) we get the major products, chiefly textile and yarn goods, cordage, automobile tire-cord, and plastic reinforcing. The linters (which are the short, cut ends removed from the seed after ginning) are a valuable source of cellulose. Cotton hulls are used for fertilizer, fuel and packing; fiber from the stalk is used for pressed paper and cardboard. From the seeds themselves (which are about 20% oil content) comes another chief by-product, cottonseed oil; an entirely separate industry has grown up around it since the late 19th century.

Folk Remedies from the Days of Slavery

In spite of its creamy white color, cotton has a somewhat dark history. Beginning in the United States with the Jamestown colony in 1607, cotton cultivation became associated with slavery and was a principal economic cause of the Civil war, which thoroughly devastated the young republic on both sides.

When these people experienced health problems they turned to plants around them for what they believed were safe and effective solutions. One plant they relied upon was cotton; the root bark, in particular, served them well for different things. The sources I consulted for the following information dealt exclusively with folk medicine of this culture:

Bep Oliver-Bever. *Medicinal Plants in Tropical West Africa* (Cambridge, England: Cambridge University Press, 1986)

William Ed Grime. *Ethno-Botany of The Black Americans* (Algonac, MI: Reference Publications, Inc., 1979)

Edward S. Ayensu. *Medicinal Plants of West Africa* (Algonac, MI: Reference Publications, Inc., 1978)

Abayomi Sofowora. *Medicinal Plants and Traditional Medicine in Africa* (NY: John Wiley & Sons Ltd., 1982)

Ordinarily, I don't often mention the references consulted if the data is not my own original research in the field. But I chose to make one of those exceptions here to enable readers to understand that scientific sources were frequently consulted in the preparation of this volume, though not always mentioned.

Cotton root bark was widely utilized by American slaves and their African progenitors as an abortifacient, an emmenagogue, a hemostatic, and an oxytocic. Besides these, it has proven to be a useful oral contraceptive *for men* and an anti-viral agent against herpes in modern times. Each or several of these will be covered separately hereafter.

A Natural Abortive

My feelings on abortion are somewhat like those of so many other religious ultra-conservatives. However, I just as vigorously beg to differ with those who carry the "right-to-life" message to dangerous extremes. I think that every woman has the inalienable, God-given right of *free agency*, and with this wonderful gift must make some hard, tough choices between the life or death of her unborn fetus. *No* democratic government on earth can legislate that right away, however terrible and sinful the act of abortion itself may be.

So with that in mind and somewhat mixed feelings about abortion in general, I undertake, for the very first time in any of my forty health books, to discuss plainly an herbal abortifacient. Specifically, cotton root bark was used by blacks in Africa and later in America and the Caribbean to abort fetuses in the first six weeks of development. A strong tea was made and consumed orally as well as used in the form of a douche. The scant historic literature suggests that a level handful of the knife *scrapings* of the root bark itself were added to about a quart of water and then boiled for about 30 minutes or longer. The remaining brew was then strained and consumed several times a day; no exact amount was ever given, but I would suspect it might be equivalent to a cup twice daily. Also, no specific length of time in which to take it has ever been discerned. But common sense would dictate that pregnant female Africans and slaves probably took it until premature expulsion of their fetuses was eventually realized.

Delayed Menstruation Helped Along

Half a century ago scientists began studying the effects of cotton root bark on delayed menstruation in African women. *Precis de Matiere Medicale*

(Paris: Maloine, 1946) by Pianchon and Bretin, explained that natives made a tea by boiling some of the bark for a while (amount and time unspecified) and then drank it a couple of times during the day in order to promote menstrual flow. Some African American women today in poorer regions of the South (Mississippi, for example), who can't afford medical care, still turn to things like cotton root bark for solving such problems.

Stops Bleeding and Hastens Childbirth

Cotton root bark makes a useful hemostatic and oxytocic for expectant mothers about to give birth. A *cold* tea of the root bark is taken 36 hours prior to a woman's water breaking and delivery ensuing. One cup in the morning and again in the evening will act as a hemostatic on the uterus, not to mention producing more uterine contractions to expedite childbirth.

To make the tea, boil one pint of water and add one tablespoonful cleaned, grated root bark of the cotton plant. Cover and simmer for 15 minutes. Strain and refrigerate until ready to use.

Birth Control for Men

Gossypol is an orange-red polyphenolic pigment which occurs as a resin in cotton root bark (between 1-2% as a rule). Gossypol is slow to be eliminated from the body and is insoluble in water, which means it won't be very effective as an oral contraceptive for men.

Studies on gossypol for human contraception were started in what was then called the People's Republic of China in the early 1970s but weren't translated into English until 1978. In 1972 semen analyses were carried out on five male subjects. After administration of gossypol for 35-42 days, at a dose of 60-70 mg. daily, four of the men were totally absent of spermatozoa in their semen, and the spermatozoa of the semen in the remaining individual was completely dead.

By 1980 more than 8,000 men in mainland China had been treated with gossypol and two other forms of this compound. The usual dose administered was 20 mg. daily for 60-70 days followed by a maintenance dose of about 60 mg. on a weekly basis. In 99% of the cases a marked decrease in sperm count, usually to 4 million/per milliliter or less of semen, was noted 2-3 months after the dosing began.

Gossypol was reported to cause a degeneration of the germ cells in the seminiferous tubules of man and animal alike when given orally, and to lead to absences of sperm production. In recent years, some scientists have begun experimenting with gossypol as a possible vaginal female contraceptive.

Successfully Fights Herpes Infection

Gossypol has demonstrated reasonably strong antiviral activity in research laboratories around the world. Influenza virus is inactivated by treatment with gossypol resulting in a 96-100% protection rate. Gossypol also displayed definite action against herpes-infected mice on both oral and subcutaneous administration. A tea (made according to previous instructions) of the root bark, taken several times daily, will help with the flu, and will control herpes.

COUCH GRASS
(see QUACK GRASS)

COWSLIP
(see MARSH MARIGOLD)

CRAMP BARK
(see HIGHBUSH CRANBERRY

CRANESBILL
(see GERANIUM, WILD)

CROCUS
(see IRIS)

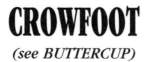

CROWFOOT
(see BUTTERCUP)

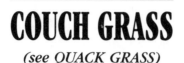

CUMIN
(Cumin cyminum)

Brief Description

The stem of this small, annual herbaceous plant is slender and branched, rarely exceeding 1 foot in height and somewhat angular. The leaves are divided into long, narrow segments, like fennel but much smaller, and are of a deep green color, generally turned back at the ends. The upper leaves are nearly stalkless, but the lower ones have longer leaf-stalks. The flowers are small, rose-colored or white, in stalked umbels with only 4-6 rays, each of which is only about 1/2 inch in length. These bloom in the summer, then eventually turn to the so-called seeds, which are oblong in shape, thicker in the middle and compressed laterally about 1/5th inch long. In some ways they resemble caraway seeds, but are lighter in color and bristly instead of smooth, and almost straight instead of being curved. Their odor and taste are likewise reminiscent of caraway, but less agreeable to the senses than caraway.

Poultice for Abdominal Pain

Soak 2-1/2 tbsp. of cumin seeds in some hot water for about 2 hours. Strain and dry thoroughly before crushing them with a heavy object (clean stone or hammer or rolling pin). Then mix them in with a little white flour and hot water—just enough to form a thin paste. Add several drops of peppermint oil to the hot water before mixing in the other ingredients.

Spread this mixture on a piece of muslin cloth and apply over the abdomen to relieve liver, stomach and gall bladder pains. A tea made by steeping 1 tsp. of cumin seeds in 1 pint of water for an hour helps relieve muscle spasms.

Marinated Delicacy

Cumin brings out the flavor in game fowl like Cornish hens and pheasants.

CUMIN-FLAVORED GAME HEN

Needed: 2-1/2 -3 lbs. of uncooked Cornish game hen; 2 tsp. sea salt; 1 tsp. brown sugar; 1/2 tsp. anise seed; 1/4 tsp. ground ginger; 2 medium bay leaves; 2 tbsp. soy sauce; 2 tbsp. olive oil; 1 tbsp. apple cider vinegar; 3/4 cup flour; 4 tbsp. olive oil; 1 1/2 cups hot *distilled* or spring water; 1 tsp. ground cumin; 4 cups hot cooked wild rice.

Wash game hens and cut into serving pieces. Combine the next 8 ingredients and bring to a boil before pouring over the hens. Cool, then cover and refrigerate overnight. When ready to cook, remove the hens from marinade, reserving it. Roll cut-up pieces of hen in flour. Brown over low heat in olive oil. Add water to marinade and pour over hens. Cover and simmer 25 minutes. Last, add the cumin 7 minutes before cooking time is up. Serve hot over wild rice. Serves 6.

CURRY POWDER

Brief Description

It is believed by many linguists that the word "curry" probably came from the Tamil (South Indian) word *kari* (meaning "a sauce"). It has become the group name for almost any hot spicy dish originating in the East. As there are hundreds of very distinct kinds of curry in India alone, it is as meaningful as an Indian calling every type of European food a "stew."

Even though curry is thought to have originated in India, surprisingly the powder mixture is seldom ever used there. Indians firmly believe that freshly ground spices are more aromatic than a premixed powder. Also, since different proportions of spices go into different dishes, the uses of it in a pre-made blend are rather limited. The closest the average Indian household gets to curry powder is in the *garam masala* which means literally "hot mixture."

Garam masala was never intended to be the entire spicing for any given dish; it is merely a base to which other spices (not a part of it) can be added later on. It is made at home at frequent intervals or sometimes bought in the local bazaar (marketplace). One type of *garam masala* might consist of half a pound of gently roasted coriander seed, half a pound of gently roasted chili and an ounce of black pepper. Another version, however, might include half a pound each of gently roasted fenugreek and mustard seeds and an ounce of ginger. These spices would be ground fine and stored in a tin with a closely fitting lid. There are many gradations of complexity from this to curry powder.

But what we are accustomed to calling curry powder was invented for Europeans. It was first made for ships and servants of the East India Company returning to their homeland. Curry powder is intended to be a complete spicing for a "curry" but as curry recipes vary depending on what part of India they come from, so also do the recipes for curry powder. It is not a standard substance. This doesn't really matter as long as it's intended just for making curry. But since it has been incorporated into European and American cooking, and is used in dishes that have nothing whatsoever to do with curries, a great deal of confusion has been produced as to exactly what comprises a *genuine* curry powder.

A Variety of Ingredients

All the common and some uncommon ingredients used in the curries of India and Southeast Asia have been dealt with in this book or two other volumes in the same series: *Heinerman's Encyclopedia of Nuts, Berries and Seeds* (Englewood Cliffs, NJ: Prentice Hall, 1995) and *Heinerman's New Encyclopedia of Fruits and Vegetables* (Englewood Cliffs, NJ: Prentice Hall, 1995). The English name is given first, followed by the Indian word for each:

allspice (kabab)	fenugreek (methi)
black pepper (kali mirchi)	ginger (fresh: adrak; dried: sonth)
cardamom (elaichi)	lentils (gram)
chilies (mirchi)	mace (tavitri)
cinnamon (dalchini)	mustard seed (rai)
cloves (laung)	nutmeg (taiphal)
coriander (dhania)	poppy seed (khus-khus)
cumin (jeera)	turmeric (haldi)
curry leaves (karipatta)	

Terrific Paste for Relieving Mosquito Bites and Bee Stings

Ayurvedic medicine is an ancient system of alternative healing, which originated in India but has recently been popularized in the West. Some time ago while I was in India I met with several Ayurvedic healers for a few days in order to learn what I could from them.

One of the local remedies involves the use of curry powder for relieving the itching and inflammation of insect bites and stings. A small pinch of any curry powder is mixed with a tiny amount of water to make a smooth, even paste, which is then smeared on the injured site and left in place. By the time it dries out, the pain and swelling have usually disappeared.

Garam Masala for Minor Burns

My Indian informants mentioned that one kind of *garam masala* (or curry) was useful in treating minor burns and sunburns. Equal parts of *fresh* ground fenugreek seed and ginger root and half as much powdered turmeric root are dry mixed by hand. A little sesame seed oil is then added to create a small, soft ball of dough. This ball is then pressed flat between the palms of both hands and then laid over the burn and left there for several hours. This curry not only draws out the inflammation, but also keeps the injured skin from peeling. Three applications or more a day for several days may be necessary. **CAUTION: Prompt medical attention is absolutely necessary for more serious burns.** *Do not* **attempt this treatment with them, but get medical help** *FAST!*

West African-Inspired Recipe

The following dish is West African-inspired. It can be served either as a vegetarian main dish or else as an accompaniment to simple roasted meats.

CURRIED PUMPKIN AND TOMATOES

Needed: 2 tsp. pure virgin olive oil; 1-1/2 lbs. pumpkin or squash, peeled and cut into 1-inch cubes (approx. 3 cups); 1 large onion, thinly sliced; 1 tomato, seeded and diced (about 1 cup); 1/4 cup curry powder, preferably Madras; a pinch of granulated kelp for flavor; nonfat plain yogurt for garnish.

In a large nonstick skillet, heat oil over medium-high heat. Add the pumpkin or squash and cook, stirring occasionally, for 3 minutes. Add the onions and cook, stirring often, for another 4 minutes. Then add the tomatoes, curry powder and 2 cups water; bring to a boil. Reduce the heat to a lower setting and simmer, uncovered, until the pumpkin or squash is tender, but not mushy, for about 23 minutes. Season with the granulated kelp (seaweed) and serve over rice, garnished with a dab of yogurt. Serves 3-4.

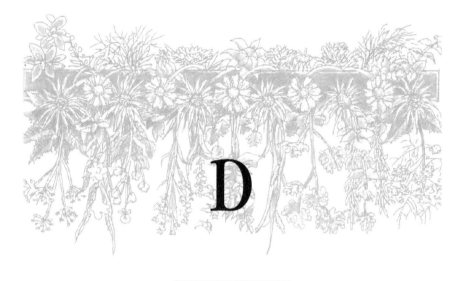

DAFFODIL
(Narcissus pseudonarcissus)

Brief Description

There are roughly a little over two dozen species of daffodil. But the species of this genus hybridize readily in nature and have been the subjects of extensive hybridization by those who grow plants for scientific or commercial purposes. It is estimated that there are a minimum of several hundred hybrids and cultivars of daffodil sold commercially. Many of these hybrids are preferred by florists for their handsome flowers. In addition many daffodils are well-suited for winter forcing of flowering and are, therefore, kept potted indoors. Daffodils are classified into 11 groups of the genus *Narcissus*. Included among these are bright yellow, cream-colored, and mixed color trumpet-shaped daffodil hybrids often used by florists.

Death in man and beast alike can result from ingestion of the bulbs, which are toxic. Nausea, vomiting, cramps, diarrhea, dehydration, weakness, and trembling are common symptoms of daffodil bulb poisoning.

Big Band Legend Glenn Miller and Daffodils

The following story has to do with Big Band legend Glenn Miller and some daffodils. Strange as it may seem, the two are connected, and the account itself quite true.

Edith Wyman and her husband Jake were just high schoolers in western New York State when the Big Bands were in vogue. Their small hometown of Wayland, located in the scenic Finger Lakes region, was a popular

198

stopover for bands as they traveled by bus from New York City to Buffalo. At one time or another, just about all the big-name bands played at Wayland's dance hall, and Edith and Jake were always there to hear them and dance to their lively beats. Edith remembers "whenever Jake and I got out on the floor to jitterbug, we'd always draw a large crowd of onlookers. We got to be so good at it that friends convinced us to enter an Arthur Murray dance contest held in nearby Bath, New York. Well, as luck would have it, Jake and I won first place! That enabled us to go on to the New York State "Shag" Championship, held at the State Fair in Syracuse in 1939.

They were up against some stiff competition from 56 other couples. But with "a lot of aerial tricks" and some hard determination, "we managed to tie for first place," she said. The prize that was awarded to them by Arthur Murray himself was $150, plus a week's engagement as the opening act for Eddy Duchin and his orchestra at a theater in Buffalo! "What a thrill it was for us to meet the members of that famous band, including singers Carolyn Horton and Lew Sherwood," Edith declared. "But we soon experienced a far greater thrill!"

In September they received a telegram from the manager of the Paramount Theater on New York's "Great White Way," offering them a three-week engagement with Glenn Miller and his Moonlight Serenaders. Edith and Jake promptly accepted without any hesitation. The Paramount billed them as "New York State Shag Champions," and they appeared along with an up-and-coming musical group known as The Four Ink Spots.

Miller's singers at that time were Ray Eberle and Marion Hutton, whose sister Betty was about to leave for Hollywood to try her luck as an actress. Edith remembers just how good a dancer Betty was: "While jitterbugging with her to the sounds of Glenn Miller's band, I accidentally twisted my right ankle. It was pretty bad and I could barely hobble around after that. Thank heavens, though, that we were near the end of our three-week engagement. Jake and I returned to Wayland to nurse my injury with enough memories to last us a lifetime."

Jack's uncle was an avid gardener, and "he had this thing with daffodils," she recalls. "One day, seeing me hobbling around with a swollen ankle, he said, 'let me try something, will you, that I think will help?' Of course, I didn't know what he had in mind, but I figured anything was better than being temporarily crippled."

The uncle dug up some of his daffodils to get the roots. He washed some off, cut them into small pieces, put them in some water and boiled them for a while until they could be mashed with a potato masher. He then spread some of these *hot* mashed daffodil roots on a clean piece of cloth and bound it comfortably around Edith's swollen ankle with some old shoelaces tied together. He then put part of the remaining mashed daffodil roots in the freezer to get cold quickly.

After 20 minutes he unbound the poultice and replaced it with another one, only this time using *cold* mashed roots instead. He kept this in place for the same length of time. Then he switched back to another *warm* poultice, then another *cold* one 40 minutes later. It took only three such treatments in 1-1/2 days before the swelling had entirely disappeared from her ankle. "I never had any more problems after that," Edith testified. Since then, she has used the same remedy on her children and some of her grandchildren for dislocated joints, pulled muscles, severe bruises and, of course, sprained ankles, with remarkable success!

DANDELION
(TARAXACUM OFFICINALE)

Brief Description

The name "dandelion" is sometimes loosely applied to other milky-sapped weeds with fluffy yellow flowers. But true dandelion is that ubiquitous weed growing prolifically in millions of lawns, backyards and pastures throughout America. This perennial herb has deeply cut leaves forming a basal rosette in the spring and flower heads born on long stalks. All leaves and the hollow flower stem grow directly from the rootstock. The creator of the comic strip "Marvin" once had his adorable diapered hero surveying a clump of dandelions and then thinking to himself, "Dandelions are Nature's way of giving dignity to weeds!"

Grandpa Walton's Wart and Liver Spot Remover

Will Geer, who portrayed Grandpa Walton on "The Waltons," was on a late-night television talk show several years ago discussing the practical uses for the milky sap contained in the stems of dandelions.

"You just take some of them, break them open and rub that juice on any wart you have," he told his host, while at the same time illustrating it by a circular motion of his fingers on the back of his hand. "You just do that two or three times a day and I'll guarantee that you won't be plagued with warts anymore."

He also confirmed that this same milky sap was excellent for reducing dark "liver spots" which generally appear on the backs of the hands of elderly people. "I just do the same thing with them that I'd do with warts," he said, "only I'd use more of the juice and rub it in more thoroughly." He then held up both his hands in front of the camera for a close-up view. From the TV monitors located in the studio, the audience was able to clearly see just how well this remedy had worked for him. Most of his liver spots had become so faded that one almost had to strain to detect any faint sign of them.

Good for Hypertension

In the spring dandelion leaves and roots produce mannitol, a substance used in the treatment of hypertension and weak heart throughout Europe. A tea made of the roots and leaves is good to take during this period, from about mid-March to mid-May. Bring 1 quart of water to a boil, reduce heat and add 2 tbsp. cleaned and chopped fresh roots. Simmer for 1 minute, covered, then remove from heat and add 2 tbsp. chopped, freshly picked leaves. Steep for 40 minutes. Strain and drink 2 cups per day.

Wonderful Liver Medicine

The late naturopathic physician, John Lust, stated in his *Herb Book* that dandelion root is good for all kinds of liver problems, including hepatitis, cirrhosis, jaundice and toxicity in general, as well as getting rid of gallstones. Bring 1 quart of water to a boil, reduce heat to low, and add about 20 tbsp. of fresh dandelion leaves, stems, and cleaned chopped root. Simmer as long as it takes for the liquid to be reduced to just a pint, then strain. Take 3 tbsp. six times daily, Dr. Lust recommended.

For those desiring something more convenient in capsule form, there is the AKN Formula from Nature's Way, which contains considerable dandelion root and other cleansing herbs. It can be obtained from any local health food store.

Remedy for Diabetes

Dr. David Potterton, a licensed, practicing medical herbalist in Great Britain, once wrote that the high insulin content of the root may be regarded as "a sugar substitute to prescribe for people with diabetes mellitus." Three capsules of the dried root each day is recommended for this. The Nature's Way brand from your local health food store is often purchased with this in mind.

Flowers Improve Night Blindness

For those with a problem of reduced vision in the dark, the substance called helenin found in dandelion flowers may be just the ticket. According to the *Journal of the American Medical Association* for June 23, 1951, which carried this report, the blossoms also contain vitamins A and B-2 (riboflavin). Steep a handful of freshly picked flowers in a pint of hot water for about 20 minutes. Drink 1 cup twice a day.

Reduces Fever of Childhood Infections

If your child or grandchild comes down with measles, mumps or chicken-pox, three common infectious diseases of childhood years, then dandelion tea is the thing to give him or her. Bring 1 quart of water to a boil. Reduce the heat and add 2 tbsp. dried, cut root and simmer, covered, for 12 minutes. Remove from heat and add 3 tsp. dried, cut leaves. Steep for half an hour. Strain, sweeten with 1 tsp. pure maple syrup or 1 tsp. blackstrap molasses per cup of tea and give to a child, lukewarm, every 5 hours or so until fever breaks and lung congestion clears up. This tea is also excellent for all types of upper respiratory infections, ranging from pneumonia to chronic bronchitis.

Homemade Wine

Delicious dandelion wine is fun and easy to make at home.

DANDELION WINE

Needed: 2 quarts dandelion flowers (make sure they're not sprayed); 1/2 gallon water; 1 orange; 1/2 lemon; 1-1/4 lbs. brown sugar; 1/2 cake yeast. Carefully remove all traces of stems. Place flowers in some kind of crockware. Add sugar, sliced orange and lemon, then pour boiling water over everything. Let set 2 days, stirring occasionally. On the third day, strain into another crock and add yeast. Let ferment 2 weeks in a warm place.

Check for Rocks

I can't help but include the following news item which appeared in the January, 1995 issue of *Health Foods Business* (p.6). It says something about the litigious society we currently live in.

A California Small Claims court recently awarded almost $2,000 to a customer who claimed he broke six of his teeth by chomping down on a pebble in bulk dandelion he ate raw after purchasing it at a Palo Alto health food store. Because it involved natural foods, the Food and Drug Administration (FDA) and the Department of Consumer Affairs took an active interest in the case. A warning went out to all California health food retailers to keep their bulk food bins clean and free of foreign objects.

But some in the health food industry with whom I spoke about this rare but unique case seemed to think that the court should have appointed a psychiatrist to check the consumer's head for "possible rocks instead of brains." They felt that such an incident was blown way out of proportion and that the real stone wasn't in the fresh dandelion but rather in the guy's head.

DAY LILY

(see LILIES)

DEADLY NIGHTSHADE

(see BELLADONNA)

DIGITALIS
(DIGITALIS PURPUREA)

Brief Description

The discovery of this beautiful but deadly herb (also called foxglove) came about in a rather remarkable way. In 1775 an English physician, William Withering, heard of an old woman in Shropshire reputed for her ability to cast spells. He was reliably informed that she had an extensive knowledge of medicinal plants. At the time Withering was treating a patient suffering from congestive heart failure who was not expected to live.

He consulted with this old hag, who gave him a curious mixture consisting of a dozen or more herbs and demanded payment. At first he hesitated, believing her price was too high. But when reminded in no uncertain terms that she had the power to put a hex on him if he kept irritating her, the good doctor quickly relented and met her price, leaving the premises with the precious herbs.

He made a tea from them and gave half-cup amounts every 2-4 hours to his patient for nearly a week. Within five days the man was considerably better and able to get up from his bed of sickness and move about. Withering carefully analyzed the unused portion of the herb mixture and finally determined it was foxglove which had helped his patient the most.

He put all his findings into a fascinating book entitled *An Account of the Foxglove, and Some of Its Medical Uses, with Practical Remarks on Dropsy, and Other Diseases* (Birmingham, England: M. Swinney, 1785). It has since been reprinted in *Medical Classics* (5:4:303-443; 1937).

Cardiotonic Drugs for the Heart

Some 220 years later doctors around the world still routinely prescribe digitalis therapy for such cardiac disorders as congestive heart failure, atherosclerosis, and hypertension (related to heart disease). Digitalis increases the contractibility and improves the tone of the heart muscle, resulting in a slower but much stronger heart beat. Digitalis slows the wildly beating ventricles to a normal level by blocking or delaying the conduction of the electric impulse through the atrioventricular node. By increasing the heart stroke, this herb is able to double or even triple the amount of blood being oxygenated by the lungs, as well as 30% with each beat. Due to this substantially improved action of the heart and blood circulation, digitalis also tends to improve kidney function, to relieve edema, and to aid the cardiac muscle to compensate for mechanical defects or structural lesions.

The magnitude of the need for digitalis therapy is reflected in the fact that over 5 million cardiac sufferers in the U.S. and Canada currently use the glycoside digoxin from one species of foxglove. And this is just one of six different glycosides from digitalis prescribed by doctors at present: digitalis leaf, digitoxin, digoxin, lanatoside C, acetyldigitoxin, and deslancside.

Because digitalis is so potent and toxic, it requires *strict medical supervision* with its use. You will need a doctor's written prescription to get digitalis from your local pharmacy; this is one herb health food stores cannot, by law, dispense.

DILL
(ANETHEUM GRAVEOLENS)

Brief Description

Dill is aromatic, somewhat like caraway, but much milder and sweeter. The taste of dill resembles fennel in some ways, but is slightly more pungent and aggressive in flavor.

The plant grows ordinarily from 2 to 2-1/2 feet high and looks a lot like fennel, although smaller but having the same feathery leaves, which stand on sheathing foot-stalks, with linear and pointed leaflets. But unlike fennel, it has seldom more than one stalk and its long, spindle-shaped root is only annual. It's of very upright growth, its stem smooth, shiny and hollow, and in midsummer bears flat terminal umbels with numerous yellow flowers, whose small petals are rolled inwards.

The flat fruits or so-called seeds are produced in great quantities—an ounce containing over 25,000 seeds. Pickled cucumbers and beets wouldn't be complete without dill seed. Nor would green apple pies, certain fish hors d'oeuvres, soups, beans, cabbage, cauliflower, peas, cottage cheese and some nut butters.

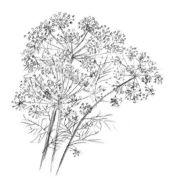

Get Your Beauty Sleep

If you have trouble sleeping at night, consider this remedy instead of over-the-counter and prescription drugs. Bring 1 pint of white wine *almost* to a boil (but don't boil). Remove from heat and add 4 tsp. dill seeds. Cover and steep for 30 minutes. Drink 1-1/2 cups lukewarm 30-45 minutes before retiring.

Increases Milk Flow in Nursing Moms

A tea made according to the above directions but using instead 1 tsp. each of anise, coriander, caraway and dill seeds is excellent for stimulating the flow of breast milk in nursing mothers, when taken daily lukewarm, 1 cup about an hour before feeding an infant.

Gets Rid of Bad Breath

Try chewing some dill seeds the next time you experience halitosis. You'll be pleasantly surprised to see how quickly they sweeten and freshen your breath.

An Interesting Salad and Dressing Idea

DILLED GREEN BEAN SALAD

Needed: 1-1/2 lbs. green beans; 1/2 cup olive oil; 1/4 cup tarragon vinegar; 1 tbsp. each chopped fresh parsley, fresh chives and dill weed; kelp to taste; small bunch of watercress. Wash and trim green beans. Boil until tender. Rinse under cold water. Drain well, patting dry with paper towel. Whisk together oil, tarragon vinegar and herbs. Season to taste with kelp. Pour over the beans and stir well. Correct seasonings, if necessary. Chill. Before serving, break watercress into small pieces and toss with green beans. Arrange on a platter. Serves half a dozen. Adapted from *Country Journal* for April 1987.

CREAMY CUCUMBER SAUCE

This light sauce makes a dandy pizza topping or lovely dressing for the preceding salad.

Needed: 1/2 cup nonfat yogurt; 2 tbsp. nonfat dry milk; 1 cucumber, peeled, finely chopped; 1 clove garlic, minced; 1/2 tsp. lemon peel, grated; 1 tsp. dried dillweed or 1 tbsp. fresh dill chopped, and 1/2 tsp. salt.

Whisk together the yogurt and dry milk until well blended. Then stir in the cucumber, garlic, lemon peel, dill and salt. Makes one cup.

Possible Protection Against Breast, Colo-Rectal, and Pancreatic Cancer

According to a recent study, limonene, an essential oil found in dill, caraway and celery seed oils as well as in citrus fruit peel oils, might reactivate a natural anti-carcinogenic process. A clinical trial started in 1995 to examine the role of the nutrient in relation to pancreatic and colo-rectal cancers.

The anti-tumor effect, with low toxicity, was first reported in rodent research in 1984. In the animal studies, limonene both inhibited tumor formation and caused regression of existing tumors. The research suggests that limonene may be able to counteract a genetic predisposition for cancer as shown in mammary tumor research in rodents. For women concerned about possible breast cancer, this should come as welcome news.

A tea made by cooking 1 tbsp. dried dill weed in 1 pint water for 15 minutes, covered, then strained and one cup drunk warm each day may help to reduce a woman's risk of breast cancer.

DOG GRASS
(see QUACK GRASS)

DOGWOOD
(CORNUS FLORIDA)

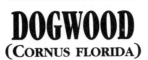

Brief Description

This can be either a shrub or small tree growing up to 30 feet in height, determined by factors such as soil, climate and elevation. It is found from southern Ontario Province in Canada and Maine south to Florida and Texas and west to Kansas. In former years when I spent a great deal of time in the Lonestar State, I experienced the advent of the dogwoods in the springtime. Or, at least, my nose and eyes did, for I sneezed like crazy and kept wiping away the tears their pollen produced.

The leaves of the dogwood are prominently veined, oval-shaped and pointed. On top they tend to be more dark green and beneath a paler green or almost whitish in appearance, with soft down on their undersides. The true flowers are tiny and greenish white, forming in a central cluster surrounded by four showy, notched, creamy white bracts that look like petals. The flowers produce red fruits.

Civil War Substitute for Quinine

During the American Civil War, ships from the North frequently blockaded many southern ports, thereby preventing the importing of cinchona bark from South America. Without this valuable bark, there was no readily available source for quinine, the principal medicine that southern doctors used to treat Rebel soldiers suffering from malaria.

Since "necessity is always the mother of invention," reasonable substitutes were looked for; dogwood bark tea became the medicine of choice for treating this disease.

One such physician who spoke highly of dogwood was Francis Peyre Porcher, M.D. In his excellent treatise *Resources of The Southern Fields and Forests* (Charleston: Evans & Cogswell, 1863; pp. 59-62), he had this to say about it: "In our present need...the dogwood bark powdered will be found the best substitute for Peruvian [bark]. Internally and externally it can be applied wherever the cinchona barks were found serviceable. The dogwood bark and root, in decoction, or in form of cold infusion, is...the most efficient substitute for quinine, also in treating malarial fevers..."

Dr. Porcher's anti-fever "tonic compound" called for *powders* of the following herbs: dogwood rootbark (6 oz.), poplar bark (6 oz.), wild cherry bark (6 oz.), and cayenne pepper (4 oz.). These were sifted through a

coarse wire screen (a flour sifter can be used instead) and then thoroughly mixed together. He would then mix one level teaspoonful of this powdered formula in 6 fluid ounces of "warm or cold water" and have each soldier drink it "three times a day, before meals."

He claimed to have never lost a patient to malaria with this simple
remedy. Over 130 years later it is still as effective for *all* fevers and fever-
related problems as it was in his day. If you have ready access to dogwoods, then I strongly suggest that you take advantage of the wonderful
healing properties in their rootbarks.

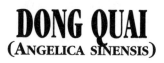

DONG QUAI
(ANGELICA SINENSIS)

Brief Description

This medicinal plant is considered by the Chinese to be the "empress of
herbs." Dong quai is a fragrant, perennial herb, with a glabrous stem that
is highly striated. The leaves and flower umbels resemble those of carrots,
celery, and parsley. The herb has a pleasant, sweet and pungent flavor similar to dill or angelica. In some other ways, the top part of dong quai
reminds one of a strange parsley.

The root is used medicinally for many things. It occurs divided into
numerous rootlets, the exterior being brownish and the interior being white
and spongy. The taste is bittersweet and the odor highly aromatic.

An Herb for the Uterus

Since 1920 research has been conducted by different Oriental scientists and
doctors on the effects of dong quai on the uterus. At that time it showed a
contractile effect when injected hypodermically into anesthetized dogs and
rabbits. The exact constituent responsible for this was never made clear.
But it stimulated uterine contractions and then assisted prolonged relax-
ation of the organ.

In cases of painful menstruation (dysmenorrhea), the herb enabled
the contractions of the uterus to be more orderly. In the opinion of some
researchers, this may be the mechanism underlying its effectiveness in treating this particular female problem. The herb, however, doesn't appear to
have any estrogenic effect.

Dong quai is frequently recommended by herbalists for women getting off birth control pills to help re-establish a regular cycle. It is considered a very useful herb for all gynecological problems that are due to deficient, poor quality or stagnant blood.

Cardiovascular Benefits

Decoctions of dong quai root were discovered to have an inhibitory effect on frog heart specimens. Alcohol extractions have a quinidine-like effect. In numerous experiments various preparations of this herb (including decoctions and alcohol extractions) have the effect of lowering blood pressure in anesthetized animals. When the dosage is small, duration is rather short and is usually followed by a rise in pressure again. Also, in controlled experiments on rats with artificial atherosclerosis, those animals fed this herb had less plaque formation than controls did.

Treatment of Pain

Injections of a preparation of dong quai root into acupuncture points of the body is used throughout China and Taiwan for the treatment of various types of pain (including neuralgia, heart pain and arthritis) with good results. In one study of 1,000 patients, over 380 were cured. In another trial of 50 patients suffering from neuralgia from the head, neck and upper back, 33 were cured and the remainder experienced some relief. This form of therapy, though, isn't used by Oriental doctors for sprains and other acute conditions or for pain from tumors or infections.

One study in a prominent Japanese medical journal pointed out that dong quai was "1.7 times stronger than aspirin" in relieving mild pain. (See S. Tanaka, et al, "Effects of Toki," in *Yakuga Zassh* 91:1098-1104, 1971).

Dong Quai Preparations

Dong quai, one of a small handful of very versatile herbs, can be consumed in many different ways. Recommended intake of the root powder is 3 capsules a day. Or, if a tea is to be made, one cup daily. To make the tea, simmer two teaspoons of grated root in 1-1/2 pints boiling water, covered, for 20 minutes on low heat. Then remove, strain and drink.

Dong quai root can also be cooked with different foods. It definitely improves the flavor of chicken or vegetable soups if some of the sliced root is added, plus it's a great way to enjoy the plant's many medicinal benefits.

Still another clever way to use dong quai is to cook one root with six jujube dates (both are readily available at oriental markets) in three cups of water. Simmer on low heat for about 20 minutes or until the amount of liquid has been reduced by half. Then strain and drink a half-cupful three times daily.

CAUTION: Dong quai is not advised during pregnancy or excess menstruation due to its blood-moving properties. It is also contraindicated in cases of fever, fast pulses, diarrhea, and abdominal distention.

E

ECHINACEA
(ECHINACEA AUGUSTIFOLIA)

Brief Description

Echinacea is a native perennial growing from the prairie states northward to Pennsylvania, but also occurs in the cooler northern regions of some southern states as well. The stout, bristly stems bear hairy, linear-lanceolate leaves, tapering at both ends. Each of the distinctive rich purple flowers features 12-20 large, spreading, dull-purple rays and a conical disk made up of numerous tubular florets that are in bloom from June - October. A weaker species (*E. purpurea*) is often substituted for *E. augustifolia* whenever the latter becomes scarce or too expensive for the herb industry's use.

The plant has a faint aromatic smell with a nice sweetish taste, leaving a tingling sensation in the mouth not unlike that of aconite or monkshood, but without the latter's lasting numbness or dangerous poison. Tasting echinacea powder is one way of determining just how fresh or old it might be. I once found some in a Gainesville, Florida health food store that was about as lifeless and dull as any herb could be. It apparently sat on the shelf for a very long time and was virtually worthless as a medicinal herb.

Tremendous Immune System Booster

Medical doctors have praised the tremendous power which echinacea seems to exert upon the entire immune system. Finley Ellingwood, M.D., a Chicago physician, some years ago (1915) published a special issue of his

211

health magazine (*Ellingwood's Therapeutist*) devoted entirely to this herb. "For 25 years," he wrote, "echinacea has been passing through critical experimentation under the observation of several thousand physicians, and its remarkable properties are receiving positive confirmation."

He noted that this herb dramatically increases the production of white killer cells in the body to help eliminate infectious diseases of all kinds. He claimed that echinacea "endows them with a certain amount of recuperative power or formative force," even going so far as to compare its effects in the body to that of the standard vaccines of the day! Various cases from tuberculosis and tonsillitis to spinal meningitis and syphilis have been successfully treated with this remarkable herb.

German scientists over the years have demonstrated echinacea's uncanny ability to reduce malignant tumors. They found that echinacea can even mimic the actions of the body's own interferon—powerful little proteins that throw up an incredibly strong wall of resistance to superinfections like the AIDS virus, for instance.

Health writer Ed Mayer explained how he cured himself of serious hospital-induced staph infection. External treatment consisted of making a potent tea by boiling for 20 minutes in 2 cups of water, 1 tsp. powdered myrrh, 1 tsp. powdered golden seal and 1/2 tsp. cayenne. He soaked his badly infected foot for about 15 minutes daily, keeping the tea as hot as he could stand it. He then applied a paste of golden seal, echinacea and water before bandaging it.

Internal treatment consisted of high doses of vitamin C, light food and plenty of fresh fruit and vegetable juices. He also drank 3 cups a day of the following tea until the infection completely cleared up: 2 tsp. echinacea, 2 tsp. burdock root and 1 tsp. sassafras simmered on low heat in 4 cups of boiling water for about 20 minutes.

Two particularly effective herbal formulas that some doctors have recommended to their patients in San Francisco as fairly good protection against getting the AIDS virus are Resist-All and Herpes, manufactured by Great American Natural Products out of St. Petersburg, Florida (see Appendix). Both products, these doctors informed me, had heavy concentrations of echinacea in them, besides other powerful antibiotic herbs like chaparral, thyme, myrrh, pau d'arco and sarsaparilla. They had their clientele take an average of three capsules each per day for maximum protection.

Protects Against Fire

Virgil J. Vogel's classic masterpiece, *American Indian Medicine*, mentioned the use of echinacea for an incredible feat of endurance in the early and mid-19th century. Winnebago medicine men would sometimes chew up the raw herb in order to numb their mouths enough so that they could insert burning pieces of hot coals as if by magic to the utter astonishment of their tribes. This amazing act without sustaining serious injury made tribal members fear their supposedly great power. The echinacea juice acted as a preventative against lengthy inflammation.

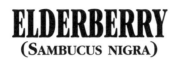

ELDERBERRY
(SAMBUCUS NIGRA)

Brief Description

Elderberries differ considerably in form and taste, growing from bushy shrubs a few feet high to trees close to 50 feet in height. Their usual clusters of aromatic, star-shaped white flowers vary from flat-topped bunches to globular arrays, maturing to berrylike, limb-sagging fruits that differentiate in color from blue, amber, and red to black and also changing considerably in taste.

Early Native American tribes employed the long, straight, hollow stems that became woodier with age for arrows and especially selected some in the springtime, dried them with their leaves on, pushed out all the soft and poisonous pith with hot sticks, and made either spouts for gathering maple and other sap or bored holes in them to fashion flutes. This gave the medicinal its added name of "tree of music." Some hunters who still use the old ways to track their game have bugled in elk with an elderberry whistle and have soon brought down a handsome buck.

Elderberries prefer rich, moist soil and are usually found in heavily forested areas, on rocky slopes, and in cool ravines. They are native to the temperate and subtropical regions of both hemispheres.

The fruit is a berrylike drupe, containing 3 to 5 one-seeded nutlets or stones. Wisdom dictates that only a few be eaten raw lest stomach upset occur. They are much better dried or cooked, but are more delicious when combined with tastier berries.

Mucus Accumulation Easily Discharged

Certain conditions bring about an excess of mucus accumulation in the lungs. Asthma, bronchitis, the common cold, influenza, and smoking or inhaling second-hand smoke can all result in a buildup of phlegm. A little bit of fresh elderberry juice, especially from the red drupes, is quite effective in promoting a discharge of such sticky yellow or green mucus from the body.

An old bachelor from the backwoods of Vermont once told me how he took elderberry juice to cough up "the stuff that rattles down below." Zeke would put several handfuls of the ripe red berries through a coarse meat grinder. He would then gather up the pulp and put it into a large piece of cheesecloth, draw the ends together and tie them, and then press out the remaining juice by pounding the packaged material with a wooden mallet. He claimed it only took two tablespoonsful on an empty stomach to get the phlegm out. He had a little rattle in his chest, probably due to his constant habit of pipe smoking. He volunteered to show me just how quickly and effectively this worked, but I declined. I told him I believed the remedy worked without having to see the actual slimy proof of the same, that would probably nauseate me for sure. He slapped his thigh, cackled a throaty laugh and took another puff. I gathered from this body English that he was probably having a good joke at my expense.

Quick Remedy for Constipation

The August 1984 edition of *Natural Foods Merchandiser* (p.54), a publication of the health food industry, featured a survey of the best-selling herbal products in several thousand of America's leading health-food stores. Of those surveyed, 50% of all herb sales were for laxative products.

In my own formulating work I've discovered also that my laxative formulas have always outsold every other product I've created, seven to one. It can truly be said that health-minded Americans have a real love affair with their colons and herbal laxatives.

Most of the herb books on the market will list a number of standard laxative agents: cascara sagrada, buckthorn bark, senna, turkey rhubarb, and psyllium seed. These are in addition to the old standby of prune juice. Granted that every one of them works within a few hours to produce the effects desired.

But what most people don't know is that a little bit of *fresh* elderberry juice will work like lightning to evacuate the bowels. Unfortunately for herbal manufacturers this isn't something you can capture and put into a bottle. It must be taken *fresh* in order to work as rapidly as it does. Amazingly enough, it's completely safe for everyone, from infants to the elderly. So says Varro E. Tyler, the retired Dean of the Schools of Pharmacy, Nursing and Health Sciences at Purdue University in his book, *Hoosier Home Remedies* (West Lafayette, IN: Purdue University Press, 1985, p. 51).

Recommended intake is six tablespoonsful of *fresh* elderberry juice on an empty stomach for *quick* results. Because elderberries are *strongly purgative* they should be used infrequently.

Migraines Gone for Good

Recurring headaches of the specific type known as migraines can be very troublesome. Not only do they interfere with the person's daily schedule of activities, often limiting what can be done, but they also create a deep sense of frustration in that nothing tried seems to work in helping them go away.

Many times the problem of repeated migraines is an internal signal that something isn't working right and needs prompt medical attention. It can be something as simple as a few chiropractic adjustments or new prescription lenses, or else something more complex in the way of surgery and specific medication before permanent relief is obtained.

An old Choctaw remedy of the early nineteenth century proved very efficacious in removing migraines from any white women who periodically suffered from them. The Choctaw formerly occupied central and southern Mississippi, with some outlying groups in Alabama, Georgia, and Louisiana. Their main economy was based on agriculture and they were perhaps the most competent farmers in the Southeast. After being forced to cede their lands in Alabama and Mississippi, they moved to the Indian Territory in Oklahoma in 1832, where they eventually became one of the Five Civilized Tribes to inhabit those parts. (The other four tribes were the Cherokee, the Chicksaw, The Creek, and the Seminole.) Here they lived for many years and peacefully practiced their way of life.

In 1889 the federal government opened the first of several strips in the western section of the territory to homesteaders. Prospective settlers lined up on the territorial border, and at high noon they were permitted to cross on a "run" to compete in finding and claiming the best lands. Those who illegally entered ahead of the set time were the Sooners. This great colonizing event has been recreated in film and a Broadway musical, *Oklahoma*, by Richard Rogers and Oscar Hammerstein.

The influx of tens of thousands of white settlers brought them into constant contact with the Five Civilized Tribes. Some, like the Choctaw, were not averse to sharing some of their remedies with their new neighbors. A few pioneer women who kept diaries of the homesteading period occasionally recorded some of these remedies. It was from one of these journals that I obtained this old Choctaw headache remedy. I've slightly revised it for twentieth century use, but it still works just as effectively as it did a hundred years ago.

One-half cup of ordinary table salt is poured into a heavy cast iron skillet, evenly spread around with a wooden spoon, and heated on a medium-set stove burner. Or the same amount of salt can be evenly spread on a cookie sheet and warmed in an oven set at 345° F. Either way, the salt needs to be quite warm, but not so hot as to scorch the skin, in order for this remedy to work.

Next, thoroughly mash 1/4 cup of fresh elderberries. Then combine them with the hot salt in a large mixing bowl. This is best done by hand, stirring vigorously with a wooden spoon. It is important to get all of the berry juice mixed in with the salt so that none of it drips out.

Fill a clean white sock with the mixture until it is pretty evenly distributed three fourths to the top. Fold a little of the top edge over and tape it down with some masking tape to secure tightly, so the contents don't spill out. Remember that the salt must still be quite *hot* for this to work. The cotton material will allow the heat to penetrate through without burning the skin.

The headache sufferer should lie down on a bed or couch, place the sock over the forehead, making sure that the salt-berry mixture is evenly distributed around inside so it doesn't bunch up on one end to form a lump. Place a small, dry hand towel over the sock to retain the heat. Keep it on the forehead until it becomes cool. By then the migraine will have ceased and comfort will ensue. This same application can also be placed on the back of the neck if necessary. The sock mixture can be reheated several times and used this way to relieve backaches, toothache, sore muscles, and pulled or sprained ligaments.

Eruptive Sores and Burns Completely Healed

The Choctaw also mixed some elderberry juice with a little boiled honey and used it as a wonderful topical application for skin eruptions and burns. The honey is primarily an adhesive agent to keep the juice from running off the skin.

One teaspoon of honey is used with two tablespoons of elderberry juice. An amount of liquid this small can be heated over a lit candle, gas burner, or cigarette lighter. The mixture is warmed only enough to loosen the honey so it can nicely blend in with the juice, which is more runny. After this, let the honey set up again before applying to the afflicted skin with a clean butter knife, popsicle stick or tongue depressor. This remedy should only be used for first-degree or minor burns. For advanced-degree burns, promptly consult a physician in the emergency room of any hospital.

Tummy Relief Just a Swallow Away After Eating Green Apples

An oldtimer by the name of Charles Wren told me this story many years ago when I was a teenager and it's stayed with me ever since. He said that "when I was a youngun, my cuzzin 'Rastus and I pigged out on a bunch of green apples in the orchard back of my grandpa's house. We felt pretty darned miserable after a spell. Started seein' things that warn't there and turning a little green 'round our gills. We both felt like pukin', but was too sick to do so.

"Well, sir, my grandma, she picked a handful of elderberry flowers she had growin' in her backyard and removed the petals from the green parts. She placed them in a pint of hot water and let them steep for half an hour. Then, she gave us each a cup of this stuff to drink slowly. Almost immediately, our sick stomachs cleared up and soon our headaches went away, too. Them elederberry flowers sure worked wonders for us two little boys. And I guarantee you, we never again ate any apples while they were still green!"

Fun Recipes

Imagine cooking with something *wild* for a change. Go ahead and dare to be different! Try these recipes using elderberries gathered from the wild for truly tasty treats.

STEWED DRIED ELDERBERRIES

Needed: 4 cups dried elderberries; water to cover; pinch of brown sugar;1 cinnamon stick; 1 tsp. cloves; 2 tsp. grated lemon rind.

Rinse the berries; place them in a pot with a tight-fitting lid. Cover generously with water and simmer briskly for 10 minutes. Then add the other ingredients and simmer 10 minutes longer.

SPICED ELDERBERRIES

Needed: 4 qts. dried elderberries; 2 lbs. brown sugar;1 pint apple cider vinegar; 1 tsp. whole allspice; 1 tsp. whole cloves; 2 cinnamon sticks.

Tie the spices in a bag. Combine sugar, vinegar and spices and boil 7 minutes. Then add the fruit and cook until the mixture has thickened. Remove the spices. Seal the mixture in sterilized fruit jars. Yield: Makes 5 pints.

ELDERBERRY RICE PUDDING

Needed: 2 cups white rice, cooked; 1-1/2 cups milk; pinch of salt; 3-1/2 tbsp. brown sugar; 1 tbsp. butter; 1 tsp. vanilla; 2 eggs; 1/2 cup dried elderberries; 1/2 tsp. lemon rind, grated; 1 tsp. lemon juice.

Combine the first seven ingredients and blend thoroughly. Then add the elderberries, rind and juice, stirring continually. Pour into a lightly oiled baking pan. Bake at 325°F. for 1-1/2 hours.

ELDERBERRY BRAN MUFFINS

Needed: 1/2 cup whole wheat flour; 1/4 cup cattail flour (see under CATTAIL on how to make this flour); 1 tbsp. baking powder (preferably aluminum-free); 1/2 tsp. salt; 1 cup bran; 1/2 cup dried elderberries; 1 egg; 1/2 cup milk; 2 tbsp. molasses; 1 tbsp. melted butter.

Cover the elderberries with boiling water and let them soak 3 hours. Sift together the first four ingredients. Then add the bran and elderberries. Beat the egg and mix with the milk, molasses and butter. Follow this by adding the dry ingredients and mix just enough to dampen all the dry ingredients, being careful, however, NOT TO OVERMIX. Fill greased muffin tins 1/2 full and bake at 400° F. for 25 minutes. Yield: Makes a dozen.

A note of thanks goes to Darcy Williamson for assistance with these recipes.

ELECAMPANE
(INULA HELENIUM)

Brief Description

Elecampane is a perennial herb common to damp pastures and fields and roadsides in the eastern and central portions of the U.S. and Canada. The plant grows anywhere from 3 to 6 feet in height, has a stout, branched stem rising from a basal rosette type of large ovate, pointed leaves, and manifests bright yellow flowerheads during mid-to-late summer. These flowerheads are usually 4 inches wide and look like small sunflowers. The root is large, heavy, long and white inside but yellow on the outside, and emits an odor similar to violets in bloom.

Bar Bouncer Finds Relief for His Aches and Pains

Some occupations by nature incur a certain amount of pain for those who work them. Furniture movers may get sore backs from bending and lifting heavy objects. Computer terminal operators and chicken deboners often get carpal tunnel syndrome because they have to move their thumbs more than the average person. Long distance truck and bus drivers are known to suffer from stiff necks from having to sit in an upright position for hours on end.

And then there are the bar bouncers—those big guys with beefy arms, brawny backs, and thick legs, who walk around bars and private clubs to see that people are behaving themselves and having a good time. Theirs is a risky profession, subject to unexpected aches and pains when a rowdy and drunken patron tries to take them on. One such bouncer I know is "Teddy Bear" Williams, a man of massive proportions, 6 foot 7 inches in his stocking feet and nearly 300 pounds. He has a chest size nearly the circumference of an oak whiskey barrel, and hands as big as skillets. He works one of the larger night clubs in a certain metropolis in Tennessee that he asked I not mention in this book.

I gave him a quick lookover and was all too eager to comply with his request. After all, only a complete fool or someone suicidal would be dumb enough to *disagree* with this monster of a man.

I asked him *very politely*, "Why do they call you Teddy Bear?"

He looked around the immense room filled with hundreds of people talking, laughing, dancing, drinking, and otherwise having a pretty good time. He motioned with a finger for me to wait for a few minutes before he answered my question.

We didn't have long to wait. A scantily clad woman at the far end of the bar shouted, "Animal!" and slapped a guy beside her in the face. The bouncer quickly eased himself through the crowd to the source of the trouble. After learning that the fellow had tried to put his hands where he shouldn't have, Mr. Williams asked him nicely to leave. Unfortunately for the other guy, a few too many drinks had filled him with a false sense of courage and he took a wild swing at the giant.

My host simply wrapped both of his gigantic arms around the other man and, ever so gently, squeezed him until he begged for mercy and promised to leave. As he relaxed his grip to let the other guy get away, he turned to me and, with a smiling nod, said, "*That's* why they call me 'Teddy Bear.'"

Now, "Teddy Bear" was raised around herbs for part of his life when he lived with his grandmother. "She taught me a great deal about herbs and such." One of those plants happened to be elecampane. She taught him how to use the root part to relieve certain kinds of pain.

According to him, she made an embrocation by soaking 1-1/2 cups of washed, chopped elecampane root in 2-1/4 cups whiskey for two weeks. She strained the liquid and put it into a dark amber bottle. Whenever she suffered from "rheumytism" (as she called it), sciatica, lumbago, or facial neuralgia, she would soak a terry cloth wash rag in hot water, then wring it out and fold it in half. Over this folded part she would next pour some of this elecampane root liniment and then quickly apply it to that area of her body which hurt the most. She would put a dry towel over this to retain the heat as long as possible. He said "she always seemed to feel better after using this remedy."

When "Teddy Bear" got hired as a bar bouncer, he sometimes found it necessary to use his grandmother's recipe on himself. Particularly after occasionally rowdy patrons tried to hit him with a chair, baseball bat, or tire iron. "Usually they end up in intensive care," he said with a broad grin, "but it leaves me a little sore, too." So, he would make up some of this same liniment and apply it to his injuries. "It always seemed to make the pain go away," he noted.

Wonderful for Asthma, Bronchitis, Chest Colds, TB, and Pneumonia

"Teddy Bear" also explained how his grandmother made a tea out of the roots for treating a number of respiratory disorders. "She would chop up enough roots to make a cup and then boil them in 3 cups of water for half an hour." She would then strain the tea and "give warm cups of it to anyone who suffered from asthma, bronchitis, chest colds, tuberculosis, or even pneumonia." My informant claimed that "everyone who took her tea for these complaints never got them again, so far as I know."

ELEPHANT GRASS
(PENNISETUM PURPUREUM)

Brief Description

Different species of elephant grass are cultivated or grow wild in tropical and subtropical areas of the world. Unlike other weeds, this perennial is a highly esteemed livestock feed in many Third World nations. It is used often in daily cuttings for fresh feed, for grazing, sometimes for silage, and is frequently included in rotation with food crops for soil improvement.

Elephant grass yields more biomass per unit area of land than any other herbaceous species used for livestock feed production *anywhere* in the world! The grass develops long roots (but not rhizomes), which is an advantage since they can penetrate deeply into the soil, thereby giving them access to more nutrients and water.

Several species of this grass are extensively cultivated in the warmer climates of North America as ornamentals. I've seen their feathery tops in many backyards of well-to-do residences in Florida, Louisiana, Alabama and Mississippi. These types of elephant grass, like all others of this genus, are easily distinguished by their cattail-like flower clusters.

Wonderful for Erysipelas

You're *not* going to find elephant grass mentioned in *any* American or European herbal book. But I've worked with elephant grass in other countries and know it to be a *fantastic healer* for some of our more complicated health problems. That's why I include it here for the very first time.

Erysipelas is an acute superficial form of cellulitis involving the skin lymphatics, usually caused by an infection by group A streptococci. The problem is chiefly characterized by a peripherally spreading hot, bright red, edema-like, brawny, infiltrated, and sharply circumscribed blotch with a raised indurated border.

A 42-year-old woman whom I'll call Renee came up to me some time ago after one of my lectures at the National Health Federation convention in Florida. She showed me her arms and part of her neck, which clearly displayed signs of erysipelas. I advised her to locate some elephant grass (which is plentiful in Florida, I might add) and make a strong tea using *only* the feathery cattail-like tops, for that is where the chief strength lies. She was to snip enough of them into small pieces to equal a full measuring cup; then she had to add this to 4 cups boiling water, covered and on low heat, simmering for 30 minutes until just *half* the amount of the liquid remained. This she was to strain and drink two cups every day, as well as to bathe the afflicted areas of her skin using a sponge.

Within days her condition started showing some improvement and by the end of several weeks it was hard to tell that she had once suffered from this embarrassing and troublesome disorder.

Seizures Reduced

In another remarkable case involving the use of elephant grass tea, a young Indian man from Madras was given 4 cups of this tea every day for several months after being diagnosed as an epileptic. The doctors, who informed me of his case, noted that considerable progress had been made because the number of seizures which he formerly experienced before treatment began to *diminish substantially* within a three-month period following the use of elephant grass. They noted that while it wasn't a cure, something in the grass itself seemed to correct the episodic impairment within the fellow's autonomic nervous system that led to such seizures in the first place.

A Great Skin Wash for Wounds, Sores, Gangrene

Many are the stories I could tell about this wonderful weed of nature. But there are still many more entries yet to cover and so little space remaining to get them all in. Therefore, the examples I've already given must suffice for now. However, I will say this: In my many travels throughout Asia and countries of the Pacific Rim, I've noticed time and again how often elephant grass tea is used to clean out old, festering wounds and sores, and to stop the progress of gangrene. It has even proven useful in Hansen's disease, better known as leprosy. In the latter instance, the diseased skin is soaked in a strong solution of the grass for an hour every day and the tea taken internally as well.

ELEUTHEROCOCCUS
(see GINSENG)

EPHEDRA
(see MAHUANG)

EUCALYPTUS
(EUCALYPTUS GLOBULUS)

Brief Description

Eucalyptus is one of the fastest growing and biggest trees in the world. It can reach heights of over 250 feet and sends out a vast network of roots, which have proven very useful in draining marshy areas. In fact, it has been of great value in eliminating malarial swamps in a number of hot, humid countries. Guatemala is one such country in Central America, where eucalyptus trees were abundantly planted for this very reason.

The tree has bluish-white, peeling bark and green branchlets. Juvenile shoots and leaves are coated with a white, waxy bloom. Young leaves are opposite, heart-shaped, bluish-green, and sticky, while adult leaves are alternate, lance-shaped, green, and smooth. When crushed, they emit a pungent odor.

Great Chest Rub for Lung Congestion

The aromatic oil contained in eucalyptus leaves is an essential ingredient in Vicks Vapo-Rub. This over-the-counter preparation has been a popular remedy with millions of people for many years for treating respiratory ailments, especially asthma and bronchitis. A little of the ointment is applied locally to the chest area and slowly rubbed into the skin in a circular motion using the forefingers. Sometimes a piece of flannel cloth will be laid over the chest to retain its penetrating warmth for a longer period of time.

Australia's "Unofficial Anthem" Recognizes the Eucalyptus Tree

From 30,000 feet up looking out of a window porthole in the Quantas jet I was in, Australia not only seemed like the flattest and driest continent (which it is), but also more like one gigantic desert than anything else. On separate trips from Darwin in the north to Sydney (a distance of 1,900 miles) and from Perth in the west to Sydney (some 2,000 miles) I never noticed a single town or anything but the most scattered and minute signs of human habitation.

The great English novelist D.H. Lawrence was repelled by Australia when he first laid eyes on it. He described it as a "vast, uninhabited land [populated] by the grey charred bush . . . so phantom-like, so ghostly, with its tall, pale trees [the eucalyptus, of course] and many dead trees, like corpses" laying about. But to Aussies born there, the bush is friendly and familiar, even if foreigners like myself or Mr. Lawrence still think it's not very pretty country. But, as one bushman told me, "the land has a unique and haunting beauty that exerts a powerful spell on all who can get to know it long enough."

Sometime in 1895 a bush poet named Andrew Barton "Banjo" Paterson visited a sheep station in the tiny Australian outback Queensland town of Winton, which had once been at the center of one of that nation's worst civil conflicts. There he composed a rather strange ballad to memorialize the efforts of workers who stood up for their rights against powerful land owners in the wool industry, which was then the backbone of

Australia's economy. This relatively innocuous ditty has since become one of the world's best known songs—it is known everywhere as "Waltzing Matilda." Written shortly after wool shearers in the continent's dry northern interior staged big strikes that turned very violent, this bizarre song tells the story of a wandering vagrant who drowns himself in a water hole rather than permit himself to be arrested. Some historians have noted that the song depicts a "supervised" suicide.

The "swagman," one of a band of unemployed men who tramped outback roads looking for work in the 1890s, jumped into a water hole after he was caught stealing a sheep that stumbled into his camp site on a private sheep station. Confronted by police and the property's owner, the swagman leaps into the water, "drowning himself by the Coolibah [eucalyptus] tree." The song says his voice is still heard there.

Bush Uses for Eucalyptus

In the brief histories which have been written about Mr. Paterson, it is said that he chose the Coolibah tree instead of some other kind to include in his ballad, because he was the most familiar with it. On one occasion this bush poet was suffering from a gum infection, and so he put a little eucalyptus oil on his forefinger and rubbed it on the gum lining. Very quickly the infection ceased. Another time one of his back molars seemed to be a little loose. So he tore himself a small, inch-square piece of cloth and soaked it with some eucalyptus oil and poked it back into his mouth, between his cheek pouch and the tooth itself and left it there for several days. The gum lining around the tooth immediately tightened up and gave him no further problem.

One historian mentioned the fact that mosquitoes and "biting black flies" were very common in those days around many of the watering holes in the outback. He claimed that Mr. Paterson would rub eucalyptus oil over the exposed parts of his body, such as head, face, arms, hands and legs to keep these biting insects away. The historian says he tried this remedy for himself on one occasion and was "very pleased to discover just how well it worked to keep the little bastards away from me."

From contacts with the colonials, Mr. Paterson sometimes contracted their colds and flus. Then he simply added *a few drops* of eucalyptus oil to a glass of whiskey, brandy, or hot water and slowly drank this down. The eucalyptus quickly removed mucus accumulation from his lungs, stopped his coughing, cleared up his fever, and removed any lingering fever. He gargled with the same application to relieve occasional laryngitis that resulted from singing too long while playing his banjo.

Other aboriginal uses for eucalyptus oil included treating stomach disorders, liver and bladder infections, wounds and sores, and (in tepid bath water) to relieve arthritis, lumbago, lower backache, and rheumatism.

Calms Nasty Cough

Stacy Chynoweth is a young high school student residing in the remote Southern Utah community of Henriville. He has been properly raised in a loving home by parents who've taught him and his younger sister well. On weekends and during the summer he works full-time on our family ranch in the wilderness about 17 miles from his home. In May 1995, he came down with a bad case of influenza that lingered on in various forms for two weeks. Hospital-prescribed antibiotics helped him over the worst of it.

But he was unable to shake a very nasty cough that left him hoarse and his vocal cords very sore for a number of days. I decided to send down some Halls Mentho-Lyptus cough drops that contain 12% eucalyptus oil, peppermint oil, and other herbs. He sucked on these periodically and soon his cough ceased entirely. These cough drops are available at larger pharmacies.

EVENING PRIMROSE
(Oenothera biennis)

Brief Description

Evening primrose is a coarse, annual or biennial plant found in dry meadows and waste places and along roadsides east of the Rockies to the Atlantic. The stem is erect, stout, and soft-hairy, with alternate, rough-hairy, lanceolate, taper-pointed leaves about 3-6 inches long. The yellow, lemon-scented leaves, 1 to 2-1/2 inches across, open at dusk and grow in spikes from June to October. The fruit is an oblong, hairy capsule.

New Hope for Schizophrenia and PMS

Sufferers who experience the socially crippling consequences of either schizophrenia or premenstrual syndrome (PMS) now have hope for a much better and brighter future thanks to oil of evening primrose. Kenneth Vaddadi, a psychiatrist at the University of Leeds in England, has achieved successful results in clinical trials on a small number of schizophrenic patients. It appears that about seven 500 mg. capsules daily in conjunction with vitamins B-3, B-6, C and zinc achieve remarkable results.

Thirty women who had severe PMS were put on 3 grams of oil of evening primrose daily from the 15th cycle day until menstruation during 2 cycles and placebo capsules for 2 cycles. PMS symptom severities, especially depression, were relieved a lot more with the oil than with the placebo. Improvement was noted during 62% of oil-treated cycles, but only 40% of the time with the placebo. Up to six capsules per day appear to give significant therapeutic benefits.

Primrose Lowers Blood Pressure

In two separate Canadian studies, the main constituent in evening primrose, gamma-linolenic acid (GLA) and the plant oil (EVO) itself, significantly reduced blood pressure. In the first study, the GLA greatly strengthened the heart's response to chronic stress, while in the second a general lowering of blood pressure in the first 18 weeks of life became evident in hypertensively-bred rats. About 4 capsules of primrose oil per day is recommended for hypertension, along with increased potassium intake (750 mg.) as well.

Relief for Chronic Disorders

While no single herb can be said to be an answer for every health problem that comes along, certain scientific research apparently justifies the use of oil of evening primrose for a host of chronic disorders. Some South African physiologists writing in the Sept. 1985 issue of *Medical Hypotheses* cited very credible evidence to support the idea that coronary artery disease, hypertension, hypercholesterolemia, allergic eczema and other atopic conditions, cancer, premature aging, and chronic inflammatory and auto-immune disorders are related to an imbalance of fatty acids in the body.

Deficiencies of GLA and another important fatty acid found in fish oils may result in the metabolic blockage of a key enzyme. This vital enzyme activity can also be inhibited by too much saturated fat, excess sugar, alcohol, high dietary cholesterol content, high levels of stress, exposure to low levels of radiation and chronic deficiencies of zinc or magnesium.

These physiologists conclude their report by suggesting that an oil of evening primrose supplement is one good means of getting around this blockage and possibly preventing and treating many chronic disorders as well. Recommended intake is 2 capsules twice daily, in the morning and again in the midafternoon for optimal health.

Utah's Senior Senator Likes Evening Primrose Oil

For several years now I've served as the editor of Utah's largest senior citizen newspaper, *Utah Prime Times*. In this envied journalistic capacity, I've
been privileged to hobnob with the likes of U.S. Senators Bob Dole (R-
Kansas), Alan Simpson (R-Wyoming) and, of course, Utah's own senior
senator Orrin Hatch (R-Utah). It is with the latter that I've formed a close
assiciation through a number of different interviews done with him for the
newspaper I edit.

Orrin Grant Hatch has been briefed on the state of the world by
Nixon foreign policy guru Dr. Henry Kissinger. He has shaken hands and
sat at the same dinner table with Chinese leader Deng Xiaoping in 1986.
He counts as close friends those of the same polititcal persuasion, such as
Marine Lieutenant Colonel Oliver North and also political adversaries like
Massachusetts' long-term democratic Senator Ted Kennedy. And he has
helped chair important Senate committee hearings on Capitol Hill, such as
the one which presided over the Clarence Thomas-Anita Hill hearings a few
years ago.

In an April 1995 interview that I had with Sen, Orrin Hatch, he made
public, for the first time that I know of, intimate details of his daily diet,
supplement, and exercise programs. This was during a break in his day-
long 9th Annual Conference on Seniors, which he and his wife Elaine host
every year in Utah for several thousand older people. He informed me that
he takes "evening primrose oil in capsule form, usually three a day, along
with vitamin C, flaxseed oil, bee pollen, lecithin, and a multi-vitamin." Of
all these, "I like the primrose oil the best. It seems to give me energy when
I need it." This is important, considering that he is a notorious workaholic,
putting in an average of 80 hours a week on Capitol Hill. "It also seems to
alleviate some of my back pain," he noted, "when I take it before doing my
exercises in the morning. I'm under a tremendous amount of stress," he
added, "and I think the primrose oil does something to help my nerves
withstand much of the pressure around me."

A Chinese Meal with Primrose

The following recipe utilizes evening primrose. It serves 4 at a Chinese
meal or 2 western style.

> *Needed:* 2 tsp. soy sauce; 3 tbsp. dry white wine; 1 tsp. sesame seed oil; 1
> tsp. cornstarch; 3 tbsp. vegetable oil; 1 clove garlic, finely chopped; 1 scal-
> lion, finely chopped; 1 tsp. fermented black beans, finely chopped; 1 cup
> evening primrose roots, scrubbed and cut crosswise into 1/8" rounds; 1 small

carrot, peeled and cut crosswise into 1/8" rounds; 1 stalk celery, scrubbed, stringed and cut crosswise into 1/8" slices.

In a small bowl combine the soy sauce, wine, sesame seed oil and cornstarch. Then heat a 12" wok or iron skillet over a high flame for 45 seconds. Then add the vegetable oil and heat for another 45 seconds. Drop in the garlic, scallion and black beans and stir-fry for 25 seconds. Add the evening primrose, carrot and celery. Stir-fry for 2 1/4 minutes or until the vegetables become tender. Recombine the cornstarch mixture and add. Stir until thick and transfer to serving platter.

Medicinal Edibles

The following recipe is a reverse of that old adage about "food also being our best medicine." In this instance, a reliable medicinal really enlivens veal cutlets. My gratitude goes to Kathryn G. and Andrew L. March for letting me borrow this from their wonderful book, *The Wild Plant Companion.*

EVENING PRIMROSE AND VEAL WITH MADEIRA WINE

Needed: 8 very thin veal cutlets, trimmed of all fat and tenderized with a mallet or dull side of a knife; some flour; 2 tbsp. butter; 16 very small evening primrose plants roots with tops washed (the roots about 1/8" diameter, or use bigger plants and parboil them); 1/4 tsp. sea salt; 1/2 cup Madeira wine; 1/2 cup water; lemon slices.

Dredge the cutlets in flour and shake off the excess. In a 10-to-12 inch skillet, over moderate heat, melt the butter. When the foam subsides, quickly brown the veal on both sides, a few cutlets at a time. Remove those browned to a plate while doing the rest. Place the evening primrose in the pan, add the salt, Madeira, water, and veal with any juices that have accumulated. Turn the heat to low, and simmer, covered, for 10 minutes until the evening primrose is tender and the sauce is boiled down. Remove to a serving platter, pour the remaining sauce over the top and garnish with lemon slices. Serves 4.

EYEBRIGHT
(Euphrasia officinalis)

Brief Description

For an herb that seems to do the eyes a lot of good, this particular medicinal plant sure grows in the darndest places. Eyebright prefers to grow in waste places, such as garbage dumps, auto salvage yards, railroad tracks, and the ground around sewage ponds and toxic waste pits. Strangely enough, it doesn't do too well in dark, loamy, healthy soil.

Eyebright is a small, delicate annual, usually between 4 to 7 inches tall, and has square, downy, branching stems. Once a garden herb, it is now abundant in the wilds of the Pacific Northwest and in British Columbia. The leaves may vary in shape, from being nearly rounded to almost narrow and pointed, and are borne in opposite pairs. Tiny red or white flowers appear in the summer months and have an upper two-lobed lip and a bottom three-lobed lip and are borne in spikes from the axils of the upper leaves.

Helpful for Some Eye Ailments and Throat Problems

Put a heaping teaspoon of the fresh or dried herb in 3 cups distilled water brought to a boil. Reduce heat, cover and simmer for 10 minutes. Let steep another 20 minutes before straining.

Fill an eye dropper half full of the strained, *lukewarm* tea and gently drop into each eye in cases of eye inflammation, eye strain, and conjunctivitis. Or drink several cups of the *very warm* tea for coughs, sore throat, nasal congestion and sinusitis. I've found it to be especially useful for hay fever and allergies to dust or cats.

Old Amish Herbs of St. Petersburg, Florida (see Product Appendix) makes a formula with eyebright called "Bright Eyes" that is useful for vision problems and night blindness.

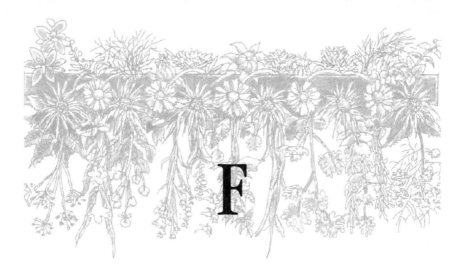

FENNEL SEED
(FOENICULUM VULGARE)

Brief Description

Fennel is a wild or cultivated biennial or perennial growing in the U.S., the Mediterranean and Asia Minor. It has a rather stiff, erect, branching stem, which bears deeply cut grayish-green flowers, followed by odd, toothed seed vessels, filled with small, somewhat compressed seeds, usually three-cornered, with two sides flat and one convex. These black or brown seeds yield a strong, agreeable, aromatic odor somewhat reminiscent of nutmegs and have a spicy, pungent taste.

Breath Sweetener

If you suffer from halitosis, just chew some fennel seeds for fresh breath. Old Amish Herbs of St. Petersburg, Florida (see Product Appendix) makes a formula for nursing mothers called "Thistle Milk." It contains fennel seed and helps to sweeten the breast milk an infant would get.

Medicinal Tea

First cook some barley in plenty of water. Strain the water and save. To 1 pint of boiling barley water, add 1-1/2 tsp. fennel seed. Reduce heat to simmer for 5 minutes; steep an extra 20 minutes. One cup taken by nursing

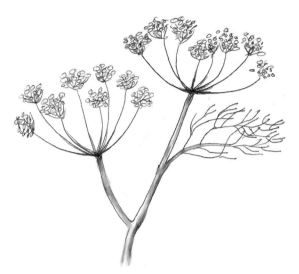

mothers will stimulate milk flow soon; 1/2 cup before a meal stimulates appetite; the eyes washed with the same strained liquid will get rid of irritation and eye strain. This same tea made with an equal amount of peppermint and given in 1-cup amounts when cool will help to calm hyperactive children.

Herbal Tea with Fennel Proves Effective in Colic

In perusing a 1993 issue of the *Journal of Pediatrics* (122: 650-652), I came across an interesting report by two Israeli doctors entitled "Efficacy of herbal tea preparation in infantile colic." These doctors were anxious to test an herbal formula containing fennel seed as its primary ingredient, along with chamomile, vervain, licorice and balm mint. They selected four primary-care community-based pediatric clinics in Beer-Sheva, Israel and conducted their experiments between June 1989 and May 1990. Seventy-two healthy infants aged 2-8 weeks, whom the parents reported to have colic, were selected as the test patients. The fennel-based tea mixture or a placebo solution was placed in the infants' bottles and administered as needed.

Of the 72 patients who entered the study, 68 (94%) completed it. Colicky symptoms such as night awakenings and crying were significantly reduced in the herbal tea group, but hardly affected in the placebo group. Four infants dropped out of the study (3 tea, 1 placebo), but not due to side effects from either preparation. The conclusion reached by these doctors is that fennel tea by itself or in conjunction with other herbs is extremely useful in reducing infantile colic in healthy babies.

Culinary Aspects

At the time of the Norman Conquest in England, fennel seed was used with all kinds of fish dishes and still is today. A real treat is to grill trout or salmon, then flame the fish in brandy on a bed of fennel seed which burns and imparts a truly indescribable flavor. The spice also goes well with pork, veal, in soups, vinaigrette sauces and salads.

ARTICHOKES WITH FENNEL

Needed: 3 large artichokes, trimmed and halved; 4 lemons, halved; 2 bulbs fresh fennel, cored and sliced (about 4 cups); 2 tbsp. each olive oil and non-fat yogurt; granulated kelp to taste.

Squeeze 2 lemons on the artichokes and rub them well with lemon halves. In a large steamer or pressure cooker, steam the artichokes for half an hour (but only 6 minutes in a pressure cooker), or until slightly tender. Steam the fennel for 5 minutes. Let cool slightly and use a spoon to remove the choke from the center of the artichokes. Squeeze the remaining lemons into a Vita-Mix whole food machine container or similar blender and combine with half of the fennel, oil, yogurt and granulated kelp until creamy. Chop the remaining fennel and mix with the fennel sauce. Spoon this mixture into the artichoke halves and serve warm or chilled. Makes 6 servings.

FENUGREEK
(TRIGONELLA FOENUM-GRAECUM)

Brief Description

The name comes from "foenum-graecum" meaning "Greek Hay," the plant being used in times past to scent inferior hay. The name of the genus, Trigonella, is derived from the old Greek name denoting "three-angled," from the form of the plant's corolla. Fenugreek is an erect annual, growing about 2 feet high, similar in habit to lucerne hay. The seeds are brownish, about 1/2 inch long, oblong, with a deep furrow dividing them into unequal lobes. They are contained, 10-20 together, in long, narrow, sickle-like pods.

Reduces Cholesterol

Mongrel dogs from a nearby pound in the French city of Villemoisson-sur-Orge were fed a standard diet supplemented with fenugreek seed meal for

8 weeks. Blood test results showed that these herb seeds reduced their serum cholesterol levels quite a bit. Based on this data, it's suggested that you might benefit from taking an average of 2 capsules per day of a formula called Cholester-Low made by Old Amish of St. Petersburg, Florida. (Consult the Product Appendix for more information.)

Great for Hay Fever

A California woman mentioned having tried everything for her allergy, but nothing seemed to work. She then decided to make a tea of fenugreek seed—8 tsp. seed presoaked in 4 cups cold water for 5 hours, the boiled for 2 minutes before straining and drinking—and consumed 1 cup per day 2 months before the hay fever season began. To her utter amazement, she didn't have any serious attacks as in previous years!

Stops Ringing in the Ear

Leota Lane of Eugene, Oregon has the perfect remedy for stopping "cricket" noises and ringing in the ear. In fact, it's the only remedy that ever seems to have helped her.

She puts about 2-1/2 full soup spoons of fenugreek seeds in 3 cups of cold water and lets it set overnight. The next morning the mixture is stirred up a little and poured off as needed. When she takes her morning cup of cold tea, she replaces it with another cup of water on top of the seeds.

In the evening she has another cup of the same tea. She follows that routine for several days until the seeds have lost most of their strength, at which time they're discarded and the process starts over again with new seeds.

She states that if the seeds are boiled, the tea becomes so bitter she can't stand it. If this is a problem, then honey may be added to sweeten to taste.

Culinary Virtues

The whole seeds may be sprouted to include in salads for a really improved flavor. Or the powdered seeds may be added to any kind of Far Eastern foods, especially Indian and Pakistani dishes, for extra tartness. When making curried rice, add some powdered fenugreek to this delicious vegetable sauce which goes over the rice.

GOLDEN FENUGREEK SAUCE

Needed: 3/4 cup cooked potatoes; 1 medium-cooked carrot; 1-1/3 cup water;
2 tbsp. chopped cashews; 1/2 tsp. sea salt; 1 tbsp. lemon juice; 1 tbsp. lime
juice; 1/2 tsp. chopped dill weed; powdered contents of 4 gelatin capsules of
fenugreek seed from any health food store.

Combine everything together in a food processor or blender until smooth
and creamy. Heat and serve over hot rice or cooked vegetables of any
kind.

FEVERFEW
(TANACETUM PARTHENIUM
OR CHRYSANTHEMUM PARTHENIUM)

Brief Description

Feverfew is a yellowish-green aromatic perennial with ridged stems, pinnate or bipinnate leaves, and the flower heads as a corymb. It grows abundantly against walls, on waste ground and long hedges.

An Unconventional Cure for Migraines
and Rheumatoid Arthritis/Osteoarthritis

This is a true story related by Mrs. Ann Jenkins, the wife of a physician in
Cardiff, England. She suffered from terrible migraine headaches from the
age of 16 until she turned 65. She finally cured herself for good by eating
three little leaves of a common garden weed called feverfew. Also, the
usual stiffness and aching pain accompanying her osteoarthritis went away
as well. Just three years later, at age 68, she was a bright-eyed, sprightly
lady with more evidence of physical activity in her movements than many
50-year-olds.

   "I have had migraines since I was about 16," Mrs. Jenkins began. I
remember that very often I couldn't do my homework or play like other
children. At first the attacks came every month to six weeks. But by the
time I was approaching 40 they had become more frequent. From the age
of 50 onwards they came at least every 10 days and lasted for 2 or 3 days.
While the migraine lasted I was laid up in bed with the curtains drawn. I
could not be bothered with anything or anybody. Even the sound of a car
driving past the house was sheer hell for me to endure.

Her ever-more-frequent migraine attacks had completely ruined all chances of a reasonable social life. Accepting invitations was a risk; if people came to her house during an attack they just had to leave very quietly. Her continued search for some relief, if not an actual cure, meant a lifetime of experimenting with this or that drug and various alternative treatments including homeopathic drugs and even acupuncture. But the side effects of some of the more conventional drugs had become nearly as painful and distressing as the migraine itself.

"Eventually I went to the Migraine Clinic in London," she continued. "There they told me that I should change the tablets I was then taking because, after more than a year, they were having no effect. They put me on a prophylactic drug which I was to take as soon as I felt a headache coming on. Of course, I had ordinary headaches as well as migraines, and I was so desperate to prevent the severe migraine pain that I took these tablets at the first sign of any headache.

"So I was really taking too many and the side effects were just horrible. I was unable to eat anything and became very billious, throwing up bile, not food. My stomach seemed to be shrinking to nothing, and in the end I could hardly keep down even a sip of water. I could no longer take the tablets because I would immediately throw them up again."

During one of her attacks her sister paid an unexpected visit accompanied by a friend. Mrs. Jenkins told them that if they wanted a cup of tea—the social equivalent of our cup of coffee—then they would have to make it themselves. She then promptly went back to bed wanting nothing more to do with them. Her curt and anti-social behavior was, unwittingly, to be her means of getting well. Her sister's friend was thoroughly shocked, not so much by the rude treatment but by the cause of it all. This friend went home and related this strange set of circumstances to her father, an old gentleman then well into his nineties. He remarked, "Why should she suffer like this? I have an herb out in my garden which is good for so many different health problems, that I believe it just might do her migraine some good."

The next day a little clump of plant complete with its roots arrived in a box by the post (the British word for mail) with enclosed instructions on how to plant it and to "take a pinch of leaf every day for your headache, dearie."

Mrs. Jenkins continued. "I took just one small leaf every day. It tasted very bitter so I took it chopped up in a bread and butter sandwich. Nothing happened, so I asked myself, 'What does the man mean by a pinch?' I then figured it might be a bit more than just one small leaf, so I started taking three leaves every day. I added a little parsley with it to take away some of the bitterness.

"I took those leaves day after day, week after week. Nothing happened for a long time, almost five months. Then I stopped being sick although the headaches went on for a little while after this. But I noticed that I was taking less and less prescription medication. Some bodily instinct told me to give the feverfew a chance to work.

"After about the sixth month I went a whole month without a headache. And when I did have one it was not as severe as they had been. After ten months there were no more headaches. Now it has been several years since I was bilious or had a migraine headache. Little headaches, yes, like we all have, but nothing ever like those horrible migraines of the past."

In the meantime she had told her physician husband, Tom, that she was taking an herb. His only reply was, "Well, you have tried so many other things, I don't suppose one more can do you any possible harm." After this, he promptly lost all further interest in the subject and went back to his usual medicinal practice.

Once Mrs. Jenkins discovered just how effective feverfew had been for her, she turned part of her garden into a feverfew nursery and began giving out free clumps to 14 other sufferers, all of whom got rid of their own migraines in 4 to 6 months.

Mrs. Jenkins mentioned another curious benefit, while on this herb for half a year. For a long time she had suffered from osteoarthritis, but considered that a minor handicap compared with the agonies of her migraine and the side effects of the drug she took. Nonetheless, her arthritis apparently vanished since she began taking feverfew—a phenomenon which, she told me, "I hardly noticed at first."

"I had always suffered from osteoarthritis," she said, "Being bothered with stiff legs, a stiff back, and aching hips. It used to take me a minute or so to get up out of an armchair." While informing me of this, she popped up and down in her armchair like a human yo-yo to prove her new found agility. "I was always dropping cups when I was washing up, and had to shake hands with my left hand because I had no grip in my right one." Her handshake with me was just as firm and strong as that of any man or woman *half her age!*

"I wasn't thinking about my arthritis, but concentrating on my migraine, so it was some time before I realized that I was able to clench my right fist for the first time in years. I used to be unable to reverse the car because I couldn't turn my neck around. Now I drive just like everybody else does. I now look and feel younger than I did when I was 50," she exclaimed. "My neighbors around here are quite amazed at the change which has come over me. And I attribute it all to this marvelous herb called feverfew."

Scientific Proof That the Therapy Works

Feverfew has had considerable writeup in the medical and scientific literature of the past decade. Two of the best articles confirming everything that
Mrs. Jenkins discovered on her own may be found in the following two references:

1. Seymour Diamond, M.D., "Herbal Therapy for Migraine: An
Unconventional Approach." *Postgraduate Medicine* 82:197-98 (July 1987).

2. E.S Johnson et al, "Efficacy of Feverfew as Prophylactic Treatment
of Migraine." *British Medical Journal* 291:569-573.

Feverfew works well for migraines in three different forms. There is,
of course, consumption of the fresh leaves each day with a little parsley.
Then there is the tea, made by simmering 5 leaves in 2 cups of boiling
water for 15 minutes and sipping 1 cup 3 times daily. Or there are the capsules—two of them twice daily in between meals for up to six months.

FLAXSEED
(LINUS USITATISSIMUM)

Brief Description

The cultivation of flaxseed reaches back to the remotest periods of history.
Both the seeds as well as the cloth woven from this plant fabric have been
found in ancient Egyptian tombs. In fact, the first linen mentioned in the
Bible has been proven by historians and archaeologists to have been spun
from flax.

The flax is a graceful little plant with turquoise blue blossoms, a tall,
erect annual 1-2 feet in height. The stems are usually solitary, quite smooth,
with alternate, linear, sessile leaves nearly an inch long. The seed vessels
with their five-celled capsules are referred to in the Bible as "bolls." When
the bolls are ripe, then the flax is pulled and tied in bundles. In order to
help in the separation of the fiber from the stalks, the bundles are placed
in water for several weeks, and then spread out to dry.

From the crushed or milled seeds comes linseed oil and meal. The oil
is applied to wood surfaces in thin layers to form a hard, transparent varnish. Internally the oil is used by some veterinarians as a purgative for
sheep and horses; a jelly from the boiled seeds is fed to young calves.

Remarkably Effective Laxative

According to Dr. Hans Fluck, A Swiss professor of pharmacology, 2 tsp. of flaxseed put into half a cup of hot water and allowed to swell for up to 4 hours and the mucilage and seeds swallowed together will produce a swelling bulk within the intestines which will provide a substantial bowel movement a few hours later.

Best Hand Lotion Around

An Oregon woman who suffered from dried, chapped hands for years had tried just about every kind of hand lotion on the market, but with no success. Then she stumbled onto flaxseed and now makes her own lotion, which she finds incredibly effective.

Her recipe calls first for whole or cracked flaxseed, about 3 round tbsp. to be soaked in 2 cups lukewarm water overnight. The next morning the mixture is boiled and strained to remove as much of the mucilage jell as possible; then the seeds are thrown away. A pint of apple cider vinegar is then added to the jell, along with 5 tbsp. of glycerin (purchased from any drugstore). The mixture is then heated again to the boiling point and immediately removed from the heat. Take an eggbeater and beat the mixture for a minute or so to keep the glycerin from separating. Bottle. Dampen hands with solution morning and evening, thoroughly rubbing the skin and letting the air dry them. You will experience a greaseless, silky feeling on your hands.

Eye Problem Corrected

The following was obtained from Violet Boyce of Logan, Utah. "I had a unique experience with flaxseed when I was a young girl. While on the train I got a cinder in my eye. I was unable to dislodge it and was suffering rather acutely. When I reached home my aunt put a single flaxseed under the lid. Sure enough the gooey sides collected the particle and it could be brushed out."

It Keeps His Machinery Well Lubricated

An old friend of mine, Saul "Charlie" Fox, lives in southern California and is an avid health enthusiast, not to mention garlic afficionado extraordinaire. Charlie has worked for many years for Wakunauga of America in

Mission Viejo, California. This company manufactures and markets the world's premier selling garlic under the trade name of Kyolic. Charlie has done numerous radio and TV appearances and public health lectures around the country on the many marvelous virtues of this herb.

But my call to him on Thursday morning, May 25, 1995 wasn't in regard to garlic, but to something else. I remembered while staying at his lovely ranch estate nestled away in a canyon somewhere, that he used flaxseed oil quite frequently. In fact, several of the large salads we shared together during my visit to his home had generous helpings of flaxseed oil as their sole dressings.

So I asked my friend, who turned 68 in 1995, why he used so much of this substance. He replied: "I depend on it to make sure that my machinery gets well lubricated. It is the only oil I ever use. I take it about 3 or 4 times a week. It happens to be one of the best sources of omega-3 fatty acids; they are essential for promoting good health and longevity. When I forget to take it, I don't feel as flexible. I take flaxseed and Kyolic Garlic EPA (about 2 capsules daily). Both give me 'power in the blood'."

Flaxseed Cuts Breast Cancer, Study Finds

Experts working to pin down a link between a low-fat, high-fiber diet and cancer prevention stated that flaxseed could reduce the spread of breast cancer in women. A recent study at the University of Toronto showed that a component of flaxseed fed to rats reduced mammary tumor growth by more than 50%.

The findings were presented at the 1995 annual meeting in Toronto, Canada of the American Association of Cancer Research. Dr. Lillian Thompson, one of the scientists involved in the study, told convention delegates that flaxseed exhibited a definite "reduction in the rate of tumor growth."

Her group suspects the lignans in flaxseed as being responsible for this. Flaxseed contains up to 800 times the concentration of them, which is more than any other food. Thompson believes these lignans may retard the growth of blood vessels in tumor tissue, thereby starving the tumor. "We now have clear proof," she said, "that flaxseed lignans have definite anti-cancer effects."

FRANKINCENSE
(BOSWELLIA THURIFERA)

Brief Description

Frankincense (and myrrh—see separate entry) are prepared from large irregular lumps of light reddish to yellowish-brown gum exuded by several species of trees. Another name for it is olibanum. Frankincense was highly regarded by Egyptians for embalming and fumigating. The gum is used in the Near East as a masticatory, to clean the mouth. Oil of olibanum is still used in some high-grade perfumes, especially for oriental and floral types.

All Aboard the "Smugglers' Express"

Amra Kevic related a story about an intriguing train ride she took some time ago on the Istanbul-Belgrade express. "As the train started pulling out of Istanbul, Turkey," she wrote, "I could hear a strange ripping sound echoing throughout the different cars. It was the sound of masking tape being torn from contraband stuck behind or below the seats, above luggage racks and anywhere else it could be hidden by enterprising Yugoslavs on their way back home. Their huge bags readily identified them as seasoned smugglers laden with bargains from Istanbul's bazaars.

She sat next to a large peasant woman of middle-age. Early attempts at friendliness were coldly rebuffed by the older woman. As the hours wore on, the occasional pieces of small talk between them both eventually warmed into a nice, glowing conversation.

The Yugoslav woman, on her back to the capital of Belgrade, was packing along with her a large supply of the dried resin of frankincense in the form of many hundreds of odd-shaped pieces in varying thicknesses and sizes.

When Ms. Kevic inquired in the Slavic tongue what she intended to do with this much frankincense, the woman replied that most of it would be going to different hospitals within Belgrade. In these health care facilities, they would be burned in some of the wards which housed patients suffering from infectious diseases, such as the tuberculosis ward.

Effective Inhalant for Respiratory Diseases

Once the Istanbul-Belgrade express entered Yugoslavia, things became pretty hectic, Ms. Kevic said. Rough looking and tough talking customs officials quickly made themselves known as they boarded the train, banging on compartment doors, yelling loud voices and cursing to high heaven.

One tall, young, uniformed man came to their compartment and yelled to both women, "Out, out, pick up your things and out, both of you, right now!"

After barely glancing at the contents of the women's four suitcases, he snapped "460 dinars [$170 at the black market rate] for the two of you." But after Amra protested that she was merely a journalist for Reuter News Service and wasn't smuggling anything in, he said very impatiently, "Then just give me 400 [$150] for both, OK?" But after this feisty reporter protested some more, the young fellow returned their passports and in a weary tone of voice ordered both women to pick up their things and get off the train.

From this train depot in an unnamed town, they had to negotiate several rides in the back of a few freight trucks to the next city, where they finally managed to catch a bus heading for Belgrade. "It was a real adventure for me," Amra said, "but I learned some interesting uses for one of the gifts that the Magi presented to the Infant Christ Child."

Her newly-made friend took her to one of the city's infirmaries which dealt exclusively with respiratory disorders. There she was shown by members of the medical staff how pieces of the frankincense were dissolved in hot water and patients suffering from asthma, bronchitis and emphysema were told to inhale its warm vapors. It took no more than 20 minutes a session and was done 3 or 4 times throughout the day.

Memory Loss Restored

At another infirmary specializing in mental disorders, equal parts of frankincense resin, whole cloves and fresh cardamoms were subjected to intense steam heat in order to draw out as much of their wonderful therapeutic properties as possible. Patients suffering from mild memory loss were instructed to inhale the vapors of this combination for no more than 15 minutes twice or thrice daily. Doctors claimed that these three aromatic spices helped to improve memory significantly in 63% of their patients.

FUNGUS

Brief Description

Various types of fungus have been used extensively throughout the Orient and some Eastern European countries for the treatment of cancer. In general, they've been pretty successful in reducing tumors, lessening pain, improving sleep habits and appetites, and increasing physical weight of many cancer patients. Some fungal growths have been clinically tested and proven valid for tumor therapy.

Fu-ling or hoelen (Poria cocos) is a fungus that grows on pine roots in mainland China and Taiwan. Fu-ling is the one fungus most frequently used in oriental herbal formulas where it occurs in over 30% of all natural prescriptions. The ancient Taoists considered this to be one of their "superior" elixirs in that it brought ease to the body and prolonged life.

An American version of fu-ling was formerly used by some Native American tribes during periods of famine as a survival food. The early white settlers called the stuff "Indian bread," while various tribes called it "tuckah," "tawking," "tuckahoe" and similar names. American fu-ling has the appearance of petrified Irish potatoes, or in its larger form, of weird-looking coconuts. It is a tuberous growth possessing a rough-textured extremity and white insides. Technically know as *sclerotia*, it grows beneath the soil where it propagates by living off tree roots and buried wood. In spite of its durable toughness when dug up, some Native Americans softened such fu-ling by burying them beneath a campfire. Sliced and sun-dried, their tuckahoes were then ready for grinding and mixing with "sorrel and meal" to make an interesting bread.

Oriental fu-ling can be taken in capsules (4 daily), small pills the size of BB shot (10 twice daily), or as a tea (2 *warm* cups daily).

Two other types of medicinal fungi, which have received considerable attention in the scientific community in the last few decades, are the reishi (pronounced REE-she) and shiitake (pronounced SHE-taw-key) mushrooms. They are venerated throughout the Orient for their marvelous healing properties, especially in the treatment and prevention of cancer. Laboratory and clinical studies done with both of them in man and beast alike have shown remarkable regression of malignant tumors, particularly through the injection method.

But intravenously or orally certainly seem to be more preferable ways of administering either of these postent mushrooms than the old folklore recipes which "call for the stewing of 30 grams [of reishi or shiitake] with the lungs and heart of a pig" for treating cancer of the esophagus!

Besides cancer, reishi (*Gandoderma lucidum*) and shiitake (*Lentinus edodes*) are also of considerable value in the treatment of Epstein-Barr Virus (EBV) which is believed to cause chronic fatigue syndrome, as well as hypoglycemia. Both are very energy-draining problems which these mushrooms seem to quickly correct. Tablets or capsules (4 daily of either) are the most convenient forms in which to take them.

I am indebted to my Canadian friend, Dr. Terry Willard, for his kind permission to make brief excerpts from his book, *Reishi Mushroom* (Issaquah, WA: Sylvan Press, 1990; pp. 131-33).

"The classical reishi mushroom...has a circular kidney-shaped cap divided by concentric growth rings and resembling a ram's horn. The cap color is a shiny, lacquered red to reddish-brown. It has a creamy white-to-yellow outer edge when young, which is the newest growth. The distinctive woody stem is attached to one side rather than in the center and is commonly the same color as the cap. The underside is covered with a white pore layer that becomes light brown with age. The sporeprint is brown.

"[Reishi] is a wood decomposer that is generally saprophytic although in some cases is parasitic. It grows on deciduous trees and stumps, especially oaks and chestnuts. Its distribution is worldwide, generally fruiting in the warm areas of the temperate zones in late summer and fall.

"Young shiitake mushrooms have a dark reddish brown cap which becomes lighter as the mushroom matures. The cap has fine white thread-like tufts or 'scales' on it, especially toward the edges. The gills are white-to-off-white and often have serrated edges. A shiitake sporeprint is pure white. The stem is typically short and very tough, is centrally attached, and is a dull white to dingy brown color.

"The shiitake is a wood decomposer commonly growing on dead deciduous trees. It derives its name from its association with the *shii* tree, but also grows well on oak, maple, alder, chestnut and beech. Shiitake is indigenous to Japan, China and other countries in the temperate zone of Indo-China. It typically fruits in the spring and fall."

I remember well some of my trips to the Orient in past years, when I've seen specimens of both mushrooms in different stages of cultivation. In 1986, I participated in a huge Joint Conference of The Second World Congress of Chinese Medicine and Pharmacy/Second International Symposium on Acupuncture and Moxibustion in Taipei, Taiwan. Dr. P.D. Lee and I co-chaired Part Six of the symposium on a Wednesday afternoon in the Sky Lounge on the 12th floor of the hotel. Our session dealt with "Chinese Herbs and Natural Products," and I gave a special lecture on the "Integration of Chinese Herbs with American Herbal Products: Several Case Studies," which received widespread media coverage in the local Taipei newspapers.

Following this, he and I were special guests of the Mayor of this capitol city. Along with several other foreign guests, I was driven to a farm on the outskirts of Taipei and shown mushroom cultivation in progress. Inside long buildings deliberately kept cool, damp and somewhat darkened, we saw numerous selections of circular oak discs which had been previously inoculated with fungal spores and were then nicely sprouting young shiitake mushrooms. The Mayor informed us that his aged mother had taken some of the processed shiitake in tablets (15 a day with meals) to shake a nasty cold and sore throat, which had hung on for some time and failed to respond to traditional therapies.

For further reading on the subject of medicinal fungi, I highly recommend the fascinating and superbly illustrated book *Icons of Medicinal Fungi from China* (Beijing: Science Press, 1987).

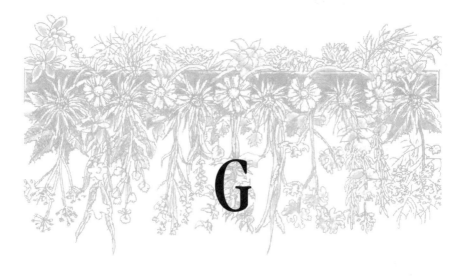

G

GARLIC
(ALLIUM SATIVUM)

Brief Description

This spice is a perennial herb whose bulb, composed of small cloves, is readily identifiable by its peculiar odor. The odor, of course, is due to the many different sulphur compounds present inside each clove. Due to the large concentration of this particularly smelly mineral, garlic has been referred to at various times throughout history as "an herb that only the Prince of Hell himself could enjoy the aroma of full time with nary a complaint."

Garlic usually grows to a height of about 2 feet and has flat, long, pointed leaves. It flowers in mid-summer and the colors range from pink to white; the flowers are quite edible.

Many varieties and cultivars of garlic exist. Some of the large, white-skinned types are referred to as American or California garlic; early and late cultivars are available. The many varieties with pink- or purple-skinned bulbs may be called Chilean, Creole, Mexican or Italian. Garlic grows well all over the continental United States, although it seems to do best in dry, mild regions. In northern climates it doesn't develop as large a bulb because of the shorter growing season. Elephant garlic (A. ampeloprasum) is a garlic relative whose prodigious heads of 4 to 6 cloves can reach the size of an orange.

Rocambole (A. sativun var. ophioscorodon) is another type of garlic sometimes seen in the gardens of garlic aficionados. It goes by other names such as Italian or French garlic and looks somewhat dramatic, with many flat leaves like those of garlic chives (A. tuberosum) appearing in spring and looped flower stalks in summer. The "flower" head of this particular garlic opens to reveal a cluster of bulbils instead of flowers. All parts of rocambole are edible and these bulbs are harvested just like those of regular garlic. According to some who have grown it, French or Italian garlic is well worth growing for different reasons. For one thing, the bulbs seem to keep very well; for another, the cloves peel a lot easier; and finally the flavor is quite good. Rocambole is available from some mail-order seed houses but is seldom offered at nurseries.

Great Flavoring Agent and Ultimate Antibiotic

Through the years I've been asked time and again which of all the herbs I favored the most. My response has invariably been that if I could have but only one herb, it would have to be garlic. I can't think of another herb which has so much versatility as this one does, and can do equal justice to both camps of food and medicine.

Garlic is probably the only spice I know of which goes well with many different dishes. You can't say that about all spices, but it certainly holds true for this herb. I would never think of going abroad without taking along a few knobs of raw garlic as well as a plentiful supply of Kyolic EPA and Kyolic Aged Garlic Extract enriched with vitamins B-1 and B-12. (The first comes in convenient capsule form and is a blend of aged garlic extract and fish oil, while the second is a liquid. Both are manufactured and marketed by the Wakunauga Company and distributed worldwide. This type of garlic is considered by many doctors and scientists who use or study this herb to be THE premier garlic supplement on the planet, but more about this later.)

Because I'm limited for space here, I'm unable to mention the many different ways in which garlic can be used for innumerable culinary purposes. Whatever is exposed to even the slightest *hint* of garlic will generally have its flavor definitely improved—unless, of course, that particular item isn't compatible with the herb (a German chocolate cake doesn't sound appetizing, does it?).

The role of garlic as an antiviral and antibacterial agent is unsurpassed. There are no....repeat, NO...modern antibiotic drugs in the entire arsenal of medical science which can even come close to doing what garlic can do. Whatever these conventional antibiotics can do, garlic can do better, cheaper, and safer. It may not always work as fast as some of these misnamed "wonder drugs" do, but garlic holds a very definite edge over all of them in one particular respect: bacteria are unable to adapt themselves to this potent spice as they have been proven to do so readily with all other antibiotic drugs.

For these reasons and many more, then, do I consider humble garlic to be *the single greatest* botanical ever. There is absolutely nothing to equal or surpass it in terms of broad application, potency and effectiveness. Trust me when I say that "garlic is the cook's and herbalist's single most precious gem in what they have to work with!

Famous Makeup Artist Relies on Garlic to Stop Skin Infection

One of America's most famous makeup artists sometimes relies upon garlic to stop minor skin infections with some of his clientele. For better than 13 years Kevyn Aucoin has been the makeup artist preferred by many famous theatrical stars such as Janet Jackson, Elizabeth Taylor, Liza Minnelli, Tina Turner, and Barbra Streisand.

They like his style, because he respects the individual woman and doesn't slap a lot of paint and powder on her to make her look good in front of a camera but nothing like herself. He tries hard not to rob these women of their character, but instead chooses to let his makeup enhance their own unique and original features.

Life wasn't always a bed of roses, though. He had a very difficult youth growing up gay in Louisiana. Other kids constantly taunted him with cruel names and would sometimes beat him up. But he rose to prominence and recently received his industry's top honor: the Council of Fashion Designers Award for makeup.

Aucoin has been familiar with garlic's virtues for years. Whenever a particular client manifests some kind of skin blemish that is attributed to an infection, he may suggest a few drops of garlic juice be applied to the area, or that a small, thin sliver of garlic clove be taped over the infection and left there for 24 hours. Invariably the problem goes away very soon.

Knowing the relative success that Aucoin has had with garlic for similar problems, I have encouraged its use for fungal infections of skin or nails. I inform my parties that they are to buy a small garlic press from a department or health food store in order to get the juice out. If none is readily available, then I tell them to peel one garlic clove and pound it with a hammer on a cutting board; they are then to lay pieces of the smashed garlic directly on the skin or nails thus affected. The procedure may need to be repeated a number of times for up to a week or more, but, sooner or later, the fungal growth will disappear.

Good for Tumors and Sexually Transmitted Diseases

Because garlic is an all-around antibiotic, it is good for just about every major kind of infection you can think of. Across the board, it fights everything from herpes simplex and meningitis to childhood and adult infectious diseases like chickenpox and shingles. Both the raw garlic and garlic supplements can be used here. If using fresh garlic, be sure to combine it with food or juice to make it more tolerable to take. The best supplement to use is Kyolic Aged Garlic Extract made by Wakunauga of America. Either the capsule (2 for a child or 5 for an adult) or the liquid (1/4 tsp. for a child or 1 tsp. for an adult) can be used daily with good results.

But two major areas of growing health concern, where garlic really seems to shine, are in various cancers and sexually transmitted diseases. There is a small but significant body of scientific evidence now to show that the spice is capable of inducing tumor regression or else halting and reversing the spread of infections such as chlamydia, gonorrhea, and syphilis. Usually the fresh *and* prepared forms of garlic are *both* used to reverse these bad situations. Generally, two raw cloves a day in meal preparation are used and up to 10 capsules of Kyolic Aged Garlic Extract taken internally; the liquid Kyolic is also sometimes used topically around the genitalia to treat sexual infections. Raw garlic is available in all grocery stores and supermarkets, while the Kyolic brand is sold in health food stores and nutrition centers. (See Product Appendix for more information on obtaining Kyolic Garlic.)

Dentist Finds Garlic Helpful for Diabetes

George Crowel D.D.S. has a thriving dental practice in the Midwest. He was diagnosed as diabetic about 7 years ago and has been taking daily insulin injections ever since. His wife heard me mention on a radio program that garlic was good for diabetes.

So she started using it more often in many of her meal preparations. She also went to a health food store and bought some Kyolic Aged Garlic Extract and had him take 5 capsules every day. After having him on this program for six months, she wrote to me, saying that "while garlic hasn't cured my husband of his diabetes, he now only needs about 6cc per day of insulin instead of the 26cc he had been taking previously. He also looks and feels much better than he did before..."

Other Things That Garlic Can Do for You

In many Third World countries the problem of intestinal parasites is constant in the local population. Many folk healers with whom I've worked have told me that they regularly encourage the consumption of garlic for those patients who suffer from roundworms, pin worms or tapeworms in the gastrointestinal tract. They are unanimous in their praise for garlic as an ideal remedy for getting rid of worms.

I noticed that when I started taking Kyolic EPA (a combination of aged garlic extract and fish oil) (see Product Appendix), both my serum cholesterol and triglycerides dropped significantly to much safer levels, and have remained there ever since. Based on what it did for me, I started recommending three capsules per day to others who had similar results. The same thing can be accomplished using fresh garlic, of course, but while your heart may be healthy the odor is liable to ruin your social life. That's why the prepared Kyolic supplement is preferred by most over the other.

Garlic is good for stopping toothache. Peel one clove and crush it. Smear some peanut butter on an inch- square piece of white bread. Lay the garlic pulp on top of it and insert into the mouth. Press it firmly with your thumb or forefinger against the gum line of the infected tooth and leave in place for several hours. The throbbing pain should cease in about 5 minutes. Repeat as needed.

Both garlic and onion juice are very effective in helping to heal *major* and minor burns. Doctors in mainland China have used them this way for severe burn cases with very good results. The garlic clove and onion are peeled and then juiced, or else run through a food processor, such as a Vita-Mix Whole Food Machine, until a thick wet pulp remains. The juice or pulp is then applied topically to the injured skin and covered with a light gauze dressing. It is changed every ten hours or so. I've been amazed at how quickly burns have begun healing using these herbs and other things like sesame seed or olive oil, calendula, and hyssop.

Cooking with Garlic

I'm grateful to Susan Belsinger and Carolyn Dille, authors of *The Garlic Book: A Garland of Simple, Savory, Robust Recipes* (Loveland, CO: Interweave Press, Inc., 1993; p.19) and their publisher for letting me include the following excerpts here. I think their ideas have considerable merit when it comes to using this wonderful spice for culinary purposes.

"The taste of garlic can be strong or gentle, pungently hot or soothingly warm... You can appreciate the differences in flavor according to season as well as cooking methods.

"Frying brings out garlic's most common, pleasantly strong flavor. Use only medium or low heat, as garlic burns easily. Even if it is not burned brown or black, garlic can become quite acrid if cooked over high heat. In Singapore, Hong Kong, and parts of Indonesia, crispy fried garlic is much esteemed as a garnish.

"Poaching garlic (cooking it in a liquid over low heat) softens it and sweetens the flavor so that surprisingly large amounts can be used. Roasting the bulb produces a complex, nutty, caramelized flavor. If you like just a whisper of garlic in a milk- or cream-based sauce, try rubbing a wooden spoon—or the pan itself—with a cut clove, then stirring the sauce. Cooking garlic in an aluminum pot gives it a disagreeable flavor, especially when it is combined with acid ingredients such as tomatoes or lemons.

"Rubbing a wooden salad bowl with garlic is not a good practice; the pungent oils will eventually turn rancid. To give a hint of garlic on salads, keep some garlic oil or vinegar on hand. These condiments are easily made by smashing the cloves and steeping them in either medium; the amount of garlic determines the strength of the flavor. We recommend making them in small amounts—no more than you will use in a month or two—because they can taste dull and musty when kept longer."

A Chef's "Secret" Recipe

One appetizer routinely served to everyone at one of Salt Lake City's more trendy eating places, Fuggles at The Brewery, is a small loaf of pagnotta bread (which is an Italian sourdough) and a saucer of specially seasoned olive oil. I spoke with Sous Chef Jason Barker about how this oil was prepared.

"There are two ways we make it," he said in a May 1995 interview. "It can be done with a hot or cold infusion. We chose the former, because it's faster. The pure virgin olive oil is heated in a stainless steel saucepan to 148° F. It is important that *no* moisture be in the pan at the time this is being done." He said that the amount of olive oil used is relative; for domestic use, he thought a pint would be sufficient.

"We take equal parts of *fresh* rosemary, basil and garlic [peeled and finely chopped] and put them into a bucket," he continued. "But if this is being made at home, an ordinary glass Mason jar will do just as well." He qualified the "equal parts" statement for home use by noting that 1 teaspoon of each of these spices should be sufficient. The last ingredient the restaurant uses is "a pinch of [fresh, chopped] red peppers." He noted that these were the *hot* peppers; for amounts smaller than the bucket sizes they make, he advised, obviously, using even *less* than a "pinch."

"Once the spices are put into the container," he went on, "the heated olive oil is poured over them. The container is left uncovered so the oil can cool. It usually takes us two days to make this oil, but sometimes we might let it go an extra day if we feel it needs a little more flavor." The oil is then strained and put into small glass decanters and served to guests with a warm loaf of sliced pagnotta bread. "This is the traditional way they eat bread in Italy," he finished. "They're not into using much butter like we are."

Other Sources for More Data

For more information on this wonderful herb, please consult two other of my books:

Heinerman's New Encyclopedia of Fruits and Vegetables (Englewood Cliffs, NJ: Prentice Hall, 1995)

From Pharaohs to Pharmacists: The Healing Benefits of Garlic (New Canaan, CT: Keats Publishing, Inc.,1994)

There is also a new Garlic Information Hotline funded, in part, by a generous grant from Wakunauga of America, suppliers of the world's best garlic preparation. This service is provided by the Garlic Information Center of the New York Hospital-Cornell Medical Center in New York City. The Center is a relatively recent component of the hospital's Nutrition Information Center, which opened in January 1995, and which provides a central outlet of accurate, reliable and updated information including a literature bank, research monitor and researchers' network.

Now consumers and health care professionals alike can dial 1-800-330-5922 at all hours to receive a brochure containing almost anything you'll want to know about garlic, including fresh garlic, cooked garlic, garlic supplements, recipes, information about garlic's potential health benefits and more. If people have specific questions, they may call the hotline Monday through Friday, 9 A.M. to 5 P.M. EST to speak directly to a nutritionist.

Because much of the information generated by other garlic companies and most health writers is often confusing, contradictory and occasionally inaccurate, Wakunauga of America and the Medical Center felt that something was needed to dispense honest and trustworthy data. Their combined efforts have resulted in this Center.

All of the services offered by the Garlic Information Center, including consumer information brochures, are available free of charge.

GENTIAN
(GENTIANA VILLOSA)

Brief Description

Gentian is a perennial herb with smooth stems reaching to a height of nearly 20 inches. The leaves are lance-shaped to oval and reach up to 3 inches in length. The small funnel-like greenish-white to purplish-green flowers that appear from August to October have purple stripes inside and are borne in dense terminal clusters.

Gentian prefers semi-shaded areas, dry coastal plains, pinelands, meadows, and open forests. It is widely distributed from New Jersey, Pennsylvania, Ohio and Indiana south to Florida and Louisiana.

Increases Stamina and Physical Strength

Gentian (also called Sampson's snakeroot) is a very popular home remedy throughout the Appalachian region of America. Residents there have sometimes carried a piece of the root to increase physical strength.

Such an incident took place some years ago in the Shenandoah Valley of northern Virginia. A young man, 6 foot 4 inches tall, weighing 230 pounds, was walking home alone one night, leisurely chewing on a piece of gentian root.

Toward the end of his journey, he was beset by a pickup truckload of hooligans. Though outnumbered 8 to 1, he ably defended himself, resulting in six of them requiring some kind of medical treatment in a nearby hospital.

This young man apparently attributed his ability, sudden burst of adrenalin and increased strength to the gentian root.

GINGER
(ZINGIBER OFFICINALE)

Brief Description

Ginger is an erect perennial herb with an aromatic, knotty rootstock that's thick, fibrous and whitish or buff-colored in appearance. The plant reaches a height of 3-4 feet, the leaves growing 6-12 inches long. It is extensively cultivated in the tropics (i.e., India, China, Haiti and Nigeria), especially in Jamaica.

Anti-Nausea Remedy

A fellow colleague, Dr. Daniel P. Mowry of the Department of Psychology at Brigham Young University in Provo, Utah, conducted an amazing experiment to show that powdered ginger root is the best remedy for nausea and vomiting, surpassing even Dramamine, the medication usually recommended for motion sickness.

Thirty-six undergraduate students were asked to take either 100 mg. of Dramamine, 2 capsules of powdered ginger root, or 2 capsules of a placebo (powdered chickweed). Then each one was blindfolded and led to a special tilted chair that rotated when the motor was turned on.

Slightly less than half an hour was allowed to elapse after each volunteer swallowed one of the above substances, before motion sickness was induced by the rotating chair. None of those who had taken either the Dramamine or placebo were able to last the full six minutes in the chair, whereas 50% of those who had swallowed the ginger capsules remained in the chair for the full time.

The ginger root group experienced no vomiting, which suggests that the herb is good to take when traveling on an airplane, train or by ship. A product made by Great American Natural Products called Ginger-Up has become very popular of late for travelers and also for pregnant mothers experiencing morning sickness, often 2 capsules at a time. (See Product Appendix for more information.)

Natural Blood Thinner

People frequently subject to blood clots are generally prescribed oral anticoagulants to help keep their blood relatively thin. One of the most commonly used drugs for this is warfarin sodium (better known as coumadin). Unfortunately, it's also used as a potent rat poison and can lead to serious internal hemorrhaging over an extended period of time. Ginger root is an ideal replacement for such synthetic blood thinners. An average of two capsules twice daily in between meals appears to have helped a small number of those with such problems.

Incredible Relief for Aches and Pains

Nothing seems to work quite like a hot ginger compress on muscular aches and pains, joint stiffness, abdominal cramps, kidney stone attacks, stiff neck, neuralgia, toothache, bladder inflammation, prostatitis and extreme body tension. But keep in mind that as wonderful a remedy as it is, time, considerable effort, patience and a certain change in lifestyle are all required in order to make it totally successful.

Dr. Koji Yamoda from Tokyo shares this cure with me.

Bring a gallon of distilled or spring water to a boil in a large enamel pot with a lid on top. Meanwhile wash 1-1/2 ginger roots, but *don't* peel them. Then grate these roots by hand, using a rotating, clockwise motion instead of the usual back-and-forth movements. This keeps those tough fibers from building up on the grater, Dr. Yamoda said.

Next put this grated ginger root in the center of a clean muslin cloth that has been cut to form an 8-inch square and slightly moistened. Then draw the corners together to form a little bag and tie the top with string, thread or fish line. Be sure to leave plenty of room inside the bag for air and water to circulate.

Before putting this ginger bag in the hot water, make absolutely certain that the heat has been turned down and that the water is no longer boiling. Now uncover the pot and gently squeeze the juice from the bag into the water, before dropping it into the pot. Cover and permit the contents to simmer an additional 7 minutes. Dr. Yamoda informed me that the resulting liquid would acquire the hue of gold and yield a distinctive ginger aroma. The bag may be pressed against the sides of the pot with a wooden ladle to turn the water yellow, if the process seems to be a little slow in happening. Remove the pot from the stove when ready and set aside.

In order to be effective, ginger compresses must be applied relatively hot, he insisted, but not so much as to seriously scald the skin of the patient. Besides being used for compresses, this ginger broth can also be added to bath water to soak an aching back or sore muscles or for soaking tired, aching feet as well. The patient should be lying flat on the floor to receive the full benefits of these compresses front or back.

A terry cloth hand towel is dipped into the pot, while holding both ends. The towel is lifted out and excess water is gently squeezed back into the pot. The steaming towel is then refolded to the desired width and applied directly to the site of pain. A second such compress can be placed immediately over or next to the first one, after which a large dry bath towel is placed over both compresses in order to retain as much heat as possible for the greatest length of time. The bath towel should be folded in half at least once before covering the compresses. Under these conditions, the compresses should remain fairly warm for up to 15-20 minutes. Dr. Yamoda recommended that another set of compresses be applied after this for a total treatment time of 45 minutes or so, and repeated again about 4-6 hours later, or as needed.

He explained that in all his years of clinical practice, nothing seems to have relieved most kinds of physical aches and pains as well as this remedy has. He has even used such ginger compresses on the chests of patients suffering from extreme asthma and bronchitis, with their mucus congestions breaking up in no time at all. Smaller wash cloth-size compresses can be applied against the side of the neck, throat or jaw to relieve neuralgia, stiffness, swollen glands and toothache.

Relief for Hypertensive Headaches

Mix enough powdered ginger and cold water together in a small bowl to make a thin, smooth paste. Then apply to the forehead and temples with the back of a large tablespoon and lie down for a while. This will help to relieve the excruciating pressure building up inside and take away that "exploding" sensation.

Breaks Fever, Eliminates Phlegm

One of the best ways to help break a high fever and get rid of mucus buildup in the sinuses, throat and lungs, is to drink some warm ginger tea. Grate enough fresh ginger root to equal about 2 level tbsps., then add them to 2 cups of boiling water and cover, steeping for 30 minutes. Drink one cup while still warm every 2-1/2 hours.

An Indian Medical Procedure for Improving Your Digestion

Ayurvedic medicine is an ancient form of healing common to the Indian subcontinent. Recently, men like Deepak Chopra, M.D. (himself an Indian) and others have helped to introduce and popularize it in the West. Dr. Chopra's book, *Perfect Health* (New York: Harmony Books, 1990; pp.249-50) recommends an old Ayurvedic procedure for improving poor appetite and indigestion due to nervousness, stress, or illness.

Equal parts (four tablespoons) of powdered ginger, brown sugar, and ghee (melted, clarified butter) are uniformly mixed in a stainless steel, ceramic or glass bowl, covered with a lid or plastic wrap and stored in a cool place. (To make ghee, gently melt one pound of unsalted butter in a quart saucepan over low heat.) Then turn it up to medium. Carefully skim off the foam that rises up. When the butter begins to boil, giving off its water content, reduce the heat again, and slowly cook for another 10 minutes. The ghee is done when all the moisture has cooked out and the milk solids at the bottom of the pan have turned light golden brown; there should be a nutty aroma, but no hint of burning. Remove from the heat, let cool, and then pour into a clean glass Mason jar. It stores indefinitely in your refrigerator.)

Dr. Chopra then advises that a small amount of this mixture be taken every morning followed by a good breakfast of hot cereal, fruit juice, bran muffins, and herb tea with cinnamon stick. The ginger mixture needs to be consumed according to this simple formula: begin with 1 teaspoon the first day and increase it by one-half every day until the 6th day; then reverse this and begin reducing the amount everyday thereafter by one-half teaspoon until on the 11th day only 1 teaspoon remains to be taken.

Dr. Chopra guarantees that appetite and digestion "should be normalized" if all goes well. But he cautions against using this procedure if abdominal cramps or stomach pains prevail. Under such circumstances, he wisely advocates "consulting a physician instead."

GINKGO
(GINKGO BILOBA)

Brief Description

Trees have long symbolized to us strength and sturdiness (as in "a strong or sturdy oak"), resilience ("the resiliance of a willow"), and resistance ("the mighty redwoods resist the elements"). The ginkgo, or maidenhair, is the world's oldest living species of tree, the sole survivor of the Ginkgolaceae family whose fossil record dates back more than 200 million years. When we think of producer Steven Spielberg's epic motion picture *Jurassic Park* (about bringing dinosaurs back to life) we should keep in mind the ginko tree, for it fits very well in this scenario.

Ginkgo trees can live as long as a millennium and often grow to heights of 100 to 122 feet. They have characteristic fan-shaped leaves that are typically bi-lobed. Once widespread in North America and Europe, it was destroyed in many regions during the Ice Age, surviving only in China where it was later cultivated as a sacred tree. Ginkgo returned to America in 1784 on the estate of William Hamilton near Philadelphia. Today, the tree is planted widely throughout America for its ornamental value and because of its incredible ability to resist insects and pollution.

Chinese Restorative for Memory Loss

The earliest mention of ginkgo as a medicine is found in the ancient Chinese materia medica *Pen T'sao Ching*, published in 2800 B.C. and attributed to China's first emperor and sage Shen Nung.

This very early text describes how some members of the royal court became a trifle senile as they advanced in years. Nothing seemed to work to help them recover some of their lost memory. One day, it is said, the emperor was looking out of his palace window for no particular reason at a ginkgo tree, when suddenly he heard a voice close to him whisper in his ear that "the tree you are now looking at will restore the minds of your relatives and friends."

So Shen Nung instructed his servants to collect several baskets of ginkgo leaves and take them to the royal kitchen, where the cooks were instructed to make them into a simple brew. Once this was done, the *warm* tea was served several times each day to those suffering from varying degrees of senility. Within weeks, the *Pen T'sao Ching* noted, everyone of them had regained much of their lost memories!

How Ginkgo Works to Increase Circulation

With almost 300 published studies and reports to its credit, ginkgo biloba extract (GBE) is the herbal medicine most frequently prescribed by alternative-minded doctors and natural-oriented pharmacists worldwide. A large German phyto-medicine company was the first to develop this standardized concentrated extract. It involves 27 different extraction steps and requires 50 pounds of leaves to yield just one pound of GBE, taking up to two weeks to complete.

The primary basis for GBE's meteoric rise in popularity over the last decade has been its ability to increase circulation, both to the brain and to the extremities of the body. Studies have indicated that GBE not only inhibits platelet aggregation (or "bunching" like with a cluster of grapes), but also regulates the tone and elasticity of blood vessels. GBE has been shown to improve both large vessel (arteries) and smaller vessel (capillaries) circulation. In fact, one study demonstrated a 57% increase in blood flow through the nail-fold capillaries one hour after administration of GBE. This positive effect on circulation has made GBE the treatment of choice in the prevention and treatment of circulatory problems in the elderly.

Other Uses for Ginkgo

Ongoing research in Europe and elsewhere has shown that the tree leaf extract is also extremely effective in prevention and treatment of *early* Alzheimer's disease, strokes, cataracts, macular degeneration, and diabetic retinopathy. The key here to its varying successes with these problems takes us back once more to ginkgo's incredible effects on blood circulation.

GBE is also licensed in Germany for the supportive treatment of asthma, transplant rejection, heart arrhythmia, heart attack, head injuries, hearing loss, tinnitus (ringing in the ears), vertigo, depression, and cerebrovascular insufficiency (originating from arteriosclerosis).

I make it a habit of taking on a daily basis a wonderful herbal formula made by Wakunauga of America. It is called "Ginkolic" and consists of ginkgo biloba extract, Kyolic aged garlic extract, and Siberian ginseng. I take 2-3 capsules with a glass of water. I've noticed that when I forget to take it, my brain function isn't up to par. (See Product Appendix for more information.)

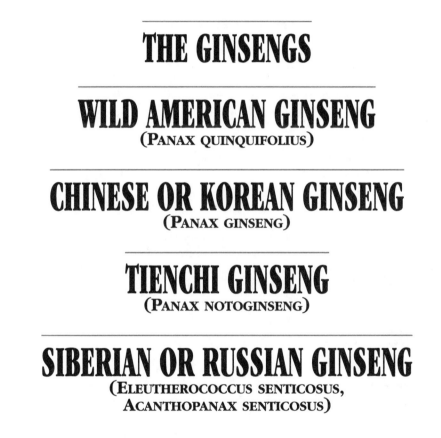

THE GINSENGS

WILD AMERICAN GINSENG
(PANAX QUINQUIFOLIUS)

CHINESE OR KOREAN GINSENG
(PANAX GINSENG)

TIENCHI GINSENG
(PANAX NOTOGINSENG)

SIBERIAN OR RUSSIAN GINSENG
(ELEUTHEROCOCCUS SENTICOSUS, ACANTHOPANAX SENTICOSUS)

Brief Description

Ginseng can refer to any of 22 different plants. Some of these are members of the same family (Araliaceae) or even genus (*Panax*). Still others are completely unrelated to ginseng either botanically or chemically and are often passed off fraudulently, trading on the good reputation and high price of the original root.

To the untrained eye, ginseng looks pretty much like any other root: brown, gnarled, and about as big as a little finger. But the root sometimes resembles part of a human body, hence its other common name of man-root.

An exception to this is Siberian ginseng, which isn't even a species of *Panax* although it is a tall, prickly shrub of the same family, Araliaceae. Siberian and Chinese ginsengs are relatively inexpensive compared to the wild American kind, which the *Wall Street Journal* said in 1983 was bought from 'seng hunters at $156.63 a pound and then resold by the ginseng brokers in Hong Kong for as much as $25,000 *per root!*

Endurance Capabilities

Ginseng is best known for its anti-fatigue, energy-giving properties. But very few people know that it must be taken for a while in order to gradually build such physical endurance, rather than expecting anything sudden to happen from only short-term use.

Soviet athletes swear by the plant to increase stamina and endurance during athletic performance. Professor A.V. Korobokov of the Lesgraft Institute of Physical Culture and Sport in Moscow has conducted experiments with eleutherococcus, or Siberian ginseng, which show indications in athletes of increased endurance, reflexes and coordination.

Soviet scientists attribute the restorative power of Siberian ginseng to the plant's glycoside content—naturally occurring chemicals which initiate the body's stress response. A minimum of 2 capsules daily with meals for several months is suggested to increase your own personal levels of physical endurance.

Protects Against Stress-Induced Problems

Siberian ginseng has achieved renown throughout Soviet bloc countries as an effective antidote to stress-related illnesses. In an interview I had with a Soviet physician during a visit to the USSR, I learned some fantastic things about this herb.

Dr. Nikolai Gurovsky was then head of the Board of Space Medicine in the Soviet Public Health Ministry. He had personally prescribed Siberian ginseng for the two Salyut 6 cosmonauts who stayed in space 96 days the year before. He related this:

> Prior to this flight, we had closely examined other cosmonauts who had returned from previous missions in space. We found that in every case, their immune systems were depleted. Some of their internal organs had been seriously weakened by constant exposure to radiation while in space. And when they came back to earth again, it took them awhile to regain their complete sense of balance.

But we decided to have our Salyut 6 team drink a special tonic of eleutherococcus we devised in the laboratory. Each day while they were orbiting in space, they took an amount equivalent to about one cup.

Upon their return, we submitted them to very intensive medical testing and found that their immunity levels were still moderately strong. Their major glands and organs also were not as adversely affected by radiation as other cosmonauts had been. And gravity didn't seem to affect their balances quite as badly either.

We attributed these differences to the herbal tonic. We intend to use it more often with other space missions in the future.

An average of 3 capsules per day of Siberian ginseng in between meals or on an empty stomach is recommended for the proper management of stress and prevention of stress-induced ailments.

Improves Mating Habits

Ginseng is considered by millions to be the world's number one, ultimate aphrodisiac. Some clinical research in this direction seems to verify this activity to a certain extent. For instance, Japanese scientists have already identified sex hormone activity in ginseng preparations given to *both* male and female rodents alike. And when I was in mainland China in 1980, I discovered a lot of women taking different kinds of ginseng to improve sexual relations with their spouses.

Male albino rats under the influence of ginseng began ejaculation earlier, mounted their female companions more often in a 45-minute observation period and performed more acts of intercourse in a 10-day period than did a control group of males without the benefits of ginseng.

The best preparation of ginseng to use for these purposes is any liquid tonic which has the root in the bottle with it. Several brands are available from larger, full-service heath food stores or local herb shops in any metropolitan Chinatown district. Drink 4 fluid ounces twice a day for at least a week in advance prior to your next sexual encounter.

GLADIOLA
(GLADIOLUS SPECIES)

Brief Description

Glads (as they are nicknamed) are everywhere cultivated for garden display and for use indoors as cut flowers. Due to extensive hybridization of *Gladiolus*, there are now so many different varieties that it is all but impossible to give them clear botanical names.

In general, glads are tender perennial herbs with long, sword-shaped leaves. They grow to four feet or more in height and produce long, dense-ly-flowered spikes of flowers in summer. Many colors are available.

Doukhobor Remedies for Dysentery, Diarrhea, and Colds

The Doukhobors were a prominent Russian religious sect in the 18th and 19th centuries. They were somewhat like the Quakers, rejecting complete-ly priesthood, sacraments, and other outward symbols of Christianity. Members came from the lower level of society, primarily farmers; they pro-moted a communal lifestyle and preached material and spiritual equality for all. Because they rejected the authority of both state and church, they were vigorously persecuted under the reign of Empress Catherine the Second. Later on Leo Tolstoy helped over 7,000 of them to migrate to Canada, where thy settled in what is now Saskatchewan. Once more their abilities produced flourishing communities, and they spread after 1908 to British Columbia.

Frugal, industrious and abstemious, the Doukhobors built their own roads and their own irrigation projects. Orchards and farms flourished. The sect became a small but important group in the development of western Canada. There were some internal strifes, however, mostly over the ques-tion of communal ownership of land. Although basically non-violent in atti-tude, they still had spectacular ways of expressing their intense displeasure toward governmental decisions. One of the more remarkable forms of dis-sent was the so-called nudist strikes, in which Doukhobor men, women, and children stripped off all their clothes and then marched in revolt into government office buildings to argue with officials.

At the time that Saddam Hussein of Iraq invaded Kuwait, precipitat-ing the Persian Gulf War, I was in British Columbia giving a summer course on herbal medicine. An instructor there who showed students how to make salves and oils in an herbal hot pot was a woman named Netta Zeberoff. She was a Russian Doukhobor by birth and recounted in private how mem-bers of her family walked "naked as jay birds" (as she so aptly put it) into a provincial government office to express their dissatisfaction with some point of law. She remembers, as a child, how the mouths and eyes of those Canadians working there, opened wide as they stared in disbelief. She still enjoys a hearty chuckle whenever relating this.

Now Netta was very familiar with many of the old folk medical reme-dies that her parents and grandparents used in Russia before coming to Canada. She told me how her folks made a tea out of gladiolas for treating dysentery, diarrhea and symptoms of the common cold. A pot of water would be boiled (about a quart) and a handful (probably about 1-1/2 cups) of cut flowers and leaves tossed in, stirred and then covered. The heat would be turned down low and the mixture brewed another few minutes (about 5, she believed). After this, the tea would be cooled, then strained, put into another container and stored in a cool place for several days.

For cases of dysentery and diarrhea, one cup of the *cool* liquid was given several times a day on an empty stomach until the problem cleared up, usually within 2-3 days. But for the symptoms of the common cold (i.e., fever, running nose, sore throat, aching muscles), some of the *warm* tea would be given periodically throughout the day, to be gargled or swallowed or both. She figures *no more* than half a cup was ever given at a time, but this repeated 4 or 5 times daily. Sometimes a folded wet cloth, dipped in the *cool* tea, was wrung out and then applied across the forehead to bring down an elevated fever.

GOLDENSEAL
(HYDRASTIS CANADENSIS)

Brief Description

Goldenseal is a small perennial plant, usually ciltivated for the mass herb product, but also occuring wild in rich, shady woods and damp meadows from Connecticut to Minnesota and southward. A thick, knotty, yellow rootstock sends up a hairy stem, almost a foot high, with a pair of five-lobed, serrated leaves near the top terminated by a single greenish white flower.

Magnificent for Eye Inflammations

In 1974, California physician Jeff L. Anderson frequently used a solution of goldenseal root in his practice to treat numerous eye ailments, especially conjunctivitis. He mixed together 1/8 teaspoon each of powdered goldenseal, comfrey and chamomile together, then added the mixture to 1 cup of boiled water and steeped it for 15 mins before straining through a sterile cheesecloth. He had his patients use the strained solution at room temperature, 2-3 drops three times daily from a sterile eye dropper.

The yellow color of the root is due to the alkaloid, berberine. The *Indian Journal of Ophthalmology* for March 1983 reported that the berberine found in goldenseal root is excellent for treating inflammations of the cornea and iris brought on by the herpes simplex virus. A solution similar to the one previously mentioned can be made for these problems, except that 1/4 tsp. of goldenseal root would be used with the other two herbs. The same directions would be followed.

Suppresses Candida, Heals Mouth Sores

A douche of goldenseal is excellent for reducing yeast infection. In an electric blender combine 3 cups of water and 1-1/2 tsps. of powdered root, then douche several times each day with it until the problem is cleared up.

A simple mouthwash made of pinches of goldenseal powder and baking soda in a little water is perfect for healing any kind of sores in the mouth or on the gums and tongue.

A Good Drug Withdrawal Program

During several trips in 1987 to Los Angeles, San Francisco, Chicago, Boston, New York City and Dallas for speaking engagements, I interviewed various alternative care doctors and holistic healers who have taken the natural approach toward helping addicts kick their extensive and debilitating drug habits. What follows is a distillation of all their combined wisdom in a simple program.

My friend, Lendon Smith, M.D., in his best-seller *Feed Yourself Right*, points out that addiction can also involve other substances we normally use on a regular basis. He then proceeds to tell the true story of what happened to a manager of a small country store in Ohio during the terrible winter of 1977/78. None of his customers ever complained as he gradually ran out of basic foods like milk, bread, fruits and vegetables. But did they *ever* get rankled and cussed him good when he ran out of Pepsi-Cola! "People can get hooked on *anything!*" Dr. Smith warns.

All of those health professionals with whom I conferred agreed unanimously that cleansing the system of drug residues is the *first and most important* step to follow.

STEP I: CLEANSING

Capsules: Goldenseal Root (4 per day for first month; reduced to 2 per day thereafter)

Chaparral Twigs (2 per day for first month; reduced to 1 per day thereafter)

Tea: 1/2 tsp. grated raw orange peel

3 tsp. dried mullein leaves

3 tsp. dried juniper berries

2 tsp. dried lemon grass

1 tsp. dried thyme herb

4 tsp. dried dandelion root

Bring 1 qt. spring or distilled water to a boil. Add orange peel, juniper berries and dandelion root. Cover, reduce heat, and simmer for 5 minutes. Remove from heat, uncover and add rest of herbs. Cover and steep an aditional 40 minutes. Strain, sweeten with honey and drink 1 cup when taking 2 capsules goldenseal and 1 capsule chaparral on an empty stomach. Repeat procedure again later the same day. A strong coffee enema 2-3 times per week for the first month is also encouraged.

The next step involves giving herbal and nutritional support to the central nervous sytem in an effort to control the ususal withdrawal symptoms (hysteria, delirium tremens, and insomnia) experienced by most addicts.

STEP II: RELAXING

Capsules: Valerian Root (4 per day)

Skullcap Herb (4 per day)

Tea: 3 tsp. dried catnip herb

2 tsp. dried peppermint leaves

3 tsp. dried chamomile herb

4 tsp. dried lemon balm leaves

Bring 1 qt. spring or distilled water to boil. Remove from heat and add all of the above ingredients. Cover and steep for an hour. Drink 1 cup sweetened with pure maple syrup 4 times daily on an empty stomach.

Supplements: Aqua-Vite from Great American Natural Products (see Appendix). (3 tablets twice daily with meals.)

Complete B-Complex (any brand) from a health food store. (3 tablets twice daily with meals.)

Vitamin C in the form of sodium ascorbate (25,000 mg. per day)

Calcium-Magnesium in the form of calcium gluconate (1,000 mg.) and magnesium sulfate (500 mg.)

Potassium (750-1,200 mg.) best taken in an 8 oz. glass of carrot juice (2/3) and mixed greens (1/3) daily with meals. Any dark, leafy greens (spinach, watercress, wheat grass, etc.) will do. Can be made at home with a juicer or obtained from some health food store juice bars.

The final part of this three-step program is rebuilding the body through sound nutrition. Evidence exists that a few prior heavy drug users experienced virtually *no* side effects when suddenly and totally withdrawing from controlled substances. The Major League baseball star, Ron LeFlore, is a case in point. LeFlore began taking heroin when he was 15 and used it every single day—both snorting and injecting it for nearly a year before being arrested and sent to prison. Much to his surprise, he experienced *no* withdrawal symptoms behind bars, even while spending time in solitary confinement. He attributes this lack of negative responses during withdrawal to his mother's good home-cooked meals, which consisted of many vegetable-meat stews, casseroles, soups, garden salads and whole-grain cereals and breads. A number of delicious recipes designed to promote good health and strength are scattered throughout this book and the reader is heartily encouraged to search some of them out as part of a very good nutrition program for recovering addicts.

STEP III: NOURISHING

Capsules: Slippery Elm Bark and Alfalfa Herb (3 of each per day with meals).

When taking them, drink only pineapple or papaya juice instead of water.

Tea: 1/2 bunch chopped, fresh parsley

1 tbsp. each of wheat and barley

1 handful cut, fresh watercress

1 tbsp. cut, dried horsetail

1 tsp. each powdered kelp and Irish moss

1 handful cut, fresh spinach

1 tbsp. each yellow dock and burdock roots

1/2 cup fresh or dried nettle

2 tbsp. honeycomb (where available)

1 small *un*peeled parsnip

Simmer everything in 1 quart of spring or distilled water in a heavy stainless steel pot, covered, for several hours until the volume of liquid has been reduced to slightly less than half. Strain and return the liquid to the same pot, discarding the rest. While still very hot, stir in 4 tbsp. of blackstrap molasses. Then allow to cool. Take 1 tbsp. of this refined tonic five times daily with meals.

All three steps of this program need to be implemented simultaneously, but emphasis can shift first to cleansing for a couple of days and after this greater attention focused on relaxing and nourishing. Since each case is different, there will be obvious variability in which steps are emphasized the most. But the point to remember is that *all* three steps must run concurrent with each other when this program is in force.

Relieves Poison Ivy Rash

Goldenseal is a blessing in disguise for those unlucky enough to encounter poison ivy. To make an effective skin wash combine 1 tsp. of powdered root with a pint of hot water and dab this solution on the afflicted parts when cool. Also 2-3 capsules taken internally will expedite healing as well.

Reduces Insulin Dependency

A small number of diabetics I've known over the years have successfully managed to lower their insulin needs by taking 2 capsules of goldenseal root per day. One fellow in Toronto, Canada went from close to 30 cc of insulin to needing injections of about half that amount each day, after taking the herb for about a month. CAUTION: Those with hypoglycemia should avoid taking the root internally, but can use it safely as a mouthwash and douche.

Incredible Sinus Relief

Changes in temperature, the arrival of spring, the growth of pollen and the aftershocks of a cold all have one thing in common: they can cause your sinus cavities to swell like a water balloon and vibrate you skull to a heavy metal rock beat. What can be done about it, besides just gulping Dristans or squirting Neo-Synephrine up your nose?

Dennis J. Partride, a long-time resident of coastal Florida, came up with one of the best remedies for relieving sinus miseries. He shared this with others in 1980. "I took the shaker of sea salt from the cupboard and rubbed 20 grains or so into my right hand, adding a pinch or two of goldenseal powder and enough unchlorinated water to form a liquid paste," he began. "I then proceeded to sniff this up my nose. The relief was felt almost immediately, because the herb was able to reach all of the mucous membranes. An ounce of the stuff usually lasts me a year and is far better than any drugstore sinus products I've tried," he concluded.

Preventing Blood Clots

The yellow alkaloid in goldenseal is called berberine. Important research conducted at the Department of Biochemistry, Second Military Medical University in Shanghai, China, demonstrated that berberine "markedly inhibited clot retraction." The research data appeared in the *Chinese Pharmacological Bulletin* (10:114-16, 1994).

Those who are prone to strokes or frequent clot formations may benefit from one capsule of goldenseal root every *other* day. However, prudence dictates that this *only* be done if they *do not have hypoglycemia.*

Goldenseal should not be used any longer than two months at any given time, as it can interfere with the colon's ability to manufacture B vitamins. And pregnant women should avoid taking it until they have delivered their newborns.

GOTU KOLA
(CENTELLA ASIATICA, HYDROCOTYLE ASIATICA)

Brief Description

This slender perennial is found throughout tropical regions of the world. Its nearly smooth surface and kidney-shaped or heart-shaped leaves accompanied by dark-purple flower petals make for a somewhat exquisite plant.

But efforts to domesticate it have often failed, because its apparent obstinance requires human persecution in order to spread. Thus, when gotu kola is sprayed with herbicides, only the leaves die, while the root actually seems to thrive on these harmful chemicals. After one good spraying, the plant usually proliferates like crazy.

Improves Mental Retardation

Very few herbs in the plant kingdom have memory-stimulating properties attributed to them, and even fewer still that can be clinically documented. Gotu kola is probably the only herb thus far that has been scientifically tested and proven to definitely increase mental activity.

Dr. M.V.R. Appa Rao and his associates administered a 500 mg. tablet of powdered gotu kola daily to a group of 15 mentally retarded children at an institution in India. As reported by the *J. of Res. in Ind. Medicine* (1973), after a 3-month trial period on this herb, these youngsters experienced "increased powers of concentration and attention" more so than did 15 other kids given a placebo. Dr. Appa Rao concluded that gotu kola "could be used for the routine treatment of mental retardation."

A gotu kola product under the Nature's Way label may be found at your local health food store. An avergae of 4 capsules per day is recommended for this.

Reduces Phlebitis, Varicose Veins

Edith Rosenbaum of Levittown, New York wrote to me some time ago about her experiences with gotu kola:

> I've been troubled with phlebitis in my legs for years. Also I've had some deep, ugly, purple varicose veins to go with it. Someone told me about this herb, gotu kola, helping them. So I figured I had nothing to lose by trying it for a while.
>
> My sister, who gets around more than I do, got me some at a health food store in Manhattan. I started taking two capsules in the morning for the first couple of days, then increased that to 4 by the following week. I'd take them about 3 hours after eating.
>
> When I began noticing my phlebitis going down a little, I decided to up the doasge to 6 capsules a day, taking 2 in the morning, 2 at noon, and 2 at night before going to bed.
>
> Some 6-1/2 weeks later, most of my varicose veins had shrunk back to a more normal size. And I didn't have so much pain in walking either. I could get around a lot easier, too. That's what gotu kola has done for me.

GUARANA

(CUPANIA AMERICANA OR PAULLINIA CUPANA)

Brief Description

Guarana is a climbing shrub native to South America and the expansive Amazon Basin. There it is cultivated for its seeds. Guarana paste (also called gum) is prepared from the pulverized and roasted seeds by mixing with water to form a paste, which is then molded into bars and dried.

Like a few other popular plant stimulants, it contains a fair amount of caffeine and traces of related alkaloids like theophylline and theobromine (which are also present in chocolate and cocoa, I might add). Following is a table summarizing the caffeine contents of some popular plants:

PLANT	*CAFFEINE CONTENT*
Coffee	1.5 — 2.5%
Guarana	2.6 — 7%
Kola Nut	1.5 — 2%
Mate (Yerba mate or Paraguay tea)	Up to 2%
Tea (black and green)	1 — 5%

World Champion Boxer Relies on Guarana for Stamina

The IBF (International Boxing Federation) World Featherweight Championshiop title fight from South Padre Island, Texas was broadcast on May 28, 1995 on "The CBS Sports Show." The 12-round fight featured defending champion Tom "Boom Boom" Johnson and challenger Eddie Croft. Both African Americans weighed around 130 pounds each.

I watched the last six rounds as both contenders battled it out. Each one held up fairly well, but the three ringside judges were clearly impressed with the continued stamina that Johnson exhibited in every round. In spite of some punishing blows to his face and midsection, he managed to stay on his feet the entire time and come back swinging at his opponent just as hard. In the end, it was a unanimous decision in his favor. This was the seventh straight win for him; overall he had won 40 fights, lost 2, and had only one bout result in a draw.

Following the fight, he was interviewed in the ring by a sportscaster. Johnson talked at length about how important conditioning was to him. "If I don't stay in excellent physical shape, then I don't win fights," he declared. Quickly concluding his interview before heading to the dressing room, he attributed determination, focused concentration, and guarana for his many boxing triumphs.

Guarana is usually included in a number of different herbal energy formulas or powdered nutrition supplements (Herbalife's NRG and Hot Stuff Double X by National Health Products are two examples). No more than 2 capsules or a level *teaspoonful* in 6 fluid ounces of liquid of any such formula should be taken in a six-hour period. Frequent use can result in caffeine dependency, wreak possible havoc with the central nervous system, and even cause blood sugar imbalances that may lead to hypoglycemia.

But like anything else, when guarana alone or in combination is used *in moderation*, it can help increase stamina for considerable physical endurance.

NOTE: Two religious denominations in America prohibit the use of *any* caffeinated foods, beverages, or herbs. These are the Seventh-Day Adventists and "The Mormons" (Church of Jesus Christ of Latter-Day

Saints). They need to do some careful label reading to make sure that whatever they're ingesting *doesn't* have any caffeine-containing substance in its list of ingredients.

GUAR GUM
(CYAMOPSIS TETRAGONOLOBA OR C. PSORALIOIDES)

Brief Description

The guar plant is a small nitrogen-fixing annual that bears fruits known as pods containing 5-9 seeds per pod and can grow to nearly 6 feet in height. The part used is the endosperm of the seed. The endosperm constitutes 35-42% of the seed; it's separated from the other components of the seed (seed coat or hull and embryo or germ) during processing. The endosperm left is then ground to a fine powder, which is commercial guar gum. Major guar producers are India, Pakistan and the U.S.

Marvelous Weight Loss

A number of obese subjects at Salgren's Hospital in Sweden were put on a long-term treatment with daily intakes of guar gum preparations, while still maintaining their normal dietary habits. In as little as 10 weeks their hunger cravings had been significantly reduced, their blood sugar and cholesterol levels lowered, and most of them had lost 10-15 lbs. of weight. An average of 4-6 capsules per day of guar gum from any health food store is recommended.

Reduces Elevated Cholesterol

Numerous sources of dietary fiber have been shown in the last decade to reduce blood cholesterol pretty well; examples include oat bran, psyllium seed hulls, xanthan gum, guar gum and others. A Finnish study which appeared in the medical journal *Atherosclerosis* (72 (88) 157-62, 1988) demonstrated the effectiveness of guar gum in the treatment of very severe hypercholesterolemia, which inevitably leads to heart disease.

Since the prescription drugs ordinarily used to treat this condition have some serious side effects, less toxic therapies should be looked at instead. Fifteen to thirty grams of guar gum per day reduced serum cholesterol 12-20%, with only the expected side effects. As with other dietary fibers, laxative effects were common, as was intestinal gas. However, since lower doses seemed to work as well as higher, these effects could be controlled. Guar gum didn't inhibit nutrient metabolism either in those who participated in the Finnish study.

I would recommend two capsules of guar gum daily with a meal and watch closely your fat intake, in order to keep your cholesterol level within a safe range.

Useful for Diabetics

Guar gum has also been recommended by some alternative-minded doctors to their diabetic patients, who also suffer from obesity. The guar gum therapy enables them to shed unwanted pounds, helps to control their cravings for sweet things and, in a few instances, has even helped to *reduce* (but not abandon entirely) their dependency on insulin. The average intake per patient whom I interviewed ranged from 2 to 4 capsules daily with meals.

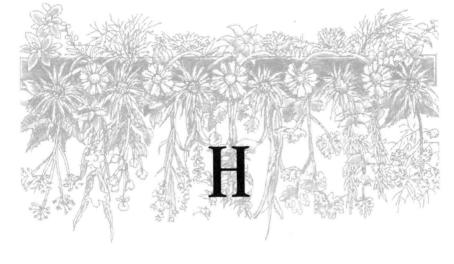

H

HAWTHORN
(Crataegus oxyacantha)

Brief Description

Hawthorns in North America consist of 100 to 200 species of small trees and shrubs, mostly in the eastern half of the United States. Their taxonomy is difficult and confusing; some 1,100 specific names have been published, but most are no longer accepted. Hybrids no doubt exist, and many varieties are recognized.

Hawthorns furnish food and cover for wildlife; species with fruits that persist over winter are especially valuable. Many species are useful for environmental plantings. Because they tolerate a wide variety of sites, hawthorns have also been planted to stabilize banks, for shelter belts, and for erosion control.

The hawthorns have thorny twigs and branches, although a few species are spineless. The leaves are single and what is known as simple, growing alternately in varying shapes and different degrees of lobing and serration. The conspicuous flowers have five creamy and sometimes pinkish blossoms and loom up importantly in this nation's history, as they gave the Pilgrims' ship, the *Mayflower*, its name. Growing in ordinarily fragrant clusters in midsummer, they usually thrive in flatish, terminal groups.

The small applelike fruit, characteristically tipped with the remnants of the outer floral leaves, are really pomes, a fleshy reproductive entity with five seeds enclosed in a capsule and an outer more or less thick, fleshy layer that differs markedly in taste on each shrub or tree, especially when it is raw. They are generally less than one-half inch in diameter and are

271

mostly reddish, sometimes yellow and rarely bluish, purplish or black, often with a high-sugar and low-protein-and-fat-content pulp.

Excellent Remedy for Hypertension

Hawthorn berry has been a very popular treatment for many heart-related problems throughout the British Isles. *The Sunday Times* magazine (a London-based paper) for May 24, 1981 cited the amazing work of a Scottish doctor some 42 years before and the incredible results he obtained with it for hypertension.

In 1939 Dr. James Graham of Glasgow University showed that a fluid extract of hawthorn berries was very effective in the treatment of 10 patients confined to bed with high blood pressure. He made his extract by combining 4 tablespoons of dried and crushed berries with 1 pint of dark mead (any dark English ale or dark German beer will do). He shook daily the flask that the mixture was kept in and did so for 15 days. He then strained the liquid into another flask and gave his hypertensive patients 25 drops of it beneath their tongues twice daily. Within a week full recovery was evident for all 10 of them.

Wonderful Tonic for Coronary Problems

The same British newspaper also reported that in 1969, medical doctors in Bulgaria were treating scores of patients suffering from coronary problems with a fluid extract of hawthorn. After 6 weeks of treatment, consisting of 15 drops beneath the tongue twice daily, three-quarters of a group of 62 patients fully recovered.

The fluid extract was made pretty much the same way that Dr. Graham made his preparation, with the sole exception of vodka used as the medium of extraction for the berries. *The Sunday Times* also explained how hawthorn berries were active in the treatment of heart palpitations, angina, and stroke. This action was attributed, in part, to the bioflavonoids such as rutin and hesperidin and vitamin C present in the berries.

A clinical report on the use of freeze-dried hawthorn berries for the treatment of heart and menopause problems in an elderly woman was given to me a few years ago by Scott Tyler, an internist then working at the Portland Naturopathic Clinic in Oregon. John Collins, M.D. was the supervising physician. I am grateful to both of them for permitting me to use the following excerpts.

Mrs. S. is a 67-year-old woman with right shoulder pain, irregular heart rhythm, mild hypertension and persisting symptoms of menopause. She had been taking Premarin for the past 15 years, on her doctor's recommendation. We felt she was experiencing multiple side effects from the Premarin and explained this to her. She decided to wean herself from this drug. Her menopause symptoms worsened almost immediately. We began a course of treatment with botanical tinctures containing female hormone precursors. The symptoms abated. The patient's shoulder pain was discovered to be due to thoracic outlet syndrome. Appropriate therapy was undertaken and the problem resolved.

The patient's cardiovascular complaints were treated also botanically. It seemed to us that we could address both the mild hypertension and the cardiac dysrhythmia (palpitations and paroxysms of tachycardia) with one botanical. [Hawthorn] solid extract was given, 3 tsp. each day in divided doses. The patient responded to the therapy well, but the expense of the product was substantial for her. When we learned that [hawthorn] was to be made available in freeze-dried form, we considered substituting it. The patient began taking 2 capsules a day of freeze-dried hawthorn berries— the equivalent of the solid extract dosage. The patient's palpitations and tachycardia were entirely eliminated by the use of the freeze-dried hawthorn berries, and her blood pressure reverted to within normal limits.

We concluded that freeze-dried [hawthorn] berries provided the same non-toxic therapeutic action as the [hawthorn] solid extract, but at a significantly reduced cost.

HENNA
(LAWSONIA INERMIS)

Brief Description

Henna is a perennial shrub common to the top part of Africa, much of Asia and some parts of Australia. It has been naturalized and cultivated elsewhere, though, in such diverse places as the American tropics, Egypt, India, and places in the Middle East region of the world. It can reach up to 20 feet in height in some places and yields fragrant white or rose-red blooms. People have been known to plant henna as an ornamental hedge occasionally.

Cosmetic Dye

The dried, ground leaves (the part actually called henna) have been soaked in water with a little lime juice since antiquity, to produce colorfast orange, red, and brown dyes. Dried, powdered leaves of henna contain about 0.5 to 1.5% lawsone, the chief constituent responsible for the dyeing properties of the plant.

Henna has been valued by the women of Egypt since the days of the Pharaohs, because of its dark dusky red, rather iron rust color. Egyptian women have always used it to stain the palms of their hands and the soles of their feet to help check excessive perspiration and prevent the sun from blistering these parts of their body. Mummies entombed for 3,000 years still retain some of their henna dye used on their nails. In Pakistan and India it isn't uncommon to find both men and women coloring their nails, fingers, hands, and hair with henna.

Adrienne's Natural Hair Coloring

A friend of mine named Adrienne Simidian, who lives by a lake in a deep wooded area near Carmel, New York, likes to use natural things wherever possible to keep herself looking young. Henna is one of these items which figures into her hair coloring to keep the gray away.

Sometime in the spring of 1995 I stayed overnight at her hideaway in the woods to visit a mutual friend of ours next day at Greenhaven Correctional Facility in Stormville. His name is Jack Madden and both Adrienne and I have come to form strong friendships with this unique individual as the years have passed.

Anyway, she demonstrated for me how she goes about coloring her hair with henna. First she mixed two cups of natural henna powder with two cups of Fuller's earth. She did this by putting them both into a bag and shaking good to mix well. She then measured out about three tablespoons of this mixture into a small glass bowl. She pointed out that if a woman is a brunette, she should use some strong, black coffee for the necessary liquid, but if a lady's hair is blonde, then she should use boiling water instead. Adrienne added just enough hot liquid to make a thick paste.

I watched as she parted her hair in different places and applied some of this paste with a pastry brush. After doing this she gently rubbed the paste through her hair with her fingertips and left it on for almost an hour. She covered her head with a plastic bag to keep the paste from drying out too soon and falling off.

She then rinsed her hair under cold, running water, dried it with a towel and brushed it back. I was amazed to see that the streaks of gray were all gone and only a dark, healthy, natural color remained. While she wouldn't reveal her exact age to me, she hinted that it was in the mid-fifties somewhere.

An Egyptian Remedy for Skin Problems

Some years ago while I was in Cairo, Egypt I had a chance to go where no tourists ever dare to venture. And this is into the stench-filled neighborhoods of the zabbaline, Cairo's traditional garbage collectors. These members of Egypt's Coptic Christian minority accept the lowly task of urban scavenging for a livelihood. The zabbaline actually pay garbage brokers for exclusive rights to certain collection routes, high-income neighborhoods being the most desirable. Men and children collect, while women stay home sifting and sorting the booty into great piles of paper, glass, textile, bones, and metals. Food waste is reserved for feeding to pigs that Coptic families raise for their main cash crop.

Considered objects of scorn by most Cairo inhabitants, the zabbaline suffer tremendous exposure to disease. As I walked among their homes and yards filled to excess with huge piles of rotting garbage, I couldn't help but notice how many of the children had open sores on their arms, hands, and legs. But upon closer examination of some of them, I was amazed to find *no* apparent spread of infection. Instead, such sores were covered with a rust-colored paste, which I later came to understand was henna powder mixed with water and applied over the sores to keep them from becoming worse. Since then I've recommended henna paste to those suffering from herpetic lesions and the sores common to AIDS patients with pretty good results in their healing.

HONEYSUCKLE

(see JAPANESE HONEYSUCKLE)

HOPS

(Humulus lupulus)

Brief Description

The hop vine is a perennial climbing plant found wild in many places throughout the world. However, it's mostly cultivated in the United States, West Germany and Yugoslavia for brewing beer. The bitter taste of beer is derived mostly from the humulone present in hops.

The vine has many angular, rough stems growing up to 20 feet in length from a branched rootstock. The leaves are rough, opposite, serrate and 3-5 lobed. Attractive yellowish-green flowers adorn the vine, with the male flowers arranged in hanging panicles and the female ones in catkins. The name "hops" generally pertains to the scaly, cone-like fruit that develops from the female flowers.

Kills Unfriendly Bacteria

Alcoholic extracts of hops in various dosage forms have been used clinically in treating numerous forms of leprosy, pulmonary tuberculosis and acute bacterial dysentery with varying degrees of success by doctors throughout the People's Republic of China. This could be due to a couple of antibiotic bitter acids, lupulon and humulon, occurring in the herb. Both kill Gram-positive and acid-fast bacteria such as strains of staphylococcus, for instance. Staph infections are evident in supporating wounds, runny sores, abscesses, boils and osteomyelitis (inflammation of bone marrow and adjacent bone and cartilage).

To make a strong extract, combine 1-1/4 cups of cut, fresh hop fruit with 2-1/2 cups of good-quality imported Russian vodka or an expensive brandy. Put into a bottle with a tight lid or cork. Shake daily, allowing the herbs to extract for about 2 weeks. Let the herbs settle and pour off the tincture, straining the liquid through a clean muslin cloth or fine filter paper. I recommend a piece of advice from an old European farm wife, if you expect a potent tincture: commence your extract during a full moon and strain off on a full moon in order that the drawing power of the waxing moon will help pull as many medicinal properties from the hops as possible.

Two tablespoonfuls each day taken orally on an empty stomach will help fight infection internally. The same amount may also be applied directly with some cotton on bedsores caused by hospital-induced staph. And clean strips of gauze may also be saturated in this tincture and then used to dress wounds so they'll heal more rapidly.

Really Gets Rid of Dandruff

After the hair is scrubbed with a strong detergent and thoroughly rinsed with plain water, some of the above tincture may be rubbed into the scalp to help control dandruff. A quicker and easier way, though, is to rinse your hair well with a can of beer each day. Any brand will do just fine.

Calms Nervousness and Insomnia

Hops has been shown clinically to exert a strong sedative action on nervous patients and to help insomniacs get a good night's sleep. Bring 2 pints of water to a boil. Add 1 heaping tbsp. each of hops and valerian root. Cover and reduce heat, simmering for 5 minutes. Remove and steep an additional 45 minutes. Sweeten with a little pure maple syrup and drink 1-1/2 cups at a time to help relax the body.

Keep in mind that since hops lose their sedative properties quickly when stored, they should always be used either as fresh as possible or pretty soon after they've been dried and cut up. An old favorite of country grandmothers used to be stuffing a cloth pillowcase with hop flowers that had been sprinkled with a little alcohol to release their precious oils.

Do Hops Contain Estrogens?

Estrogens are hormones which exert a variety of biological activities within the body. These include bone growth, preventing or stopping production of breast milk, suppressing ovulation, relieving cancer of the breast and prostate gland and stimulating sexual heat in women to permit intercourse with men.

Several studies cited in Vol. 11 of *Food & Cosmetics Toxicology* indicated an estrogenic activity in hops ranging from 20,000 to 300,000 I.U. (International Units) per 100 grams of herb. This is comparable to, or even higher than, the daily intake of estrogens by women taking certain oral contraceptive preparations. This may help to explain why some old herbalists have recommended hops tea for sexual stimulation.

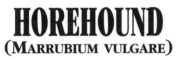

HOREHOUND
(MARRUBIUM VULGARE)

Brief Description

Horehound is a perennial found in waste places, in meadows and pastures and along railroad tracks and roadsides in coastal areas of the U.S., Canada, Great Britain, France and Germany. A tough, fibery rootstock sends up many bushy, square, downy stems. The leaves are somewhat distinctive, being wrinkled, rough on top and wooly-like underneath.

Real Congestion Buster

Nothing breaks up severe mucus congestion quite like horehound. In fact, I've found it to work a lot better than even coltsfoot, another congestion buster, does. One cup of warm horehound tea will instantly loosen impacted phlegm in the throat, lungs and sinuses, like you wouldn't believe, and relieves a great deal of the misery attending a sinus headache.

To make the tea just bring 1 pint of hot water to a boil, then add 2 1/2 tsp. of the fresh or dried herb. Remove from heat, cover, and steep 45 minutes. Drink while still lukewarm with a squeeze of lemon juice in it and sweetened with a touch of blackstrap molasses. Makes a real gutsy brew that will just about knock any cold unconscious.

Horehound candy makes a super remedy for sore throat and inflamed lungs due to cold, flu, allergies or smoking.

Needed: 1 oz. fresh horehound or 1/4 cup dried; 1-1/2 cups water; 2 cups honey; 1 cup blackstrap molasses.

Boil water in small saucepan. Add horehound and simmer 10 minutes. Allow to stand off heat for 5 mins., then strain liquid into large, heavy 5-qt. pot. Add honey and molasses to pot, mix and cook at medium heat until the temperature slowly reaches the hardcrack stage: 300-310°F. on a candy thermometer. Scum that forms can be scooped off and thrown away before the candy reaches the high temperature. Don't stir mixture while cooking even though it foams up. Pour into a greased 9 X 13-inch pan and score into pieces before it sets but as it cools. Mixture will settle and harden as it cools. Refrigerate. Suck on a piece of this horehound candy to relieve nagging coughs.

HORSEMINT
(see BERAMOT)

HORSERADISH
(ARMORACIA LAPATHIFOLIA)

Brief Description

Horseradish is a perennial plant native to southeastern Europe and western Asia, and occasionally is found wild but usually is cultivated in other parts of the world. The long, white, cylindrical or tapering root produces a 2- to 3-foot-high stem in the second year.

The dried, powdered root found in many herb formulas today is practically worthless. The real benefits lie in the freshly dug root. When grated, however, the strong volatile oils are released, so it's necessary to cover the grated root with apple cider vinegar and refrigerate it in a glass jar with a tight-fitting lid. It will keep for at least 3 months this way or the entire root can be packed in damp sand and kept in a cool corner of your basement or garage. Keep sand moist.

Great Massaging Oil

A very stimulating massage oil to relieve muscular aches and pains and help break up chest congestion can be made by steeping a small amount of freshly grated root in some cold-pressed oil of your choice (wheat germ, sesame, olive).

Cosmetic Benefits

Horseradish vinegar lightens the tone of the skin and gets rid of freckles and blotches. Also makes a great hair rinse and really enlivens a dead scalp. Cover grated root with apple cider vinegar and permit to set on a sunny windowsill for 10 days. Vinegar is then strained and stored in an airtight glass bottle.

When using on the skin, dilute with at least 50% water. Can be added to milk to bring more color to the face and to help relieve the itching of eczema. Soak 1 tbsp. freshly grated root in 1 cup of buttermilk for half an hour before straining. Dab on face and allow to remain for 15 minutes before rinsing with water. Refrigerate the rest for later use.

Warm Up Tea

During the winter or when an older person experiences cold sensations in the hands, legs and feet due to poor circulation, a nice "warm up" tea can be taken to relieve some of this hypothermic feeling. Bring 1 quart of water to a boil. Add 1 tbsp. each grated ginger root and grated horseradish root. Cover and reduce heat, simmering for 10 minutes. Remove from heat, uncover and add 2 tbsps. each fresh or dried mustard greens and watercress. Cover and steep for an hour. Flavor with a pinch of powdered kelp and dash of lime juice. Drink 1 cup lukewarm every few hours.

Postnasal Drip Cured

There is an effective folk remedy marketed by some of the Florida Amish in the form of an encapsulated product called "Old Amish Sinus-Stop." Those who've used it report that many of their sinus problems cease or eventually clear up. This includes postnasal drip, sinus infection, and sinusitis. The formula includes a mild horseradish, echinacea, and other herbs and spices. It may be ordered by mail from Old Amish Herbs of St. Petersburg, Florida (see Product Appendix for more data).

Sauce Recipe

Here's a favorite horseradish sauce that's been in the Heinerman family for almost 200 years and was brought to America by my grandmother, Barbara Liebhardt Heinerman from the old country (Temesvar, Hungary) at the turn of the century.

It delivers full flavor and body, but without the unpleasant bite.

MY GRANDMA'S BASIC HORSERADISH SAUCE

Needed: 1/4 pint plain yogurt; 1/4 pint homemade mayonnaise (see recipe below); 2-1/2 tbsps. grated horseradish; 1/2 tbsp. each of lemon, lime and grapefruit juices. Mix everything together in blender or by hand. Goes great with fowl, fish, and beer.

GOOD HOMEMADE MAYONNAISE

Needed: 1 cup sour cream; 1/4 cup plain yogurt; 3 tbsps. of pressed onion juice; 1/2 tsp. pure maple syrup; 1/4 tsp. ground ginger root; 1 tsp. dillweed; 1 tsp. each very finely minced French tarragon and chervil (both fresh). Mix everything in blender until a smooth and even consistency has been reached. Makes 1-1/2 cups.

Horseradish, a Part of the Jewish Passover

The ritual of the Passover, in which horseradish plays an integral part, celebrates the Jews' flight to freedom from slavery under the Egyptian Pharaoh Ramses II, with the parting of the Red Sea by Moses. The Hebrew word for Passover is Pesach, which signifies the "passing over" of the Jewish homes by the angel of death sent from heaven to slay the firstborn of Egyptian families, in retaliation for Pharoah hardening his heart and refusing to release God's people from bondage.

During the eight days of Passover, Jews eat only unleavened bread (called matzo) to commemorate the frantic exodus from Egypt, when there was not enough time for their bread to rise. Jews say "Kiddush" and drink kosher wine during Passover to praise the glory of God, who created the fruit of the vine. During this special celebration, also known as the festival of the unleavened bread, Jews are asked to sacrifice by eating only this "bread of affliction."

On the first night of Passover, which begins at sundown the day before Friday, Jews sit down at the Seder dinner table, reading from the Haggadah— a special book recalling the story of the first passover—and partake of symbolic foods, representing the horrors their ancestors endured as slaves in Egypt, and the joyful coming of spring. A ceremonial plate, prominently set in the middle of the table, displays the Passover symbols— a burnt shankbone, reminiscent of the lamb that was sacrificed in the Holy Temple, then roasted and eaten for the main meal. It is the primary symbol of redemption from bondage. Lamb is often served at Passover feasts.

Parsley is universally a symbol of spring. But at the Passover table it is dipped in salt water, to remind Jews of the tears shed in slavery. Morar, or *the bitter herb, is represented by horseradish*, which is the symbol of the bitterness at the servitude of the Pharaoh. Charoset, a mixture of grated apples, chopped nuts, and wine, represents the mortar and mud bricks used by the Isrealites to build Pharoah's cities. During the ceremony, it is combined with the morar between two pieces of matzo to symbolize the oppression and optimism of the Jewish people.

A roasted or hard-boiled egg is part of the ceremonial plate, too. It symbolizes rebirth and spring. Wine is critical to Passover—four cups are called for during the long ceremonial dinner, and people spill 10 drops onto their plate, one droplet for each of the 10 plagues visited upon Pharoah by God for refusing to free the Isrealites. This is the religious feast of the Jews in which horseradish plays an integral part.

HORSETAIL OR SHAVE GRASS
(EQUISETUM ARVENSE)

Brief Description

This perennial plant is common to moist loamy or sandy soil all over North America and Eurasia. It is a strange-looking sort of plant with creeping, stringlike rootstock and roots at the nodes that produce numerous hollow stems, which are of two types. A fertile, flesh-colored stem grows first, reaching a height of 4-7 inches and bearing on top a conelike spike which contains spores; this stem quickly dies. A green, sterile stem grows up to 18 inches high and features whorls of small branches. In the dinosaur era, horsetails reached incredible heights of up to 40 feet or more and resembled skinny lodgepole pines, but lacking the green boughs. During the Middle Ages clumps of the plant were often used as scouring pads to clean iron cookware and pewter dishes due to a high silicon content.

Heals Fractures, Torn Ligaments

No other herb in the entire plant kingdom is so rich in silicon as is horse-tail. This trace element really helps to bind protein molecules together in the blood vessels and connective tissues. Silicon is the material of which collagen is made. Collagen is the "body glue" that holds our skin and mus-cle tissues together. Silicon also promotes the growth and stability of the skeletal structure.

A few European clinical studies have determined that fractured bones heal much more quickly when horsetail is taken. The incidence of osteo-porosis is, likewise, more greatly reduced when some horsetail is added to the diet. A few folk healers I'm aware of have recommended this herb to athletes who've suffered sprains, dislocated joints, pulled hamstrings or torn ligaments. Generally three tablets or capsules daily has been the rule-of-thumb until total healing has resulted of the injuries sustained.

An Internal Cosmetic

Horsetail is that kind of rare and unique cosmetic agent which beautifies from the inside out rather than just externally. It improves the texture and tone of hair, nails and skin, and greatly strengthens bones and teeth. Some even ascribe to this herb a certain hidden "youth factor."

A special type of horsetail, grown, harvested and processed in Europe, has become the favorite of many American consumers. This for-mula is marketed in local health food stores under the name of Alta Sil-X Silica and was developed by a Pasadena, California naturopathic/homeo-pathic physician, Dr. Richard Barmakian. His formula contains an extract more easily assimilated by the body without some of the harsh complica-tions attending other horsetail products and found in the whole herb itself. An average of 2 tablets each day has been prescribed by him to a number of his patients for revitalizing externally and rejuvenating internally.

Reduces Bleeding, Good Diuretic

A tea made of horsetail helps to reduce minor edema. Half a cup internal-ly every 45 minutes works well to stop bleeding in the urine and the stool. Some powder from an empty capsule or a crushed tablet can be sprinkled on a minor cut. Horsetail is a reliable diuretic for all urinary problems. In 1 pint boiling water, add 2 tbsps. herb and steep for 30 minutes. Drink 3 cups daily or 3 tbsps. every 1-1/2 hours. Dr. Barmakian's Alta Sil-X Silica from any local health food store or obtained directly from Alta Health Products is just as effective as well.

HO-SHOU-WU
(POLYGONUM MULTIFLORUM)

Brief Description

Ho-shou-wu is a perennial herb that can grow anywhere from 23 to 33 feet in length. The leaves are petiolate, about 2-1/2 inches long and 1-1/2 inches wide. The tip is acuminate, the base cordate. Flowers are white and appear in September and October.

The tuberous root is often irregularly shaped, reddish brown, and bitter and astringent to the taste. The larger the root, the more effective and valuable the plant. Oriental herbalists highly prize thicker, older roots of ho-shou-wu. In some of the market places in Taiwan or mainland China (especially down by Hong Kong), I've been reliably informed by some herb doctors that slices of the very old roots are darker in color and more potent than younger ones, which are streaked with white and usually of lower quality. One way of determining quality is to see *how* the tuber has been cut. If the root is neatly sliced, this is a good indication that it is of higher grade.

Base Ingredient for Many Herbal Tonics

Ho-shou-wu is quite renowned throughout the Orient, and used by tens of millions of people regularly to help develop their Ch'i or life energy force. It is often taken in conjunction *with other herbs*, but sometimes can be used alone.

Ho-shou-wu has acquired a wide reputation through the centuries as a preserver of youthfulness and as a sexual rejuvenator, ideal for old age or for crippled sexuality or impotency. It also works to improve heart function and reduce elevated serum cholesterol levels.

Either the tablet/capsule or tea may be taken. Of the first, an average of two per day is suggested. For the second, about half a cup twice daily is advised. Bring 1/2 pint water to a boil; add 2/3 tsp. chopped, dried root; cover and simmer 10 minutes; strain and drink.

HYSSOP
(HYSSOPUS OFFICINALIS)

Brief Description

Hyssop is a perennial shrubby-looking herb with slender, stiff stems that can get almost a yard tall. The opposite leaves are narrow and pointed. Blue to purplish-blue flowers appear from July to October in small-one-sided clusters along the upper portion of the stems. Its range is from the Canadian province of Quebec to the "big sky country" of Montana, and as far south as the Carolinas.

Great American Poet Used Hyssop to Treat Respiratory Ailments

The first great major poet to create a truly American vision and style was Walt Whitman (1819-92). Ironically, though, he wasn't fully appreciated until a century after the publication of his masterpiece, *Leaves of Grass.* He was a key inspiration to the Beat Generation of the 1960s. ("Beatniks" as they were called in Greenwich Village in New York City, were the predecessors of the seventies' "hippies.") Beatniks were hopeless idealists and were more into poetry writing and reading, usually accompanied by the soft beat of a pair of bongo drums, than anything else. Whitman the man has been summarized by Allen Ginsberg, Galway Kinnell, and Donald Hall as being democratic, homosexual, lover of the human voice, purveyor of liberation, and a staunch believer in progress.

Because he used his voice a lot, Whitman sometimes suffered from periodic lung inflammation, sore throat, tender vocal cords, laryngitis, and occasional coughing spells. As a remedy, he resorted to hyssop quite frequently by making an infusion of the plant, then sipping one or more cups of the *very warm* tea.

Bring one pint of distilled water to a rolling boil. Then add two heaping tablespoons of hyssop leaves, cover, and let steep away from the stove for 30 minutes. Strain and reheat, if necessary, before *slowly* drinking. Up to four cups a day may be necessary if the problem is severe enough.

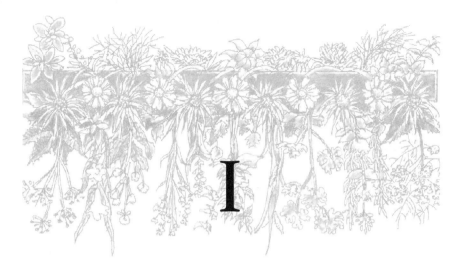

I

ICELAND MOSS
(see MOSS)

INDIAN TOBACCO
(see LOBELIA)

IPECACUANHA
(CEPHAELIS IPECACUANHA)

Brief Description

Ipecacuanha, commonly referred to as ipecac, is a tropical, perennial, herbaceous plant that grows to 1-1/2 feet high. It has a slender, cylindrical, corky, underground stem from which extend several horizontal roots. When mature, the roots have from brick-red to dark-brown "bark," that is smooth or somewhat prominently transversely ridged or ribbed. They have a musty odor and a bitter taste.

Ipecac is native to the humid forests of Bolivia and Brazil, especially around Mato Grosso and Minas Gerais. Most of the roots originally used for this drug came from wild plants, but in the mid 1960s experimental cultures of ipecac were begun in Bolivia and Nicaragua. Within a decade several large plantations were underway in South America that were capable of growing a half million plants each per year to supply the nearly 83 tons of roots needed for harvest annually.

Chief Antidote for Some Types of Poisoning

One of the most popular uses for ipecac, in the form of a syrup, has been as an emetic to stimulate the vagus nerve, which induces vomiting and empties the stomach of poisons. Medical doctors and hospital emergency rooms still routinely prescribe it for food, mushroom, plant and some chemical poisonings (except for lye, petroleum products, or strychnine). It has also been successfully administered to relieve tachycardia (excessively rapid heartbeat). Ipecac syrup is generally included in poison antidote kits because of these emetic properties. Also included is some activated charcoal to be used as directed by a physician to counteract the effects of different poisonous substances. Each kit usually contains a half-ounce bottle of ipecac syrup and a 5-gram container of activated charcoal packaged in a plastic box.

Some years ago, when I was an assistant scoutmaster, I had to use the contents of such a kit when one of our Boy Scouts accidentally sampled what he thought were "safe" mushrooms; as luck would have it, they weren't. I gave him 15 milliliters of the syrup and then followed this up with enough water from my canteen to equal about 1-1/2 glasses. Within about 5 minutes, we had success, which probably saved his life.

Syrup of ipecac is available at your local pharmacy as an OTC (over-the-counter) drug. The average dose for a child under 13 who has been poisoned is one teaspoonful; for teenagers and adults, about one tablespoonful, in each case with 1-2 glasses of water. Vomiting will generally be induced within a matter of minutes. If not, then the same procedure should be repeated again in 20-minute intervals until stomach contents are totally evacuated.

IRIS
(Iris species)
(also see BLUE FLAG)

Brief Description

It has been estimated that there are more than 200 species of Iris and even more hybrids. Nearly all of them may be used as cut flowers and some can be grown as potted plants. Irises ordinarily grow from either a thickened underground stem called a rhizome or a bulb and are available in a vast variety of colors and flower forms. The leaves of nearly all species and hybrids are linear or sword-shaped.

The rootstocks of some iris species and hybrids (particularly *I. germanica, I. florentina,* and *I. pseudoacorus*) have demonstrated the presence of certain glycosides and resins that can induce intestinal miseries, if consumed in a fresh state. It is much more advisable to cut the bulb into pieces and dry them out for a week before ingesting them. You can also gently pound the fresh bulbs to a slightly pulpy mass and then soak them in some wine for a few days before using them internally. Either way will render the bulbs more tolerable to the gastrointestinal tract.

Good for Dry Coughs and Hoarseness

When iris bulb is dried and ground into a powder, it yields a pleasant violet-like odor. One-half teaspoonful of this powder stirred in two-thirds glass warm water and slowly sipped will stop an annoying dry cough. If the same tincture is gargled before being swallowed, it will relieve hoarseness of the throat due to excessive use of the vocal cords.

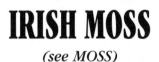

IRISH MOSS
(see MOSS)

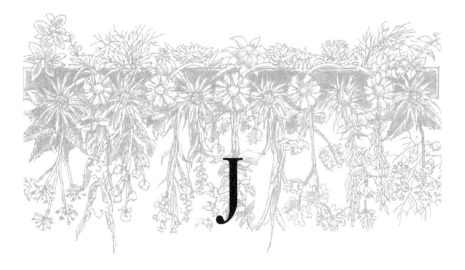

JAPANESE HONEYSUCKLE
(Lonicera japonica)

Brief Description

More than a few horticulturists have described this plant as having a dual personality. For where else could you find in the same plant something that cloaks a front porch with fragrance and protects a steep bank from erosion, while at the same time brutally invading woodlands by climbing up large trees and eventually smothering them to death?

Though nurseries still offer it as a flowering vine and fast-growing groundcover, in many people's eyes Japanese honeysuckle has earned its bad reputation as one of the most pernicious weeds around. As a competitor it has few equals. One plant may produce 30 feet of vine in a single year. The root system of an established plant may be six feet across and three feet deep. Additional roots are produced readily at the nodes along the stem, providing an even greater supply of water as well as insurance that the vine will continue to spread if something should happen to the mother plant.

The foliage of this plant is semi-evergreen. In mild winters it retains a significant portion of its leaves, and even when winters are more severe it leafs out nearly two months ahead of most deciduous species, giving it a vegetative jump on the season. The two-lipped tubular flowers open white in May and may even be tinged with purple. As the summer progresses into fall they deepen to a soft yellow. The flowers are an absolute delight to young children, who enjoy pulling out each pistil to sample the drop of sweet nectar at its base. New blossoms open at dusk, which facilitates visits by night-flying hawkmoths, and the fragrance is strongest in the evening, when you are most apt to detect that distinctive sweetness carried by a warm breeze.

Bluebirds, juncos, purple finches, robins, and white-throated sparrows all eat the shiny black fruits and distribute the seeds over a greater distance, thereby assuring the Japanese honeysuckle's prolific spread.

Relieves Nervous Tension and Anxiety

One of the most unique applications I've ever found for this vine was in relieving anxiety and nervous tension in individuals who were hypersensitive to stressful situations. Some people often experience a tightening feeling in their chests or throats; they clear their throats, are rather fidgety, and become easily paranoid over things that the rest of us might ignore.

A tea is made of the leaves and vine stem. Bring a quart of water to a rolling boil; add 1-1/2 cups cut leaves and stems. Cover, lower the heat and simmer for five minutes. Then turn off the stove and let the contents steep for 40 minutes. Strain, sweeten with honey, and drink one cup of *warm* tea every 4-6 hours on an *empty* stomach. In most cases the Japanese honeysuckle brew will help to ease the mental and emotional tensions of those who suffer from constant anxiety.

Interestingly enough, this is also one of the important flower remedies developed over 60 years ago by Dr. Edward Bach, a renowned London physician.

JASMINE
(JASMINUM OFFICINALE)

Brief Description

This vinelike plant is indigenous to the warmer regions of the eastern hemisphere and is currently grown in some gardens throughout the southern United States. Some species of jasmine also appear as evergreen or deciduous shrubs. The vine leaves are usually opposite, dark green and pinnate. Both the vines and the shrubs produce extremely fragrant flowers which are of considerable value in the perfume industry.

The unique aroma has been described as being a "delicate, sweet odor so peculiar that it's without comparison one of the most distinct of all natural odors."

Overcomes Sexual Frigidity

In parts of China and India, the oil extracted from the flowers of jasmine has often been used to arouse erotic emotions in those who may experience frigidity during sexual engagements.

For those who can afford to purchase jasmine oil from specialty shops, they may find that massaging certain areas of the body, such as the abdomen and groin, with a few drops mixed in with some sweet almond oil should help to promote sexual stimulation.

It is also said that a few drops rubbed on the upper lip below the nostrils contributes to this heightened stimulation.

JEWELWEED
(IMPATIENS PALLIDA)

Brief Description

In Mother Nature's wisdom, she seems to have always provided a handy remedy somewhere nearby for a very real problem. In my various herb treks through the Appalachias from North Carolina south to Georgia and in Glacier National Park in northwest Montana, I've never ceased to be amazed at finding this lovely and useful plant located not very far from poison ivy or poison oak. Knowing that some of us would probably encounter the latter, Mother Nature placed an easy cure within our reach in the former.

Jewelweed has succulent, transparent and watery stems, leaves that look silvery when held beneath water, and pale yellow and spotted flowers that are horn-shaped and closed at the bigger end. I discovered to my own amazement that if you reach out and gently touch one of the plant's urn-shaped flowers, it will immediately jump from its position and shoot out a couple of inches; hence, the other common name of "spotted touch-me-not."

Blackfoot Cure for Poison Ivy/Oak Rash

Once when I was in Montana on the Blackfeet Indian Reservation, I had an old medicine woman show me how she had often used this herb on others unfortunate enough to have encountered poison ivy or poison oak. She picked a generous handful of the jewelweed and plunged it into a small pail of water, then took it out and shook it hard. She next rubbed half of this amount between the palms of both hands until the stems were fairly well broken up. She then handed the plant material to me and told me to rub it all over my face, neck, arms, hands, chest, abdomen, thighs, legs, and feet, while she used the rest of it to rub all over my back. My first-hand experience with jewelweed convinced me that it is the *single best cure* for many different types of skin maladies where serious inflammation and painful itching are involved.

Also, some crushed jewelweed held on an insect bite or sting or where the skin has made contact with stinging nettle, briars or brambles, will quickly deaden the pain and stop the itching sensation.

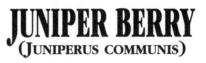

JUNIPER BERRY
(JUNIPERUS COMMUNIS)

Brief Description

Those who imbibe gin have only to take a whiff or sip of it to be able to discern the scent and taste of juniper berry. Although it also grows as a tree, one usually thinks of the juniper as a low, scraggly, creeping, prostrate evergreen with miniature vinelike needles instead of leaves, and fragrant blue berries that provide a nourishing and pleasant nibble.

Our family ranch in the Painted Desert wilderness of southern Utah is just below and east of Bryce Canyon, a world-famous national park noted for its beautiful towering sandstone formations. Juniper trees, wild Oregon grape shrubs, and sagebrush dot the landscape everywhere. It is a tree we have come to love and respect.

The common juniper is a low evergreen shrub between 12 and 30 feet high, growing low and spreading upright. The bark of the trunk is reddish-brown and shreddy. The pine-family needles are straight, sharply tipped, ridged, and nearly at right angles to the branchlets.

The male flowers are yellow and form a short catkin; the greenish female flowers are composed of three to eight pointed scales, some or all of which bear one or two ovules.

Scales of the female flowers become fleshy and fuse to form small, indehiscent strobili commonly called berries, which ripen the first, second or occasionally the third year, depending upon the species involved. When I was in the former Soviet Union in 1979, various plant scientists with whom I discussed juniper used the term *aril* instead of berry for these fruits. They informed me that the immature berries are generally greenish; ripe berries are blue-black to red-brown and are usually covered with a conspicuous white, waxy bloom. I've discovered in my own investigative work that the fruit coat may be thin and resinous as in eastern red cedar, Rocky Mountain, and one-seed juniper, or nearly leathery or mealy as in the Utah juniper.

There are usually one to four brownish seeds per fruit; rarely will you find as many as a dozen seeds. The seeds are rounded or angled, often with longitudinal pits. The seed coat has two layers—the outer layer is thick and hard, the inner thin and membranous. Embedded within the fleshy, white-to-creamy-colored endosperm is a straight embryo with two to six cotyledons. However, many seeds from a given tree may lack endosperm or embryo.

Sometimes berry crops will be heavy throughout a woodland; other times few berries are ever produced throughout a large geographic region. Almost every year a tree can be found in a stand that is so loaded with berries it appears covered with wax; such trees are popularly known as candle trees.

In the western United States, juniper also goes by the name of cedar; hence, a reference to "cedar berries" can also mean "juniper berries."

Antiseptic Aerosol for Lung Disorders

I'm intimately acquainted with juniper berries since I've used them for many years in treating a wide range of health problems. They are particularly efficacious in certain lung disorders.

An elderly lady residing in Hurricane, Utah was suffering from bronchial asthma. She had been under doctors' care for some time and on just about every current medication, but with little relief or benefit. Both she and her family were getting very discouraged with her lack of progress.

The matter was referred to me by one of her daughters. I recommended the use of juniper berry oil in an electric vaporizer. I instructed the daughter to have her mother mix 15 drops of juniper berry oil with 3/4 cup distilled water and then put this in a vaporized setting on a nightstand by her bed and turn it on. The patient was then to lie down on the bed and inhale the antiseptic aerosol given off for a period of 1 hour. This treatment would enable her to breathe better for up to 4 hours, after which time the process would need to be repeated again.

I explained to her how to make the juniper berry oil as well. Ripe juniper berries (one full cup) are lacerated and pounded in a stone mortar and pestle. (If such items aren't handy, then use a cutting board and wooden mallet.) Add the pulpy mixture to two pints of pure virgin olive oil and allow the entire solution to set in a glass Mason jar in a warm place, with the lid lightly screwed on for three days. After that the oil is strained, bottled, and labeled.

The daughter reported to me some time after this that her mother's condition had vastly improved by weeks on this treatment. The treatment is also recommended for emphysema, sinusitis, head cold, and influenza. The use of juniper berry incense or the aerosol oil also helps to disinfect a room previously contaminated by germs emitted from a sick person's breathing, coughing, nose blowing, talking or laughing.

I probably should mention in passing that in the preparation of juniper oil, some of the needles can be crushed with the berries to increase its strength.

Natural Birth Control Potential

India is a very crowded country with a huge population expected to top *one billion* by the middle of the next century. Most of its people, who are resigned to a life of virtual poverty, never practice any form of birth control, which explains this explosive growth.

Medical researchers, therefore, have a strong incentive for finding natural means of birth control from the plant kingdom that could be given to the population without any religious or social hindrances. The journal *Fitoterapia* (65:248-52, 1994) recently reported "potent antifertility activity" from an extract of dried juniper berries. Adult female rats given 300-400 milligrams of the berry extract per kilogram of body weight experienced considerable interference with their progesterone activity. This antihormonal activity prevents the females from becoming fertile. Further studies are currently underway to determine juniper's role as a possible natural birth control agent for women.

Knocks the Flu for a Loop

When influenza hits, it usually spells a long period of aggravating miseries, which seem to change with the infection going through its several different stages of activity. The worst part about the flu, however, is that it usually tends to linger for days, even weeks, after the worst symptoms have passed.

There are a number of herbal remedies for coping with the flu. But none of the herbalists I know or the books they have written have ever suggested hot juniper tea for this problem. In fact, I didn't even know myself just how good it was until an old Navajo shaman years ago acquainted me with it when I was an invited guest in his hogan, located out in the middle of nowhere.

I somehow picked up the flu "bug" before I got there, and it didn't take very many hours to aggressively dominate my body. In plain words, I felt like hell! But my friend, Ned Many Sheeps, boiled me up some tea by throwing a handful (probably one-half cup) of juniper berries into an old coffee pot sitting on top of an old iron stove situated in the center of the dirt floor and filled with one quart of boiling water. A series of black stove pipes snaked their way up through a hole in the rounded clay roof firmly packed down on top of sawed juniper planks laid next to each other in a circular fashion and expertly supported together in the middle without the benefit of a center column.

Between the strong juniper scent and the hot tea he kept pouring into me every couple of hours, I got better in a big hurry, I can assure you. The warmth of the tea felt good going down and induced the perspiration I probably needed to throw off the excess poisons within me. The strong disinfectant properties within the berries themselves went a long way in killing the viruses responsible for my miseries.

Not only did I quickly recover, but I fully recuperated. I'm not being redundant with this statement. Remember earlier how I said that remnants of the flu usually tend to hang on for days or weeks after most people have gotten over the worst parts of their infections? Well, in my case, there was *no* additional evidence of anything lingering; when I got well, that was it, *period.*

Stops Internal Hemorrhaging Quickly

Here's an herbal math equation for emergency situations: juniper astringency times internal bleeding equals first-aid *coup d'etat.* You see, when juniper berries (1/2 cup) are simmered in hot water (1-1/2 pints) for a while (25 minutes), certain important constituents from their oils are extracted that help to hasten the coagulation process when taken internally.

The tea must be warm, however, for this to work. Half-cup amounts should be slowly sipped every 1-1/2 hours when the stomach is empty to do the most good.

CAUTION: Juniper berry is contraindicated in pregnancy and in cases of kidney inflammations.

An Important Role in Diabetes

Researchers in the Department of Pharmacology with the Universidad de Granada in Granada, Spain recently tested a decoction of juniper berries on diabetic-induced female Wister rats. Each rat was given the decoction at a dose of 125 milligrams of the total berries per kilogram of body weight, for 24 days straight. Every rodent drinking the juniper tea, according to a report published in *Planta Medica* (60:197-200, 1994) "showed significantly reduced blood glucose levels, lost less weight, and had a significant lower mortality [death] index compared with untreated diabetic rats." Autopsy results afterwards on all of the test animals showed that the hypoglycemic activity of the berries was due to an increased consumption of peripheral glucose, and/or an increased glucose-induced insulin secretion.

To make a decoction of juniper berries, bring one quart distilled water to a boil, then add one-half cup berries. Cover, lower heat and simmer for 50 minutes. Let cool before straining; store in refrigerator. Drink one cup three times daily with meals.

CAUTION: Excess or prolonged consumption of juniper berry tea can irritate the kidneys and urinary tract. Also, this *isn't* a cure for diabetes, merely a natural way to help control it better and *decrease* but *not* entirely eliminate, daily insulin dependency.

I am grateful to Mathew King, a Lakota (Sioux) spokesman for the more traditional members of the Pine Ridge Reservation in South Dakota, and Beyond Words Publishing of Hillsboro, Oregon for the following true story which appeared in *Wisdomkeepers: Meetings with Native American Spiritual Elders* (Hillsboro: Beyond Words Publishing, Inc., 1990; pp. 31-33).

> Once, while I was up on the mountain, I prayed to God to give us a cure for diabetes. And while I was there, somebody said, "Turn around." So I turned around and there was the most beautiful Indian woman I'd ever seen. She had long black hair and the most wonderful face. She was holding something out to me in her hand. It was those little berries of the cedar [or juniper], the dark blue berries on cedar [juniper] trees. She held them out, but before I could reach out my hand she disappeared.

> I know who she was. She's the one who brought the sacred Pipe to our people. We call her White Buffalo Calf Woman. God sent her to save the Indian people. [But] that was long ago...So, I knew when I saw her up on the mountain that this was the same woman. But she disappeared before I could take those blue berries from her hand.

> Later on, when I got diabetes, I forgot about the berries. They sent me to White Man's doctors. They gave me pills. Every morning I had to take insulin. I spent a lot of time in the hospital. Then I remembered White Buffalo Calf Woman and those little blue cedar [juniper] berries. I picked some, boiled them, strained the juice, and drank it. It's so bitter it took the sugar right out of my body. The doctors checked me and were amazed. They said the diabetes was gone. *I didn't have to take insulin any more!* They asked me how I did it, but I didn't say. God gave us medicine to share with people, but if the White Man gets his hands on it he'll charge you a great price and will let you die if you don't have it. [But] God's medicine is free. God doesn't charge a fee. We don't give money to God. We give him our prayers, our thanks.

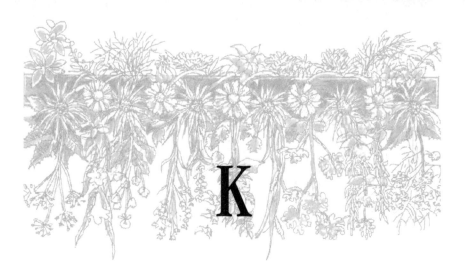

K

KAVA KAVA
(PIPER METHYSTICUM)

Brief Description

This tall, leafy shrub of the South Pacific has been used for many centuries among the islands of Oceania as a social beverage for many different occasions. The infusion prepared from the rhizome or stem of the plant is still used in many social ceremonies—to welcome visitors, commemorate marriages, births and deaths and to remove curses.

Polynesian Relaxant

A recently published study in the *Journal of Ethnopharmacology* reported that the pyrones in kava kava helped reduce anxiety and fatigue as well as relaxing twitching heart muscles and calming hysteria.

Other researchers who've worked with kava kava have described its effect upon the central nervous system as being "placidly tranquil." In a study with rats, they found that while this herb truly relaxed the rodents, yet in no way did it affect their overall mental or physical performances.

Hence kava kava can be taken on a regular basis without interrupting one's ability to work. In fact, it will probably help ease some of the stress that accompanies most jobs these days. The best brand of kava kava can be purchased in any health food store under the Nature's Way logo. An average of two capsules twice daily (late morning and late afternoon) on an empty stomach is recommended.

KELP
(Fucus vesiculosus)

Brief Description

The common name of kelp applies to a broad range of seaweeds of many different species. But for major users of herbs, kelp probably refers to seaweeds of the brown alga order Laminariales which possess large, flat, leaflike fronds. A class of brown algae called bladderwrack is generally used most often for producing kelp products.

Iodine Content Controls Obesity

Kelp has many medicinal uses and claims attributed to it. One of the more popular is in controlling obesity, probably because of its iodine content which is believed to stimulate production of iodine-containing hormones that help keep you slim. Doctors recognize that the thyroid gland is the body's own pace-setter, either having our cellular engines merely poke along or else race at breakneck speed. When thyroid activity moves at a snail's pace, fat isn't burned rapidly enough, and, therefore, accumulates in the body. However, when the thyroid accelerates, fat disappears more quickly before it can form deposits in body tissue somewhere.

Recommended intake of kelp tablets or capsules for weight control under the Nature's Way label from your local health food store is at least two per day with a meal. If you are on a sodium-restricted diet, you should monitor intake with care.

Great Seasoning

Kelp is an ideal substitute for table salt and black pepper and should be used wherever these other two seasonings are called for since it's healthier and far less problematic.

KOLA NUT
(Cola acuminata)

Brief Description

The dried seed or cola nut comes from evergreen trees with long, leathery leaves and growing up to 66 feet in height. They are native to western

Africa, Indonesia and other tropical climates. The fruit consists of 4-5 leathery or woody pods each containing 1-4 seeds. The seeds are dried and their outer coats removed. Although not actually a nut as such, it resembles a nut in appearance due to its hard consistency when dried.

Eliminates Fatigue

In small doses kola nut produces a passing excitement on the central nervous system, increases blood pressure slightly, and elevates the strength of the heartbeat. This is due to the presence of 1.5-2% caffeine and lesser amounts of theobromine, both natural stimulants to the body. Mental activity is likewise increased due to the considerable amount of fructose occurring naturally in kola nut, which reaches the brain to nourish it.

A leading health magazine, *East West Journal*, did a survey of herbal energy stimulants currently available in the market place and concluded that one product called Super Energy had the highest amount of kola nut, making it extremely effective. An average of 2 capsules daily from Great American of St. Petersburg (see Appendix) is the amount generally taken by thousands of consumers.

Helps Drug Withdrawal

The *Journal of the American Medical Association* (Nov. 4, 1974) recommended kola nut for sustaining the body during symptoms experienced when withdrawing from alcohol, tobacco and drug addictions. Great American also has another product called Kola Nut that is particularly useful in these cases (see Appendix). Up to 4 capsules daily as needed in such cases.

Diet Coke as a Contraceptive

Kola nut occurs in all cola beverages, but in varying concentrations. Diet Coke appears to have an unusually high concentration of kola nut. Researchers at Harvard Medical School studied the effect of Diet Coke on sperm motility and reported their findings in a 1985 issue of the *New England Journal of Medicine*.

They found that Diet Coke had the "most pronounced spermicidal action" of all the cola beverages. That is to say, Diet Coke killed all of the active sperm in the vagina when women used it as a douche immediately following sexual intercourse. Doctors speculate that it may have some as yet undiscovered value as a potential birth control agent in the near future.

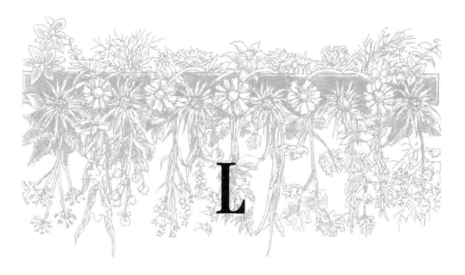

LAVENDER
(LAVANDULA OFFICINALIS)

Brief Description

Lavender is common to all portions of southern Europe, but is extensively cultivated elsewhere including in many of the southern and western United States. It prefers dry, sunny locations as a rule.

This small shrub with a woody stem averages between 6 and 24 inches in height, and has many branches. The leaves are opposite, very narrow, anywhere from 3/4 to 2 inches in length, are gray-green in appearance, and more or less tomentose.

Lavender flowers appear from June to September, but stay in bloom a little longer with one species (*L. latifolia*). They are small, baby-blue in color, strong-smelling, and culminate in spikes at the end of long stalks. One species in particular (*L. angustifolia*) has the finer odor. However, the flowers of all lavender species yield a highly perfumed, colorless, volatile oil that contains linalyle acetate and an hydroxycoumarin called herniarin.

First Aid for Minor Burns

James Lattimer of New Jersey considers himself a "holistic paramedic" with the local ambulance service for which he works. In cases that are not life-threatening and where the subjects don't object, he will use natural remedies wherever possible. "They're just a lot better for you than drugs are," he told me when we met at an alternative health convention in New York City.

Here is the simple treatment James uses for minor burns. First, he has the person hold the injured body part under running cold water for about 12 minutes, unless the skin is broken. Then he uses hydrogen peroxide and iodine tincture on the area to prevent infection from setting in.

The next procedure is to apply lavender *oil* promptly to the burned tissue. He recommends that a piece of gauze be used to cover it, securing it at the edges with only some strips of adhesive tape. This procedure is repeated every two hours for 24 hours, but without changing the gauze. If for some reason the burn has failed to completely heal in that length of time, he advises diluting 6 drops of lavender oil and 2 drops of geranium oil in 1 teaspoon olive oil. This mixture is then gently spread over the affected area. The process is repeated four times a day until it has totally healed. However, he was quick to caution that medical care should be sought IMMEDIATELY if the degree of burn is severe.

Relieve the Inflammation and Itching of Insect Bites/Stings

James has a good way of dealing with insect bites and stings. He suggests first removing the bee or wasp stinger very carefully with a pair of tweezers. Then apply one drop each of lavender and tea tree oils to the stung or bitten area. Repeat every hour on the hour until inflammation and itching symptoms subside. For subsequent applications, use four drops of lavender and tea tree oils diluted in a teaspoon of extra virgin olive oil. Apply twice daily until symptoms have cleared.

Wonderful Agent for Emotional Problems

James is a great believer in aromatherapy. He knows from personal experience how the essential oil of a particular plant can sometimes be better for a situation than using the entire herb or parts of it. He noted that in aromatherapy, inhalation, application, and baths are the principal methods used to encourage essential oils to enter the body.

He has employed the essential oil of lavender for a number of emotion-related problems, because it is "uplifting and soothing." He finds it ideal for "alleviating anxiety, depression and stress" as well as being "good for insomnia and migraines." Some drops of the oil can be used in an inhalation, a vaporizer, a bath, or as a topical application with good results.

The Ultimate Aphrodisiac

During early 1995, several national network news programs featured interesting research recently conducted by scientists in Chicago. Allen Hersch and his team, who are affiliated with the Smell and Taste Research Institute, discovered that certain smells dramatically increased the penile flow in healthy male volunteers more than other aromas did. Lavender flowers and pumpkin seed oils gave 40% more erections in men between the ages of 20 and 39 when they were told to sniff small swatches of material containing tiny amounts of either oil.

Interestingly enough, the smell of pure vanilla had more of a sexually arousing effect on older men (over the age of 45) than it did with younger ones. One of the conclusions reached from this fascinating piece of research is that certain aromas may have beneficial effects on men experiencing vasculogenic impotence. As one female television commentator wondered aloud, "Perhaps the real way to a man's heart is through his nose instead of his stomach."

Television comedian Jay Leno of "The Tonight Show" also added his own brand of humor to this story. "I just read an article in the newspaper the other day," he began, "which said that men got sexually stimulated when they smelled pumpkin. The scientists doing this study noticed that whenever male volunteers were exposed to the smell of pumpkin, they soon got strong erections. H-m-m-m, now I know why those carved jack-o-lanterns at Halloween are wearing those silly grins; they're probably up to something I can't mention on the air."

Great Cough Suppressant

If you ever have one of those coughing spells that sounds like the barking of a dog, then here is something to quell it in minutes. Take one-half cup of fresh lavender flowers and cover them with two cups of brandy or rum in a fruit jar with a screw-on lid. Store in a cool, dry place and shake twice daily for 5 days; try to do this at midnight when a full moon is present. I know this sounds like folklore, but it *really does* make for a much *stronger* tincture. Strain and store in another receptacle of some kind. Take one tablespoonful every 1-1/2 hours.

The other method is to add one-half cup *dried* lavender flowers to two cups boiling water. Cover, remove from heat, and steep for 30 minutes. Strain and sip a cup of the warm tea through a plastic straw, if necessary, every 3 hours.

My "Instant" Headache and Tension Reliever

There are very few things in nature that can work as quickly as their synthetic drug counterparts do. You have to take *a lot* of white willow bark tea or capsules in order to achieve the same effects that two Bayer aspirins or Tylenol capsules can deliver within minutes following consumption.

But there is *one* thing that works almost *instantaneously* to relieve headaches and muscle/nerve tension. Bear in mind that I'm a trained scientist (medical anthropologist) and my academic background has always taught me to stay on the conservative side, so I'm not exaggerating in the least when I say that. I'm speaking, of course, about a remarkable headache and tension relief remedy that I developed some years ago and, only until now, have kept pretty much a secret. But what good are secrets that can help, if they're not shared with others? They do nobody any good when the one keeping them takes them to the grave. So for that very reason, I've now decided to include it in this book for *the very first time!*

To begin with, it is *absolutely* essential that you work with *fresh* lavender flowers; dried ones simply won't do. Cut enough lavender flowers to fill one cup full. Then in a stone mortar and pestle, gently macerate and pound them well. Or use a rolling pin or a small ball-peen hammer on a cutting board or a table or countertop.

Then put these crushed flowers in a fruit jar and cover them with 1 to 1-1/4 pints olive oil, sesame seed oil, macadamia nut oil, or avocado oil. Set in a warm place for four days, shaking morning and night. Strain and add about 800 I.U. vitamin E oil to help preserve the other oil. Store in a cool, dark, dry place thereafter.

Whenever a headache comes on, just rub some of this oil across the forehead, on the sides of the temples, and the back of the neck. For other parts of the body, do the same thing, remembering always to rub in a circular motion using the tips of the three middle fingers. You'll be astonished at how quickly and effectively this simple remedy removes your aches and pains.

Infantile Colic Corrected

As you can probably guess by now, lavender happens to be one of my favorite herbs, judging from the length of this particular entry. The following true anecdote was related to me by Glen Harvey, then an Amtrak conductor on the Desert Wind train which ran from Salt Lake City to Los Angeles from midnight to the next afternoon.

"My son Ian was born on July 10, 1986. Early on he developed a very bad case of what the doctor termed 'infantile colic.' He had it from two days of birth to six months. We went to five different pediatricians. They just kept prescribing different formulas, none of which seemed to help our boy very much.

"By now I was getting pretty fed up with doctors in general. I said to my wife, 'You mean to tell me that with all of the medical doctors out there, no one seems to have a cure for this?' I mean, I'm telling you that our poor kid screamed so bad, my wife would have to take him to the park in our old VW [Volkswagon] van and let him bawl and scream so I could get some sleep during the daytime [he always worked the midnight shift].

"I went to work one night as usual in a grouchy mood 'cause the kid had kept me up part of the day. Our train engineer asked me what the matter was and I told him all about my kid's colic. He told me that his mom used lavender flower tea on her kids for this same complaint and he had used it on his own kids successfully. So sometime later when we were both off work, I went to his house in West Bountiful [Utah] to get some of this tea. We gave some of it warm in a bottle to our kid. I swear that the minute my kid starting drinking this stuff, he began looking and feeling much better. In two days, what the doctors couldn't cure, the lavender did—his colic disappeared and never came back again. I've had it with doctors, but have become a devoted disciple of herbs!" he concluded matter-of-factly.

Tea and Cake

Try some of this cake with some warm chamomile tea. You're in for a real taste treat and scrumptious snack delight.

WHOLE WHEAT LAVENDER CAKE

Needed: 2 eggs, separated; 1/4 cup hot water; 1 tsp. real vanilla; 3/4 cup brown sugar; 1/8 tsp. salt; 1 cup whole wheat pastry flour; 1 to 1-1/4 tsp. baking powder (preferably aluminum-free); 3 tbsps. lavender jelly; lavender berries and flowers for garnish.

Preheat oven to 325°. Pan spray an 8-inch round cake pan. In a large bowl, beat together egg yolks, water and vanilla until nicely thick and pale. Slowly beat in 1/2 cup sugar; set aside.

In a medium bowl, beat egg whites until foamy, add salt, and continue beating until they hold soft peaks. Gradually add remaining 1/4 cup sugar and beat until stiff peaks form.

Stir 1/4 cup of the whites into the yolk mixture. Spoon the remaining whites onto the yolk mixture and sift the flour and baking powder on top. Carefully fold until blended. Spoon into the pan and bake for 25 to 30 minutes, or until a toothpick comes out clean. Invert pan onto a rack and let the cake cool completely before removing pan.

Split the cake into layers and sandwich together with lavender jelly. Decorate with lavender berries and flowers.

Lavender Jelly

Needed: some cheesecloth; 4 tbsps. dried lavender flowers; 4 tbsps. powdered pectin; 3 cups apple juice; 2 tbsps. lemon juice; 3 cups brown sugar.

Line a small sieve with double thickness of cheesecloth. Cut a 5-inch square of cheesecloth, put lavender flowers in the center and tie up ends to form a small bag. In a 6-quart saucepan, combine pectin and apple juice, stirring until the pectin is dissolved,

Set the pan over high heat and bring to a boil, stirring constantly. Stir in the lemon juice and sugar and drop in lavender bag. Boil for 2 minutes, stirring constantly. Remove bag. Strain through cheesecloth-lined sieve into sterilized empty baby food jars. (To sterilize jars, immerse them in boiling water for 11 minutes.) Yield: Makes 3 8-ounce jars.

LEMON BALM
(MELISSA OFFICINALIS)

Brief Description

Lemon balm is a hardy lemon-scented perennial that was a favorite with bee-keepers in ancient times. They would rub some of the crushed fresh leaves on beehives to encourage bees to return to their hives and bring others with them. In fact, the generic name *Melissa* comes from the Greek word for bee; another common name for it happens to be "bee balm."

Lemon balm has upright, hairy, branching stems that reach a yard in height. Light green toothed ovate leaves grow in opposite pairs at each joint. White or yellowish two-lipped flowers appear from June to September and form in small loose bunches at the axis of the leaves, which emit a strong lemon scent.

Warm Tea Soothes Menstrual Cramps and Relieves PMS

Eleanor Hawkins is an executive secretary in California. Due to job stress, poor diet, and little sleep, she used to suffer frequently from menstrual cramps and other symptoms of premenstrual syndrome.

But when she started drinking some lemon balm tea, her problems cleared up. She began sleeping and eating better, too. In one cup boiling hot water, she would steep one teabag of lemon balm for 5 minutes before drinking. You can also put 1-1/2 tablespoonfuls of the leaves in one pint boiling water, cover, remove from the heat, and steep 15 minutes before straining and drinking.

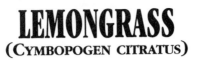

LEMONGRASS
(CYMBOPOGEN CITRATUS)

Brief Description

Lemongrass is common to the tropics of Southeast Asia, even though it is grown as well in India, Africa, Australia, the United States, and parts of the South American continent. The herb is characterized by a strong citrus flavor.

The most important constituent in the leaves is citral, which varies in amount with the locality in which the lemongrass is grown. Citral is used extensively as a fragrance component in soaps, detergents, creams, lotions, and perfumes. Lemongrass oil is used in most major food categories, including both alcoholic and nonalcoholic beverages, frozen dairy desserts, candy, baked goods, gelatins and puddings, meat and meat products, and fats and oils.

Relief for Aches and Pains

Lemongrass oil is sherry-colored with a pungent taste and lemon-like color. Three to six drops of the oil on a sugar cube or in one teaspoonful of real vanilla flavor provides wonderful relief from intestinal gas, colic, and obstinate vomiting. Ten or fifteen drops of the same oil can be rubbed into the skin to relieve lower backache, sciatica, lumbago, sprains, tendinitis, and rheumatism.

A tea can be made by adding one-half cup dried lemongrass leaves to two pints water, covering and simmering on low heat for about 10 minutes before straining. One cup every four hours is recommended for fevers.

An Unusual Insect Repellant

A related species of perennial grass called citronella (*Cymbopogon nardus*) is cultivated extensively in Sri Lanka, Malaysia, Indonesia, Africa, and Central and South America. The oil has been reported to have antibacterial and antifungal activities in vitro, being as active as penicillin against certain Gram-positive bacteria. As with lemongrass, citronella oil has been used as a fragrance component in soaps, brilliantines, disinfectants and perfumes, including almost the same foods uses cited for the former. But one area in which it is outstanding is as a major component in certain insect repellant formulations.

During a warm June evening in the summer of 1995, the Hansen family of Salt Lake City went for a picnic in City Creek Canyon. Others were there for the same purpose, but the gnats and mosquitos proved very annoying. In fact, several parties packed up their things and left earlier than expected. However, Mrs. Hansen came prepared. She had bought a unique product at a local supermarket that would save them from having to leave, too.

She removed from the package several flat, small candles containing citronella oil, placed them in candle holders, and lit them. The aromatic fumes kept *all* winged insects away, so they could enjoy their evening. The name of the product Mrs. Hansen used is *Off!*, made by Johnson Wax.

Cook's Choice

Lemongrass improves the taste of curries, soups, stews, and casseroles, especially those made with chicken and seafood. Here's something different for your next light meal.

HOT AND SOUR SHRIMP SOUP

Needed: 5 cups chicken stock; 4 scallions, white and green parts, chopped; 2 tbsp. chopped fresh cilantro; 1 small fresh hot green chili, seeded and chopped; 3 lemongrass stalks, cut into 1-inch pieces; pinch of salt; 1-inch piece lime peel; 2 tbsp lime juice; and 1 lb. shrimp.

In a saucepan, combine all the ingredients except the shrimp. Bring to a simmer, cover, and cook over low heat for 25 minutes to nicely blend the flavors. Strain and discard the solids. Return the liquid to the saucepan, add the shrimp, and cook until the shrimp are just heated through, no more than 1-1/2 minutes. Yield: Serves 4.

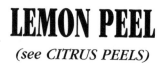

LEMON PEEL
(see CITRUS PEELS)

LICORICE ROOT
(GLYCYRRHIZA GLABRA)

Brief Description

Licorice is a perennial plant found wild in southern and central Europe and parts of Asia, and cultivated in the U.S. and Canada, to some extent. The woody rootstock is wrinkled and brown on the outside, yellow on the inside, and tastes sweet.

Heals Peptic Ulcers

Certain constituents found in human saliva and licorice root have nearly identical actions in healing peptic and duodenal ulcers. More remarkable still is the fact that these several constituents bear an uncanny resemblance to each other when examined under a high-powered electron microscope. Two capsules daily are useful for relief.

Treats Emotional Imbalances and Hysteria

Michael Tierra, a southern California practicing herbalist, really believes in the tranquilizing influence of licorice root on the nervous system. He often adds small amount of licorice to balance many of his formulas, harmonize the action of the herbs in them and to avoid potential side-effects later on. He calls licorice root a "peacemaker" type of herb.

In his book, *The Way of Herbs* (Santa Cruz, CA: Unity Press, 1980), Michael Tierra recommended this herb along with something like hops or skullcap or valerian to calm the nerves in cases of hysteria and mental or emotional instability. Two capsules daily are suggested.

Good for Addison's, Graves', and Parkinson's Diseases

Addison's disease is an autoimmune-induced destruction of the adrenal cortex that results in dangerously low blood pressure, weight loss, anorexia, weakness, and a bronzelike hyperpigmentation of the skin. Addison's is usually the fatal end of extended and untreated hypoglycemia. Graves' disease received media prominence during George Bush's presidency; his wife, Barbara, suffered from it. It is a thyroid disorder common to women.

Parkinson's is a slowly progressive disease characterized by a tremor of the resting muscles, a slowing of voluntary movements, hasty gait, peculiar posture, muscle weakness, excessive sweating and feelings of heat.

In every one of these health situations, licorice root will be of definite benefit. To what degree, though, depends on the length and severity of the illness involved. An average of three capsules each day (one per meal) or one cup of licorice root tea daily will lessen many of the symptoms connected with them, improve appetite and digestion, and stabilize muscle and nerve functions.

LILAC
(Syringa vulgaris)

Brief Description

The lilac can be either a shrub or small tree and is a member of the Oleaceae or Olive family. It is widely cultivated as an ornamental. Since colonial times, the common lilac has been one of the best loved of the flowering shrubs in America, meriting its favor by its cone-shaped masses of lavender or white flowers, its fragrance, and its ease of cultivation. The purple flower clusters of the lilac are the floral emblem of the state of New Hampshire.

Applications for Lilac

Some years ago I was a speaker on the medicinal folk applications for this shrub at one of the lilac festivals held annually in Rochester, New York. An attendee heard me mention my special "lilac tonic" for acid indigestion and decided to give it a try. She followed my instructions by adding one-half handful of lilac flowers to almost 2 pints of boiling water, covering, setting aside and steeping for 40 minutes. She strained and drank one cup of cool tonic with each meal and was amazed at how quickly her acid indigestion cleared up.

Another attendee used some of the shrub bark on one of her school-age children suffering from the fever that always accompanies measles, mumps, or chickenpox. She used a small pair of pruning shears to cut enough of the stems and bark to equal a handful, which she then added to 2 1/4 pints boiling water. She covered the pot and simmered the contents on low heat for 25 minutes. She strained the tea and gave half-cupfuls of the *warm* tea every 3 hours to her six-year-old son; his fever left him by the next morning and his condition was much improved thereafter.

Lilac tea is also good for gout, abdominal cramps, and rheumatism.

LILY
(LILIUM SPECIES AND HYBRIDS)

Brief Description

Lily is the common name for the Liliaceae, a plant family numbering several thousand different species of as many as 300 genera. They are widely distributed over the earth's surface, especially abundant in warm temperate and tropical regions. Most species are perennial herbs characterized by bulbs (or other forms of enlarged underground stem) from which grow erect clusters of narrow, grasslike leaves or leafy stems. A few are woody, and some are even small trees.

In an evolutionary sense, the lily family is without doubt the most basic monocotyledonous stock, its ancestors having given rise to the majority of contemporary monocots like the orchids, the palms, the iris and amaryllis families, and probably the grasses, too.

Many common flowers belong to the lily family: asphodel, brodiea, camass, Canada mayflower, dogtooth violet, greenbrier, lily of the valley, Solomon's-seal, Star of Bethlehem, and trillium. Because of the showy blossoms characteristic of the family, many species, including several of those already cited, are cultivated as ornamentals. In fact, this seems to be the chief economic value of the Liliaceae; over 160 genera are represented in the American trade alone.

Types of hyacinth, lily, meadow saffron, squill, and tulip constitute the bulk of the "Dutch bulb" trade in the Netherlands. It may surprise those who use the next two herbs a lot to know that both yucca and aloe species are popular lily succulents. And even more interesting is the fact that asparagus and plants of the onion genus are the only liliaceous food plants of commercial importance

Sego Lily Saved Mormon Pioneers from Starvation

The white-blossomed sego lily (Calochortus nuttalli) is the official flower of the "Beehive State" of Utah (so nicknamed because of the old-fashioned cone-shaped beehive which is the centerpiece of the state seal). This dainty plant with the trumpet-shaped flower and velvety-white petals rests on an 8-to-10-inch stem. The petals themselves are marked with orange and yellow colors near the yellow stamens which stand in its center.

Come every spring, tens of thousands of these exquisite botanical gems decorate the foothills all along the Wasatch Front, from Ogden on the north to Provo on the south. But in a moment of crisis nearly 150 years ago, the sego lily's bulb, with its distinctive nut-like flavor, served as a temporary means of food to keep the Mormon pioneers from literally starving to death.

In May of 1848, a "very severe frost" nipped all of the vegetables which the early settlers had just planted a month or so earlier. Another "cold, dry spell" in June did the grain in. By the time fall harvest came, "there was a veritable famine" throughout the territory, noted one historian. With the absence of flour, fruit, vegetables, and sugar, there was nothing left to fall back on save beef and the products of the cow—milk, cheese, and butter. Even these were in short supply, and couldn't feed the multitudes continually immigrating into the valleys.

As a last resort, thousands of Mormon pioneers took to eating sego lily roots, pigweeds, Canadian thistles, and stinging nettle. A favorite "soup" with many families was a pot full of water, chopped sego roots, and any old piece of rawhide or leather goods (boot, belt buckle, hat, glove, chaps, etc.) added for flavoring; everything was boiled over the fire until ready and then consumed with considerable relish. It may not have been your upscale *cuisine* for the gourmet crowd, but it certainly was better than mass starvation and death.

Bible's "Lilies of the Field" Had Reference to Stomach Tonic

The Bible has immortalized one species of lilies. Matthew 6:28 says: "Consider the lilies of the field....." He also stated that King Solomon, in all his magnificence and glory, "was not arrayed like one of these" (verse 29). Solomon had lived a sophisticated life, which was totally out of touch with the Kingdom of Heaven. But the lilies of which The Master spoke were simple, yet elegant, common, but extraordinary in their beauty.

Some Biblical scholars have pointed out in their writings that these particular "lilies of the field" were gathered in ancient times by the people and used for medicinal purposes. The beautiful flowers were steeped in hot water for an unspecified length of time, strained through cloth material, and then the tea drunk with meals to help settle an upset stomach.

Australian Red Lily Remedies Daydreaming and Indecisiveness

A book I picked up a few years ago in Australia mentions a singular application for another type of lily. Entitled *Australian Bush Flower Essences* (Moorebank, NSW: Transworld Publishers Pty. Ltd., 1991) and authored by Ian White, a highly respected naturopathic practitioner, it explains how the essence of red lily has been successfully used to treat negative mental functions such as indecisiveness and daydreaming.

Dr. White states that this flower essence (similar to the Bach Flower Remedies) is for those who "are up in the clouds, daydreaming...[who] lack an interest in worldly events and the present, and tend to fantasize and live in the future." Furthermore, he says, red lily essence is for those who "often lack concentration because their minds are elsewhere"; it is chiefly intended for those who "are very absent-minded and impractical, and live in thought rather than action."

He also claims that red lily can be employed by those "who are suffering from the detrimental effects of taking drugs, especially hallucinogens such as LSD or 'magic' mushrooms."

Red lily flower essence is taken morning and evening by putting 7-10 drops under the tongue or by adding the same number of drops to *distilled* water and taken over a two-week period. Some health food stores carry these flower essences. To receive more information or order products, write or call:

The Australian Bush Flower Remedy Society

P.O. Box 531, Spit Junction

New South Wales 2088, Australia

Tel: 02-972-1033

Star of Bethlehem Neutralizes Shock

Periodically throughout this book I've mentioned several of the Bach Flower Remedies. This was a method of treatment developed by a prominent London physician, Edward Bach. In addition to his 38 *single* remedies, there was a 39th which he termed Rescue Remedy. It is a composite formula of five other individual flower remedies:

Star of Bethlehem, for shock

Rock Rose, for terror and panic

Impatiens, for mental stress and tension

Cherry Plum, for desperation

Clematis, for the bemused, faraway, out-of-the-body

The Rescue Remedy is very simple to prepare. First, you need to purchase separate bottles of each of the previously mentioned remedies from any health food store, herb shop, or direct marketing company (Nature's Sunshine, Inc.) distributors that carry them. Next, add two drops from the stock bottles of each of these five other Bach Flower Remedies to a one-ounce (30cc.) bottle filled with brandy or rum; cork well or screw lid on tight and carry with you at all times.

Dr. Bach claimed that his "Rescue Remedy could well save a life during an emergency when seconds count, and before qualified medical help arrives." Add three drops of the Rescue Remedy to a glass of water. Have anybody who is experiencing mental and emotional traumas slowly *sip* this (preferably through a plastic straw). Or, if the person in shock is unconscious, then rub some drops on the lips, the gums, behind the ears, on the sides of the temples, and on the wrists.

You will be amazed (as I was when I first used it years ago) at just how efficiently it works on such trauma cases. The one in shock or experiencing severe panic, fear, or desperation will soon begin calming down and regaining his or her composure. "The Rescue Remedy has no ill effects, yet it is quite capable of saving a human life pending the arrival of a qualified physician," Dr. Bach stated.

In addition to this, Bach Flower Remedy Number 30, which consists of the Star of Bethlehem by itself, is of considerable therapeutic value in treating mental, emotional or physical shocks of any kind. This member of the lily family "quickly neutralizes the effects" caused by shock, Dr. Bach claimed. In his landmark study, *Handbook of the Bach Flower Remedies* (edited by Philip M. Chancellor) (London: C.W. Daniel Co. Ltd., 1971), seven case histories are presented in which Star of Bethlehem was successfully used to treat nervous tension, "utterable grief," insomnia, mental depression, deep anxiety (due to substantial financial misfortunes), nervous exhaustion, and hopelessness.

Remedy Number 30 is basically applied the same way as is the Rescue Remedy: 3-5 drops in one glass of water, or the same amount of drops rubbed on key nerve points around the head and face, in the mouth, and on the wrists.

Another Lily Member Counteracts Poison Ivy, Wounds, and Bruises

Solomon's seal (Polygonatum multiflorum) grows in woods and thickets all along the Atlantic Seaboard. This perennial herb has a thick, horizontal, scarred rootstock, which has been found to have suitable medical applications in treating poison ivy, wounds and bruises. The fresh root is dug up with a shovel, thoroughly cleaned under running water, and then pounded to a pulp with a hammer on a heavy cutting board or work bench. The mashed root is then spread out on a clean cloth and bound to the site of a wound or bruise and left for 24 hours before being changed. To counteract the effects of poison ivy/poison oak, boil one cup of the chopped root in 1-1/2 pints distilled water, covered, for 15 minutes. Allow the liquid to cool, then strain, and wash the afflicted skin with this tea.

LIME PEEL

(see CITRUS PEELS)

LOBELIA

(LOBELIA INFLATA)

Brief Description

This North American plant can be either annual or biennial. It grows wild in pastures, meadows, and many cultivated fields throughout the Midwest and eastern United States as well as the Rocky Mountain region and Pacific Northwest. Lobelia has an erect, angular stem and can reach upwards of a yard in height, is hairy and yields a milky sap when broken open or cut. The delicate leaves are light green, alternate, hairy, ovate, and bluntly serrate. The top is adorned with many small, two-lipped, blue flowers that grow in spike-like racemes in the last six months of the year.

Tried and True Remedy for Smoking Addiction, Whooping Cough, Asthma, and Erysipelas

Over 150 years ago lobelia was the mainstay of an eclectic botanical healing system developed by Samuel Thomson, known as Thomsonian Medicine. Once extensively employed in midwifery to eliminate the rigidity of pelvic muscles in childbearing women and for respiratory and inflammatory disorders, it has pretty well fallen out of favor at present except with a small number of those who still practice classical herbal medicine. They find that the herb is quite effective as a smoking deterrent, as a antispasmodic for whooping cough, for diphtheria, tonsillitis, and as an anti-inflammatory in cases of erysipelas.

The herb works best when used either as a tincture or tea. To make the tincture, mix 3/4 cup of cut fresh or powdered lobelia herb with one pint Russian vodka, English brandy, Southern gin, or Jamaican rum. Put in a glass fruit jar with a screw-on lid. Shake twice daily, in the morning and again at night, for sixteen days. Let the mixture settle before straining through cotton cloth or a paper coffee filter. Do this *during a full or new moon* so the potency of the tincture is stronger. This isn't only folklore but *scientific* fact! Take 5-7 drops beneath the tongue once or twice daily for 3 weeks or longer to curb nicotine cravings. Put 10-15 drops in one-half cup *distilled* water that is *lukewarm* and slowly sip to alleviate whooping cough, asthma, and tonsillitis.

To make a tea, bring 1 pint water to a boil and then add 2/3 cup cut fresh lobelia plant, cover and simmer on low heat for 10 minutes; set aside and steep 30 minutes more. Strain when cool and drink one-half cupfuls every four hours for dysentery or erysipelas, as well as bathing or sponging the skin with this tea for the latter condition.

LOOSESTRIFE
(see PURPLE LOOSESTRIFE)

LOVAGE
(LEVISTICUM OFFICINALE OR LIGUSTICUM OFFICINALIS)

Brief Description

Lovage is a perennial plant which grows between 3 and 7 feet tall and populates gardens, meadows and hedgerows in Great Britain. In some ways it closely resembles a few poisonous members of the carrot family, such as water hemlock, poison hemlock, and idiot's parsley (so named because only a stupid person would eat it). Its tiny pale yellow flowers are arranged in dense, umbrella-like clusters atop a thick, hollow stem. The leaves are divided several times, with lobed or sharply toothed leaflets. The lower leaves may grow as much as 2-1/2 feet in length. The plant emits an unmistakable celerylike aroma.

This One Is a Real Gasser

Lovage is of wonderful therapeutic benefit for relieving abdominal pains due to gastrointestinal gas and even in reducing the amount of what is passed. But more about that later. Right now, I want to talk about gas. Gastrointestinal gas, if you will. A former deputy director of the prestigious bank of England (who's story appears in this section) preferred to call it "breaking wind." But over here in America it's usually called flatulence by better educated folks, or just plain farts by the working class.

Terry Bolin, an Australian gastroenterologist, practices and teaches at the University of New South Wales Medical School in Sydney. In a phone call to him recently, I asked two of the most popular questions that have probably been on people's minds from time to time.

Q. "Why do beans cause so much gas?"

A. "Because they have lots and lots of fiber."

Q. "Why does gas sometimes smell so bad?"

A. "Because it usually contains high amounts of sulphur dioxide or hydrogen sulfide."

Yet, he explained to me, the production of odorless methane and sulphur dioxide is as normal a bodily process as blinking the eyes. Ironically, he noted, abundant gas production is, without a doubt, a sign that you're doing something right.

"Gas is the penalty you pay for eating a healthy diet," Dr. Bolin said. "Farting's a normal part of life. The more fiber you eat, the more gas will be produced, and the more you'll fart. A survey we did sometime ago showed a very nice correlation between increasing fiber and increasing farting in both men and women. By the way, advise your American readers that 'down under' [meaning in Australia] here, we consider the term 'farting' to be as socially acceptable as your term 'flatulence' up there."

Each of us is a walking gas factory, he went on to say, producing each day anywhere from 400 to 2,100 milliliters, with the average of 1,500 milliliters; this includes methane, ammonia, carbon dioxide, hydrogen, hydrogen sulfide, nitrogen and sulfur dioxide. This is enough gas to half-inflate a balloon for your little kid. "But," he hastily added, "If you're going to quote me direct, remind your readers that I was only using this as a mere illustration and didn't intend for it to be any kind of suggestion."

Most of the gas passed "is produced in the colon by bacteria as they break down some kinds of complex carbohydrates and most types of dietary fiber," he explained. "These good and useful bacteria grow and multiply by using the gases produced as a source of energy for themselves. Producing gas isn't abnormal at all. Just as some people have blue eyes and some brown, the bacteria in some people produce more foul-smelling sulphur dioxide and hydrogen sulfide in their gas than others have. In fact, if you *don't* produce very much gas, then there is probably something dreadfully wrong with you," he added.

"Holding gas in may be the polite thing to do," he pointed out, "but it isn't too good for the colon. The lower bowel is blown up like a balloon, creating a great deal of pain and pressure inside. And that gas needs to come out in a hurry. So better to be socially impolite than to create discomfort for yourself. By the way, a sitting posture always tends to produce a louder noise than standing does.

"People seem to give a lot of unnecessary attention to smell. Men definitely have, how should I say it, a more *aromatic flavor* than women. Women are inclined to hold theirs in, whereas we men just let it rush on out. Nothing much can be done about the aroma, though. Just as some people have blue eyes and some brown, the bacteria in some people produce more foul-smelling sulphur dioxide and hydrogen sulfide in their gas. Meat eaters always tend to smell up things more than vegetarians do, when they cut a 'ripe one.'

"Learn to like it and live with it. Think of gaseous emissions as a sign that the bacteria that live inside your colon are doing their jobs, breaking down your food and nourishing your body," he concluded.

Bank of England Official Drinks Tea to Help Relieve His Gas

As I promised you at the start of this section, there would be included here a true account of how one prominent London banker coped with his awful flatulence problem.

The 300-year-old Bank of England, which prints Britain's money and regulates its finances, stands in decorous splendor on Threadneedle Street in the heart of London's business district. Every morning, promptly at 8:30 a.m., its heavy doors are swung open by comical-looking guards in pink frock coats and black top hats. When I questioned one of them about his uniform, he took me aside and whispered in my ear that "I feel like a bloody fool wearing it, but it's part of me requirements for me weekly paycheck."

Once a week, the bank's august governing body, the Court of Directors as they are properly called, meets in an ornate lime-green room decorated with medallions of England's kings and queens. And ever since the beginning of the 18th century this venerable financial citadel has been called the Old Lady of Threadneedle Street.

A former deputy director of the place, who had been in charge of discipline and bank personnel, gave me a "royal tour" of the establishment, but asked that I not mention his name in connection with his use of lovage. Following a hearty lunch, we returned to his somewhat elegant office, where he proceeded to make both of us some lovage tea.

He put one level teaspoon of the dried root into each of two empty cups, followed with boiling water poured over them. These he let steep for about 15 minutes until they had sufficiently cooled, then took one himself and offered me the other cup. "It tastes much better if you leave the root in," he hinted with a smile, and we merrily sipped and chatted the hour away.

My host explained that he always drank a cup of lovage tea following every meal to "help reduce my breaking wind so frequently." He said that on one occasion, when rushed because of some bank business that needed his immediate attention, "I forgot to drink my tea, and soon everyone around me almost knew what I had for lunch." After that embarrassing experience, "I never failed to drink my three daily cups of lovage tea."

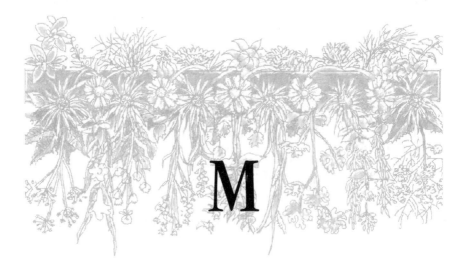

MAGNOLIA
(MAGNOLIA GLAUCA)

Brief Description

Magnolia is a genus of ornamental, widely cultivated evergreens or decid-uous shrubs and trees of the family Mangoliaceae. There are close to 40 dif-ferent species native to America, Japan, China, and India. Magnolias are pretty common from New England to those southern states encompassing the Gulf of Mexico.

They are marked by large alternate leaves, very fragrant flowers either white, purple-green or yellow, and usually red, decorative fruit that is always cone-shaped. Magnolia can vary in height from a mere 6 feet to five times that, getting upwards of 30 feet in the south, but much less than that from Ohio to Massachusetts.

Tonic Tea for Heart Disease and Cancer

The following tea has proven to be very useful in the treatment of heart disease, hypertension and malignant tumors. Put 1-1/4 tbsps. of cut or gran-ulated magnolia bark in 2 pints *distilled* boiling water, cover, reduce heat to lower setting, and simmer for 35 minutes. Then set aside and cool for 20 minutes. Drink half-cupfuls every four hours 4-6 times daily. The cool tea is also a useful scalp tonic to prevent hair loss.

MAHUANG
(EPHEDRA SINICA)
(Also see BRIGHAM TEA)

Brief Description

Since mahuang closely resembles Brigham Tea in so many ways, it is unnecessary to repeat the description here (consult BRIGHAM TEA).

Using Mahuang Safely

Mahuang is widely used in many OTC (over-the-counter) drugs and herbal supplements for energy and weight loss. It is the source of the natural constituents ephedrine and pseudoephedrine which are used for upper respiratory ailments. The latter variant of ephedrine is the chief ingredient in Sudafed, Actifed, Contac, Robitussin-PE, Sinutab, and others.

Mahuang is the main factor in numerous herbal energy formulas and dietary supplements marketed by the powerful health food and herb industries. Consumers should read the labels of such products to see whether or not they contain mahuang.

The FDA (Food and Drug Administration) has warned the public that over-consumption of herbal energy stimulants containing *both* mahuang *and* kola nut or guarana can induce heart attacks and damage nervous systems. Also, doctors warn that those with general weaknesses, the tendency to perspire, poor digestion, hypertension, nervousness, insomnia, cardiac arrhythmias and heart disease should *avoid* using mahuang.

No more than one capsule of an energy stimulant or two capsules of a weight loss aid containing mahuang should be taken in one day. And these should only be used for *short-term* periods and always taken *with food* to avoid complications. When taking mahuang-containing products avoid drinking coffee, black or green tea, or using the herbs guarana or kola nut.

In 1995 at least two states had commenced legal action to restrict the sale of natural food supplements and drugs containing mahuang or ephedrine. According to the *Fort Worth Star-Telegram* for Monday, March 20, 1995 (Section A, p. 14), the Texas Board of Health took steps to prohibit the further sale of food and dietary products containing ephedrine, except in naturally occurring amounts (such as in mahuang or Brigham teas). And the January 1995 issue of *Health Foods Business* (p. 6) mentioned that the Ohio State Board of Pharmacy had enacted regulations to restrict sales of ephedrine to pharmacists as well as to block sales of the herb from which it is derived. Several other states had similar legislation pending as of mid-1995.

MAPLE
(ACER CAMPESTRE)

Brief Description

There are close to 100 different species of maple and several types of shrubs that make up the family Aceraceae. They constitute one of the most widely useful genera of trees, extensively propagated for ornamental reasons.

One of the best known, most widely planted and important species in eastern North America is the sugar maple (A. saccharum). It abounds from the province of Quebec in Canada through Maine and Vermont and southward to the mountains of Georgia. When this large maple is tapped it yields between 3 and 6 pounds of sap annually. Genuine maple syrup is unsurpassed in flavor and nutrition.

New York and Vermont are the principal states producing maple syrup and maple sugar. The latter is used for flavoring confectionery and tobacco. Maples are popular shade trees and can be easily distinguished by their brilliantly colored foliage in the autumn.

Tonifies the Entire Body

Maple is probably one of the most neglected of all medicinal trees. It is seldom mentioned in most of the modern herbal books, and then only very briefly. But I have found it to be an extremely useful agent for tonifying the whole body. A tea made from the leaves and inner bark is, in fact, good for major organs like the lungs and heart, the liver and spleen, the kidneys and pancreas, the nerves and the adrenal glands.

It is hard to describe precisely what the tea does internally except to say that it greatly *invigorates* all of these organs and seems to invest them with renewed life. Peel away with a sharp hunting knife some of the exterior tree bark. Turn it over and scrape away the *inner* bark with a small pocket or paring knife. Put 2/3 cup of this *inner* bark in 2 1/2 pints boiling water, cover and simmer for 12 minutes on low heat. Remove the lid and add 1/2 cup finely cut maple leaves; cover and simmer again for 5 more minutes. Set aside and steep for another 40 minutes. Strain, bottle and refrigerate. Drink one *warm* cup of this tea 2 or 3 times daily in between meals; the tonifying results it works on the body are nothing short of amazing!

Helpful for Boils, Sores, and Wounds

A tea made just from the leaves makes a good poultice or wash for boils, sores, wounds, and other skin afflictions. Make the tea as previously indicated, only omit the first part involving the bark; cool and then strain. Soak a clean, folded cloth in the tea, wring out the excess liquid and apply as a poultice, or else just wash the skin. Either way works well.

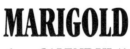

MARIGOLD

(see CALENDULA)

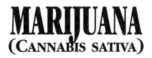

MARIJUANA
(CANNABIS SATIVA)

Brief Description

Marijuana is the drug obtained from the flowering tops, stems and leaves of the hemp plant. It has been used as an agent for achieving euphoric pleasure since the time of the Egyptian pharaohs. It was cultivated extensively during World War II when Asian sources for hemp were cut off. It was probably introduced into the U.S. in the early part of this century by Mexican migrant workers, Latin American mariners, and emigrants from Jamaica and Haiti. In the 1930s the American government conducted a vigorous campaign against it, decrying the dangers against what then became known as "reefer madness." However, in recent times, a growing number of doctors and scientists believe that the drug's medical merits greatly outweigh its hallucinogenic effects. Unfortunately that view still isn't shared by law enforcement officers, who enjoy arresting and confiscating the personal property of those who grow, sell, or use it.

The resin found on flower clusters and top leaves of the female hemp plant is the most potent drug source and is used to prepare hashish, the highest grade of marijuana. The primary active component is tetrahydro-cannabinol or THC. President Bill Clinton made headlines several years ago, when he openly admitted to journalists that during college he once tried smoking a marijuana "joint" (slang for cigarette), but claimed he did-n't actually inhale it. This left most reporters very skeptical and he became the focus of many TV and nightclub comedians' jokes because of this statement.

Breathe This Air and You're Apt to Get a Gratuitous High

Scientists at Spain's Cordoba University advised the public in the south of the country sometime in the latter part of June, 1995, that a bumper crop of marijuana across the Mediterranean Sea in Morocco was sending clouds of cannabis pollen into the region. A persistent sirocco wind over the past few weeks blew the particles from the Atlas Mountain hemp farms to the cities of Malaga, Estepona, Cartagena, Cordoba, and even Madrid. Residents in some of these places had reported feeling "deliriously joyful" (as one metropolitan newspaper described them) after inhaling some of this mari-juana-tainted air.

Marijuana for Cancer and Glaucoma

A recent survey conducted by Harvard University Medical School discovered that 40% of cancer specialists have advised their chemotherapy patients to smoke marijuana joints to relieve the excruciating pain, nausea and vomiting accompanying medical treatments for their disease. Some time ago I spoke with respected AIDS researcher Donald Abrams of the University of California in San Francisco about this very thing. For the past 4 years he has sought federal approval to conduct a clinical trial to determine whether smoking marijuana can help patients overcome the deadly AIDS wasting syndrome. He boldly declared: "This trial will advance forward in that science manages to survive the self-righteous and self-serving politics of the Republican Party."

Despite the federal government's obvious reluctance, it has been forced to admit that some individuals have a true, legitimate medical need for this very useful drug. I spoke with Bob Randall a few years ago when I was in the nation's capitol attending a garlic research conference. At that time he was still driving a cab and took me across the Potomac River to my destination. Bob is one of *just eight* people in the entire country who can legally smoke marijuana. In fact, Uncle Sam (our government) has been supplying him with it for two decades now.

Bob told me that in the early 1970s he was diagnosed with glaucoma. By accident, he discovered that smoking marijuana reduced the pressure and halted the deterioration of his sight. After prevailing in court, Bob, then 43, was permitted to start smoking between 8 and 12 joints a day. And what about this presumed "reefer madness" that the government claimed many years ago would be caused by smoking a lot of marijuana? "Look at me," he said. "Do I look like I'm crazy? Do I look like I have the shakes?" as he extended a steady hand in mid-air. "I'm telling you, man, it's like this. I still have my eyesight because of this illicit weed. If our society was sane, which it isn't," he quickly noted, "the prospect of an easy-to-grow weed that could ease human suffering and prolong life would be a cause for great celebration."

The *Journal of the American Medical Association* (*JAMA* 273:1875-76, June 21, 1995) recently carried an editorial authored by two Boston doctors, entitled "Marijuana as Medicine." The authors, one from Harvard Medical School and the other from the Massachusetts Mental Health Center, made an earnest plea for politicians, physicians, and the public to reconsider this substance as a valuable medical drug. They noted that marijuana is "useful as an anticonvulsant, as a muscle relaxant in spastic disorders, and as an appetite stimulant in the wasting syndrome of human immunodeficiency virus infection. It is also being used to relieve phantom limb pain, menstrual cramps, and other types of chronic pain, including . . . migraine." They rightly point out that a number of public polls and voter referenda "have repeatedly indicated that the vast majority of Americans think marijuana should be medicinally available." But their best reason for wanting it medically legalized is because it is "a remarkably safe" medicine. "There is no known case of lethal overdose," they wrote. And "marijuana is far less addictive and far less subject to abuse than many [legally prescribed] drugs [now are]." Hopefully, the time will soon come when medical doctors are able to utilize this wonderful plant as a valuable therapeutic agent in the treatment of their patients.

Because marijuana continues to be illegal, I cannot recommend known sources for it. Nor do I intend to give any recommendations on how to use it. But I will say this: the federal government has been allowing serious medical cases such as Randall's to be *legally* treated with marijuana under a doctor's strict supervision. Hiring a good attorney and getting an open-minded doctor on your side increase your chances of getting marijuana the right way. There are, of course, other alternatives that are much easier but are illegal. You may wish to experiment with catnip (see CAT-

NIP), which *is* legal and may be of some benefit when smoked for cancer or glaucoma.

Marijuana Jeans, Shirts and Dresses—
The Latest Fashion Craze

The American Hemp Mercantile in Seattle, WA, Head Case in Jersey City, NJ and The Hempstead Co. in Costa Mesa, CA have started utilizing hemp as a natural fiber fabric in the same way that other manufacturers might use cotton. There are now marijuana jeans, shirts and dresses that look like silk. Recently I saw in Englewood Cliffs, NJ a young male in his early 20s sporting a cap that read: **"WARNING! DO NOT SMOKE THIS CAP!"** What's next? Marijuana pj's embroidered with the mind-altering slogan: **"DREAM THE NIGHT AWAY WITH US!"** (For more information read Robert A. Nelson's fascinating work on "the world's most extraordinary plant," *The Great Book of Hemp* (Park Street Press, 1994).

MARJORAM AND OREGANO
(ORIGANUM MAJORANA, O.VULGARE)

Brief Description

Sweet marjoram is a tender, bushy perennial herb with wooly-hairy leaves, which gets up to 1-1/2 feet in height. The herb is native to the Mediterranean countries, but is cultivated as an annual in colder climates. The dried flowering herb yields a faint, sage-like odor and leaves a slightly minty aftertaste in the mouth.

Oregano, as such, is not just one or two well-defined species but rather any one of over two dozen known species that yield leaves or flowering tops having the flavor recognized as oregano. European oregano is a hardy perennial herb with erect, more or less hairy, branching stems and hairy leaves. The herb can grow to over 2 feet tall, and is acrid and pungent with a strong, sage-like aroma somewhat reminiscent of thyme.

Fevers, Cramps, Epilepsy

In my work entitled *The Complete Book of Spices,* I discuss at some length a myriad of uses for both culinary herbs. When made into a tea and consumed warm to slightly cool, they help reduce fevers and relieve cramps; they are also effective in treating bronchitis, childhood diseases such as

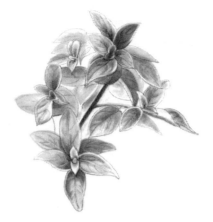

measles and mumps, and irregular menstruation. And when Oil of Oregano (obtainable at some pharmaceutical houses) is applied to the neck, spine, throat, chest and temples, and rubbed into the skin of a person having a seizure, it will often help in bringing that individual out of his or her attack a lot sooner and with very little trauma.

To make a tea, simply bring 1 pint of water to a boil. Remove from the heat and add 1 level tsp. each of marjoram and oregano. Stir well, cover and let steep for 30 minutes or so. Strain and refrigerate, warming slightly on the stove only that amount to be consumed at any given time. Generally one cup two to three times daily is suggested.

Culinary Uses

Marjoram is used as a flavor ingredient in most food categories, including alcoholic (bitters, vermouths, beers, etc.) and nonalcoholic beverages, frozen dairy desserts, candy, baked goods, gelatins and puddings, meat and meat products, condiments and relishes and others. Sweet marjoram is also used in baked goods, meat and meat products, condiments and relishes, soups, snack foods, processed vegetables and others, with highest average maximum use level of about 1% in baked goods.

European oregano is used extensively as a major flavor ingredient in pizza. The more spicy Mexican oregano is widely used in Mexican dishes (chili, chili con carne, etc.); it's less preferred for use in pizza than the milder European type. Oregano is also widely used in other foods, including alcoholic beverages, baked goods, meat and meat products, condiments and relishes, milk products, processed vegetables, snack foods, fats and oils, and others. Highest average maximum use level reported is about 0.3% in condiments and relishes and milk products.

MARSHMALLOW
(ALTHAEA OFFICINALIS)

Brief Description

Marshmallow is a perennial plant growing to a height of nearly 4 feet in some cases. It is both cultivated as well as found growing wild in damp and wet places everywhere. The rootstock is white and sweetish like a parsnip, but with considerable mucilage to it. The plant sends up several unbranched, wooly stems with serrate, pubescent leaves. The axillary flowers are about 2 inches in width and can be either light red to white or royal purple in color.

Formula for Healing Hernias

The late Utah herbalist, Dr. John R. Christopher, developed a special formula for helping knit together torn ligaments and herniated muscles. His formula consisted of marshmallow and comfrey roots, slippery elm and white oak barks, some mullein leaves and calendula flowers, along with lesser amounts of skullcap herb, black walnut hulls and a tiny amount of gravel root.

A mother in Orem, Utah had a teenage son who accidentally sustained a hernia in his groin through the improper lifting of weights. She told me that she had met Dr. Christopher earlier at an herb lecture and had explained the problem to him, saying that doctors were recommending surgery for her boy which she rejected.

He told her about his special BF&C formula and gave her instructions on how to use it. She purchased it from his family-owned herb company and had her son take 4 capsules three times daily on an empty stomach, with additional supplements of calcium, horsetail and zinc in unspecified amounts. Each time he would also drink a full 8-oz. glass of papaya juice made from liquid concentrate. He also refrained from strenuous exercising. According to what the mother told me, her son's hernia healed within 2-1/2 months; a later physical examination and further X-rays by their family doctor confirmed this to, indeed, have been the case.

Nature's Way later obtained this BF&C formula from Dr. Christopher and currently markets it to most health food outlets nationwide. The formula is good for sprains, too.

A Wound-Healing Ointment

To make a marvelous ointment for helping heal facial sores, skin eruptions, leg ulcers and ugly-looking wounds a lot faster, lightly crush approximately 1 gallon each of fresh marshmallow leaves and elder flowers. Then scatter them around evenly in a large roast pan and ad about 2-1/4 cups of melted lard or Crisco shortening and 1-1/2 lbs, of beeswax. Stir thoroughly with a wooden ladle, cover, simmering in a 150° F. oven until the herbs are fairly crisp, easily crumbling when touched. Strain mixture through a wire mesh strainer and continue stirring with a wooden ladle until entirely cold. Half a cup of glycerin or 2/3 cup powdered slippery elm can be added to help preserve ointment from rancidity later on. Put into clean jars while still relatively warm and allow to become somewhat firm. Seal with tight lids and store in a cool, dry place until needed.

Curing Cystitis

Cystitis is an infection of the bladder accompanied by a burning sensation during and following urination. As the female urethra is only 1-1/2 inches in length and the male urethra is 8 inches long, it is much easier for the germs to reach the female bladder; therefore, women are 20 times more likely than men to get this problem.

An herbal combination routinely used by Manhattan-based holistic practitioner and health educator Martin Ravitzky to treat cystitis employs marshmallow and several other herbs. He claims that his formulation "will be safe and effective in preventing and treating cystitis." Furthermore, he declares that it "will also soothe, strengthen, tonify and protect the whole urinary system from the kidneys to the bladder."

Like myself and other traditional herbal experts, he believes that this particular herbal combination (as well as many others) "is most effective when *taken as a tea*." But that's not always an easy task convincing many people who've been in the habit of taking most of their herbs in capsule or tablet forms. "It is best," he said, "to boil the roots and berries but steep the leaves of the herbs involved. Add one teaspoon of the combined marshmallow root and juniper berries to one cup of water and boil for 15 minutes. Then put the entire contents into a teapot that contains the remainder of the formula: one teaspoon of the combined leaves of buchu and uva ursi, and steep an additional 15 minutes. Drink two cups a day on an empty stomach. These herbs can all be bought at a health food store or an herb store. Be sure to buy organic herbs wherever possible."

MELALEUCA
(MELALEUCA ALTERNIFOLIA)

Brief Description

Species of melaleuca are common from the Philippines and Malaysia to Indonesia and Australia. Under normal circumstances it is usually a large bush or small tree, and with a rather dense, narrow crown and a stout, often twisted trunk. The bark is spongy and peels off in layers. The young leaves and twigs are silky. The leaves are thin and leathery, alternate, lanceolate and pointed at both ends. The flowers have a fine hairiness to them and are white and fragrant. The fruit is small and grayish-brown with a narrow groove around the top surrounding a small, craterlike cup marked with five radial grooves.

In the Philippines, Malaysia and Indonesia it is also known as the cajeput tree, and in Australia as the tea tree. In that part of the world it is often planted along broad avenues as a handsome ornamental and comforting shade tree. It also produces good firewood, and the papery bark has been used in the past by Malaysians for caulking their boats. But it is the peculiar oil with its turpentine-like smell that has made this species of trees highly desirable. Several enterprising individuals have capitalized on the oil's many virtues and have earned themselves some small fortunes by selling it through direct or multi-level marketing schemes.

But the melaleuca isn't favored everywhere. In Florida it is now considered to be "one of the three most environmentally dangerous plants" which threaten the entire state, according to an article in *The Orlando Sentinel* (Sunday, April 21, 1991, pp. K-1; K-4). With an alarming headline that referred to "monster" trees, the article described damage already done by trees growing near the lakes surrounding the small community of Belle Isle. Melaleuca was described as "sucking up water faster than a thirsty construction worker..... depleting neighboring plants' water supplies, and turning marshes into dry land." So obnoxious have they become that even devout nature lovers and hard-core environmentalists have taken to cutting them down with a vengeance, using chainsaws, hatchets, machetes, and even regular wood saws.

One such nature enthusiast by the name of Kay Jones admitted with some reluctance that "this innocent-looking thing . . . is a monster," and said she never imagined herself being put in the position of having to *destroy* something in the very nature she so ardently and passionately defends. But "they're just taking over and they've got to be stopped," she said, with iron-like determination.

Animal Groomers Discover Healing Benefits of Melaleuca Oil

Angie and Annie operate a very successful animal grooming service in Salt Lake City's trendy and upscale east bench. I took my office cat Jake (a five-year-old part Persian-Siamese male) to their business to be washed and groomed. When I returned several hours later to pick him up, Angie Armstrong spoke with me while her partner talked on the phone with the anxious owner of a very distraught poodle.

"She thinks her pooch is paranoid," Angie said with a nod of her head in the direction of the telephone. "She wants to give it some Prozac and Annie is trying her best to discourage her. We don't believe in giving *any* drugs to our animals and try to use only natural products whenever we can."

As I picked up my elegantly groomed tomcat, my nose detected a slight camphor odor about its head. I inquired what the aroma was and it led to a discussion between Angie and me on melaleuca or tea tree oil. "I dipped a pair of Q-tips in some and cleaned out Jake's ears; we do this all the time with every cat we groom. We find it is good to get rid of any mites that may be in a cat's ears."

Angie then held up her left hand and pointed to a very faint semicircular scar. About a year ago, she said, a feisty cat she was attempting to shampoo reacted violently to its bath by suddenly biting her hand. She had scrubbed her wound, applied some hydrogen peroxide, and then poured a little melaleuca oil on the injury. "It didn't sting but felt cool," she said. "I could tell the healing process was setting in because my wound had an itchy feeling to it. By the next day it was completely healed. There was *no* infection and *no* swelling of any kind. I was able to go back to washing cats and clipping poodles again."

Angie and Annie use melaleuca oil as well to help heal wounds and sores on animals they groom, and to keep fleas and ticks off. They believe it is truly "a miracle remedy from Mother Nature."

Indonesian Applications

In 1984 and again in 1986 I spent some time touring the different islands which comprise the populous nation of Indonesia. I interviewed a number of folk healers and scientists who've devoted their careers to the study of *jamu* (the Indonesian word for traditional herbal medicine). I learned from all of my sources a variety of uses for "cajeput" or melaleuca oil. Two drops of oil in some lukewarm water, shaken well, and given to an infant in a plastic feeder bottle will relieve the worst case of colic. A few drops rubbed across and on the sides of the forehead and on the back of the neck will relieve the worst migraine imaginable, A cotton ball soaked with some of the oil and packed next to a sore tooth will stop it from hurting. A couple of drops put into the ear with an eye dropper will help to get rid of an earache. By rubbing 4-5 drops on the calves, leg cramps will soon disappear. Minor burns heal more quickly when some melaleuca is applied to the surface of the injured skin. Bed sores, herpes lesions, and sores from sexually-transmitted diseases respond well to applications of melaleuca.

MEXICAN YARN
(see WILD MEXICAN YARN)

MILFOIL
(see YARROW)

MILK THISTLE
(SILYBUM MARIANUM)

Brief Description

Milk thistle can be either an annual or biennial plant. It grows to 6 feet in height and has coarse, lobed, prickly-shaped leaves streaked with conspicuous white veins. The flowers appear in May and June, are born in solitary heads, a couple of inches wide, crimson to reddish-violet in hue, and surrounded by prominent, spiny bracts.

Natural Treatment for Cirrhosis, Hepatitis, Chemical Poisoning, and Other Liver-Related Problems

In the early 19th century a famous German physician by the name of Rademacher developed for his liver patients a tincture made from the seeds of milk thistle. The product bears his name (Tinctura Cardui Mariae Rademacher) and still shows up in some European pharmacopeias today. In more recent years, however, the active principle has been isolated and its chemical constitution well established; it is a new kind of flavonol called silymarin. The German researchers Wagner, Hoerhammer and Muenster were the first to describe it and showed through numerous animal experiments that it is safe even if given in large doses, and with virtually no side effects. Currently the literature on silymarin and milk thistle seed in general has already reached incredible proportions. It is *the* preferred liver medicine throughout much of Europe today.

Milk thistle seed comes in several different forms. Herbal capsules or tablets contain anywhere from 20-35 mg. of silymarin. In cases of cirrhosis of the liver or chronic hepatitis, between 2-4 capsules or tablets are prescribed by German doctors three times daily after meals, for periods lasting anywhere from 4 to 6 weeks. After this, the dose is usually reduced to just one capsule or tablet 3 times daily. Treatments often last a full six months, even with the reduced amount.

Liver poisoning due to man-made chemicals, such as carbon tetrachlorides or things found in nature like the death cap mushroom, can be helped with *regular* consumption of milk thistle seed: 2 capsules or tablets 4 times daily; 2 ampoules (containing 50 mg. silymarin) every 4 hours for the first 48 hours; 20 drops milk thistle seed tincture 4 times daily; or 3 cups *hot* tea 3 times daily and 30 minutes before a meal. To make a tea put one tsp. of the seeds in boiling water, cover and let steep 20 minutes and drink while still hot. A pinch of peppermint leaves can be added to improve the flavor and effect of the tea; or 20 drops of milk thistle seed tincture can be added to a cup of warm peppermint tea instead.

I translated and adapted much of the foregoing data from the German publication *Lehrbuch der Phytotherapie* (Stuttgart: Hippokrates Verlag GmbH, 1985) by Rudolf Fritz Weiss, M.D.

MINTS

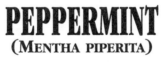

PEPPERMINT
(MENTHA PIPERITA)

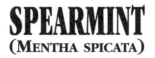

SPEARMINT
(MENTHA SPICATA)

Brief Description

Both kinds of mints are closely related perennial aromatic herbs with runners by which they are propagated. The leaves of spearmint are sessile (no petioles), while those of peppermint are petioled. Both grow to about 1

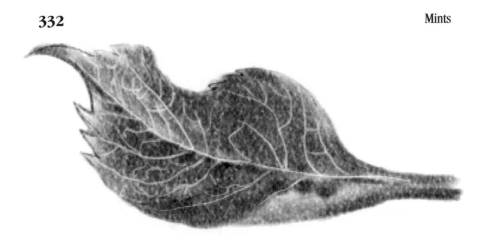

yard high and are cultivated worldwide. Each species has numerous varieties that produce essential oils, which yield a menthol aroma and taste to varying degrees.

Relieves Migraines

Peppermint tea is excellent for relieving the pressure of migraine headaches. Bring 1 pint of water to a boil. Remove from heat, adding 2 tbsps. of fresh or dried mint leaves. Cover and steep for 50 minutes, then strain. Drink 1-2 cups of cool tea when a headache occurs. Also rubbing a little peppermint oil on either side of the temples and toward the back of the neck gives additional relief as well.

Calms Digestive Disorders

General nervousness and stomach disorders may be effectively treated by drinking several cups of lukewarm peppermint/spearmint tea sweetened with a little honey. This combination of equal parts of both mints is pleasantly soothing to the nervous system. The tea can be made according to the previous instructions given.

Digestive disorders of various kinds may be greatly relieved by taking a presteeped water extract in capsule form or powdered form as a tea. This European-made extract is only available under the Alta Health Products label from most health food stores or may be ordered directly from the manufacturer in Mission Viejo, California (see Appendix). Dr. Richard Barmakian, a renowned southern California naturopathic/homeopathic doctor, has included in his special formulation other herbs, besides peppermint, such as alder buckthorn, marigold flowers and marshmallow leaf.

Called Can-Gest, this pure herbal digestive extract helps to relieve heartburn, indigestion, abdominal cramps and other gastrointestinal discomforts. Some have reported no further need to rely on antacids once they've begun to use Can-Gest. Recommended intake suggested by Dr. Barmakian to many of his patients is between 1-3 capsules per meal as needed or 1/2 tsp. of the powder made into a tea.

Inhibits Herpes

Peppermint is strongly antiviral and may be used with good success in helping to inhibit the further progress of herpes virus. It works best in tea form, however, since the gelatin capsule tends to nullify its strong antiviral properties. Two cups of warm tea a day are suggested during those periods when the herpes virus is the most active. Dr. Barmakian suggests emptying the contents of about 3 capsules of Can-Gest into a cup of hot water sweetened with some honey, then sipping slowly when lukewarm.

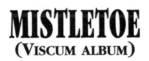

MISTLETOE
(VISCUM ALBUM)

Brief Description

Mistletoe is a spherical shrub belonging to the Loranthaceae family. It is a parasitic plant growing on deciduous trees, spruce and pines, but very rarely on oaks. The stems branch in two ways in a regular fashion normally seen in lower plants such as algae. The flowers are yellowish-green and barely worth noticing. The white berries, on the other hand, are quite important. They are filled with sticky mucilage, which makes them adhere to the feet and beaks of birds and results in their distribution over a wide area. The leaves grow in opposite pairs, are yellowish-green and persist through the winter.

Mistletoes are widely used for Christmas decorations worldwide. The custom of kissing under a branch of mistletoe is thought to have originated with the ancient Druid priests of old Celtic Britain, Ireland and Gaul, as far back as the 3rd century B.C. The mistletoe most widely sold in America is *Phoradendron flavescens*, but it is the *true* mistletoe of Europe that holds the best medicinal properties and should be used.

Dead Men DO Tell Tales

What I'm about to share with you is worthy of an investigation by the great Sherlock Holmes himself. Mistletoe has been used since the time of Christ for alleviating the symptoms of hypertension. But the evidence doesn't come from ancient Celtic inscriptions painted on a broken pottery shard or stiff piece of leather; instead it comes from the stomach of a very water-logged and mummified ancient Briton.

In 1984 a remarkably well-preserved body was found during peat-cutting at Lindlow Moss, 10 miles south of Manchester, England. The body seemed to be in such good condition that police initially feared it might have been a modern murder victim. So, very carefully lifting it in the enveloping block of peat, the excavators transferred the corpse to a hospital mortuary where experts could determine its age by radiocarbon-dating techniques. The body proved to be ancient, *almost 2,000 years old*, and was sent for scientific study to the British Museum. Lindlow Man (as he came to be tagged by the news media) was a sensational discovery, because his natural "coffin" of waterlogged, partly rotted, oxygen-free vegetation had *preserved the soft tissues astonishingly well*, including not only skin but hair and even fingernails. Internal organs were also in a remarkable state of preservation.

Lindlow Man lived around the end of the Iron Age, probably the first century A.D. Scientists subjected him to a painstaking series of investigations over a period of many months. Removal of the peat in the laboratory revealed the remains of a bearded adult male, naked except for a fox-fur band around the left arm and a cord around the throat. It soon became evident that this well-fed young man had met a homicidal, horrifically brutal end. He was struck twice or thrice on the head by a narrow-bladed axe. He lost consciousness, but didn't die instantly, because the wound swelled, indicating that his heart was still beating. Next a cord was tied about his neck (where it remains today), and then a stick inserted at the back and twisted to tighten what was, in effect, a garrote. The strangulation was done with such violence that it snapped his neck. This was the moment of clinical death, but the Lindlow Man's killer or killers weren't finished with him yet. They cut his throat from ear to ear and soon afterward dumped his remains into a pool in the bog.

However, there was also more positive evidence of how he had lived. Because many of his internal organs were still in near-perfect condition, it was possible for doctors and scientists to determine that he suffered from malignant hypertension in life. Autopsy results showed vascular exudative and hemorrhagic lesions, medial thickening of small arteries and arterioles, and left ventricular hypertrophy of the heart—all indicative of a severe hypertensive state.

But what really fascinated this medical investigative team were the contents of his stomach. Inside were found grains of pollen from mistletoe berries. They concluded that not only must Lindlow Man have chewed some of these berries, but also quite possibly have drunk a beverage made from them as well.

For many centuries, herbalists throughout Europe had relied on a tea and tincture of the berries to treat some of the symptoms associated with raised blood pressure: headaches, dizziness, loss of energy, irritability, etc. So from the grave has come one ancient remedy for a very serious medical condition.

European herbalists have a couple of different ways of using mistletoe as a heart sedative and antihypertensive. One way is to take equal parts (about two tablespoons each) of mistletoe and hawthorn berries and lemon balm leaves and steep them in two pints of boiling water for 25 minutes. One-half cup of the *warm* tea is taken morning and evening. The other way is to soak 4 teaspoons of chopped mistletoe in 1-1/4 pints of cold water overnight, and take one cup of the cool beverage first thing the next morning.

WARNING: Ingestion of the raw berries may produce gastric upset, nausea, vomiting and diarrhea.

MORMON TEA

(see BRIGHAM TEA)

MORNING GLORY
(IPOMOEA PURPUREA)

Brief Description

Although there are many kinds of morning glories, this particular species is quite common throughout the U.S. and Canada, often growing more as a nuisance weed in damp waste places or cultivated ground such as garden plots or farmers' fields. Its creeping, spreading vinelike stems can cover an area up to 7 feet in circumference. The leaves are usually alternate and the trumpet-shaped flowers, while of different hues, generally are white.

Flower Tincture for Sore Eyes

A tincture of morning glory blossoms is useful for getting rid of a headache and to relieve inflamed eyes. Combine 1-1/2 cups of finely snipped flowers in 2 cups of gin. Put in a jar with a tight-fitting lid, and set on a window sill for about two weeks. Be sure to shake the contents twice daily. Strain through several layers of cheesecloth or gauze.

Soak a clean cloth with some of this tincture, wring out the excess and apply to the forehead or over closed eyes for relief. A small hand towel may be applied over the cloth to prevent the rapid evaporation of the alcohol.

Antidote for Insect Bites

If you should be outdoors and get bitten or stung by an insect such as a horsefly, mosquito or wasp, then just look around for some morning glory. Pick a small number of the leaves, crush them with a smooth stone or hammer and then rub them on the afflicted site, retaining in place either by holding them or else by covering with a small, square piece of gauze and adhesive tape.

Bathing Sores and Wounds

In the Bahamas local practitioners skilled in folk medicine make a tea out of the leaves and flowers of morning glory. They use the resulting liquid for bathing herpes lesions, diabetic leg ulcers, gangrene, syphilitic sores and wounds. Bring 3 cups of water to a boil and add 1 cup of cut flowers and leaves. Cover, remove from the heat and steep for 45 minutes. Strain and use.

An Effective Poultice for Boils

Throughout Jamaica and Brazil, morning glory leaves are used as effective poultices for drawing the purulent matter out of serious abscesses and boils. The quickest way for making such a poultice is to throw a handful of picked and washed leaves into a food blender with 2 tablespoons of ice water, and puree. Apply this thick pulp directly to the boil or carbuncle previously lanced with a sewing needle that has been sterilized over an open flame. Cover with some gauze and secure with adhesive tape. Change every 45 minutes or so.

MOSS

Brief Description

Moss is any species of the class Bryopsida. Mosses (along with liverworts) comprise the division Bryophyta, the first green land plants believed to have evolved several hundred million years ago. It is thought that they developed out of certain very primitive vascular plants and have not given rise to any other type of plant. Their rootlike rhizomes and leaflike process-es lack the vascular structure of the true roots, shoots and leaves found in higher plants. Although limited to moist habitats because they require water for fertilization, bryophytes are usually extremely hardy and grow every-where except in the sea.

Mosses grow vertically rather than horizontally, like the liverworts. The green moss plant, being visible to the naked eye, seldom ever gets over six inches in height. Except for the commercially valuable sphagnum or peat moss, mosses are of little direct importance to humans except in extreme survival conditions. They are of some benefit to soil formation and as fill for barren habitats prior to the growth of higher plants; they also pro-vide food for certain animals.

There are certain unrelated higher plants which share the name "moss"; these include club moss, flowering moss, Irish moss or carrageen (an algae), reindeer moss (a lichen), and Spanish moss (a plant parasite).

Moss and Bugs Saved Downed U.S. Pilot from Starvation

During the first ten days of June 1995, media headlines focused on the loss and then later rescue of a 29-year-old American fighter pilot from a wilder-ness area in Bosnia-Herzegovina (part of the former Yugoslavia). Captain Scott F. O'Grady's jet fighter had been cut in half by a Serbian missile over Bosnia on June 2nd. As his broken craft tumbled earthward, he managed to tug the ejection lanyard and parachute down into Serb-held territory.

For the next six days, he managed to survive in a sparsely populated area of pinelands while always evading the searching enemy. He remained hidden by day, but ventured out at night to catch succulent bugs and eat them for protein. He also made ample use of moss growing on wet stones near a cleft in some rocks. These he scraped off with a 5-inch survival knife and methodically chewed bite-size pieces to quench his thirst (he was unable to find the source of the moisture). He eventually ran out of can-teen water and the daytime heat made his mouth very parched, so he sometimes kept a small plug of moss inside next to his cheek to help keep his tongue from swelling.

On the following Thursday morning two helicopters packed with U.S. marines landed near the captain's lookout, as yellow signal smoke pointed them in the direction of his hideout. Above them hovered two AH-1 Cobra attack helicopters, gunships bristling ready for a major fight with the Serbs in the surrounding territory below. Further up in the sky were two AV-8 Harrier jump jets on tight patrol, ready with even more awesome firepower in case it was ever needed.

At precisely 6:44 a.m. the fugitive pilot emerged from the pine forest and was pulled up into the cockpit of one of the choppers, firmly in the hands of a Marine colonel. The pilot was then whisked aloft and covered with a blanket. He was handed an M.R.E. (military parlance for "meal, ready to eat") and promptly wolfed it down, exclaiming at the same time that he didn't "ever again want to see any more bugs, moss or grass," if he could help it. As the air convoy moved out, rescuers took note of a ground-to-air missile that narrowly missed them and some gunfire that grazed a helicopter without effect.

He was taken aboard the *USS Kearsarge*, which was then sailing in the Adriatic Sea, for routine medical treatment. Upon hearing the good news of O'Grady's safe rescue, President Bill Clinton stood on the Truman balcony of the White House in the early morning dark and lit up a victory cigar which he jubilantly smoked. Sometime later O'Grady publicly thanked God for delivering him from danger and the Marines for rescuing him.

Thus, we may learn from Capt. O'Grady's nearly week-long ordeal that even something as lowly and awful-tasting as moss can be quite helpful in emergency situations.

Moss Poultice Stops Bleeding

Some years ago I took three teenage Boy Scouts on an overnight outing in the mountains near Salina, Utah. One of the youngsters accidentally hurt himself with a hatchet while attempting to chop firewood. Although the wound was not serious, the bleeding didn't stop even with an applied tourniquet. So I got my hunting knife and scraped off a handful of moss from the wet surface of a flat stone. This I applied directly to the open wound and instructed the kid to hold it in place. In about ten minutes the continued trickle of blood ceased completely.

MOTHERWORT
(LEONURUS CARDIACA)

Brief Description

Motherwort is native to the European continent, but has been naturalized throughout North America, ranging in geographical extent from Novia Scotia to Montreal and south to Texas and North Carolina. It prefers vacant lots and similar waste places.

Motherwort is a perennial herb growing to five feet. The leaves are shaggy-appearing and to some extent resemble a lion's tail, which explains several of its other common names: lion's tail, lion's ear, lion's tart. Each leaf has three lance-shaped lobes. The tiny flowers bloom between June and September and are pink, white, or purple and grow in clusters.

Neuritis, Neuralgia, Sciatica, and Rheumatism

Patricia Kenney is a practicing herbalist of West Roxbury, Massachusetts. My full telephone interview with her on Tuesday, July 11, 1995 appears in full in one of my other books, *Heinerman's Encyclopedia of Juices, Teas, and Tonics* (Englewood Cliffs, NJ: Prentice Hall, 1996) under WOMEN'S PROBLEMS.

One of her very favorite herbs is motherwort. She likened it to "going back to your mother for consolation and comfort." She said, "I have recommended it consistently to many women for problems associated with menopause, premenstrual syndrome, hot flashes, mood swings, heart problems, and blood clots. The form in which it works best for these various disorders is as a tincture. I recommend a standard dosage of 40 drops in one-half cup warm water three times daily." (She uses the tincture extract of motherwort made and sold by Gaia Herbs of Harvard, Massachusetts. Call 508-456-3049 for more information.

MOUNTAIN MAHOGANY
(CERCOCARPUS SPECIES)

Brief Description

Mountain mahogany grows on dry, rocky slopes up to the 9,000-foot elevation and is rarely encountered in flat terrain. It is found on nearly all mountain slopes of the American West and Southwest. The bush attains a height of 6 to 10 feet, although some species have been known to grow 20 feet tall in favored locations with a trunk circumference of one foot.

The leaves, borne on little spurlike branchlets, resemble those of birch. They are alternate and have a rather pronounced center vein with many small side-veins branching off. The inner margins are straight, forming a fanlike right angle, and the outside margins are sharply notched, coordinating with the side veins. The various species have nearly round to oval lance-shaped leaves. The bark is usually reddish but can occasionally be gray. The dense inner heartwood is a dark reddish brown. The flowers are small, single, and without petals, the buds starting in late winter in the axils of the evergreen leaves, the calyx forming a little flared-out tube containing numerous stamens. Altogether it resembles a rose missing all of its petals. The blossoms mature into a single fruit with a long feathery whip extended 1 to 4 inches, which serves both to disperse the fruit in the wind and to help it adhere in moist dirt.

Herbal Remedies of a 106-Year-Old Paiute Indian Medicine Man

In the summer of 1966 I traveled with a friend to the Duck Valley Indian Reservation in northeast Nevada. There I was introduced to Pa-Mo-Tau (or Willie Dorsey, as he was known to the non-Indian world). He was then in his 106th year and had lost his sight, but was still quite conversant. From the time he was 14 years old, he had practiced folk medicine among the northern Paiute members of his tribe at his Miller Creek residence. He was reported to be the greatest Indian shaman in the West at that time. I interviewed this remarkable man with the deeply lined, heavily tanned face and incredible knowledge of herbs. Fortunate that I did, for he died the following March in his 107th year.

One of his favorite plants was mountain mahogany, which is prolific throughout the Intermountain West and California. He remembered how useful the whole leafy branches were for warding off bedbugs, for he used to place some of them under his mattress every so often and never once was bitten.

Over the years, he said, hundreds of older white men had sought him out for help in treating their many cases of prostatitis, enlarged prostate, or cancer of the prostate gland. He only used one herb: his favored mountain mahogany. His instructions: take a generous handful of the shrub twigs and boil them, uncovered, in a coffee pot holding a pint of water for 40 minutes. He didn't believe in straining anything, but leaving the twigs with the liquid until it was all used up (he thought it made for a stronger tea doing it this way). Men were told to take 3 cups of this daily before meals—in the morning, at noon, and again at night. Every man who did this faithfully discovered that his prostatitis cleared up or that his enlarged prostate gland returned to normal within several months. Only in *advanced* cases of prostate cancer did the tea fail to always work a healing miracle; but, at least, it substantially reduced the pain and made the last weeks or months of the patient more comfortable. However, if taken in the very early stages of cancer and continued for up to 5 months thereafter, the tumor would usually recede and there would be no further recurrence.

Pa-Mo-Tau also recommended the same tea to those who were severely constipated or else suffered from hemorrhoids. In the first instance, two cups taken an hour apart would invariably invoke a very healthy bowel movement; and in the second instance, the piles would shrink and go away. The tea wouldn't work well, though, on bleeding hemorrhoids.

The same tea formula was routinely prescribed for the common cold and influenza. For lung problems such as asthma, bronchitis, emphysema, and tuberculosis, he made a stronger tea from the scrapings of the second or *inner* bark. He would peel away the outer bark of branches with a pocket knife, but leave the second skin on. This he would later scrape away carefully and let it dry in the sun. Afterwards, he pulverized it in the bottom of an old cast-iron frying pan using the end of a Coke bottle; then he would sift the powder and store it in an empty Diamond match box. To make a tea, he told his patients to add one-half teaspoon of the powder to a cup of very warm water, stir it with the forefinger or a spoon, and then drink it down in two large swallows. He had them do this 5 times daily on an empty stomach. Those who adhered to his medical advice soon got well; but those who didn't continued to suffer or eventually died from their respiratory problems.

The same tea was sometimes used as an eyewash for conjunctivitis, inflamed eyes, or "cloudy vision," as he described it (probably *early* cataract formation).

MULLEIN
(VERBASCUM THAPSUS)

Brief Description

Mullein is aligned with snapdragon in the same family of *Scrophulariaceae.* Mullein flowers are stalkless with their sulphur-yellow corollas forming irregular cups an inch across, having five rounded petals enclosed in wooly calyxes. All manner of insects are attracted to this plant due to the easy accessibility of the nectar. By this means the plant is able to propagate itself elsewhere.

The unique leaves are large and numerous, 6-8 inches long and 2-1/2 inches wide, becoming smaller as they ascend toward the stem. Mullein can reach heights greater than the average man and prefers clearings, fields, pastures and waste places from the Atlantic to the Pacific. This herb is a common sight along many of our nation's highways and railroad tracks, but shouldn't be picked in these places due to frequent spraying with noxious chemical herbicides.

Cure for Asthma

A woman from Indiana had spent large sums of money on various medications prescribed by her doctors for her asthma, but found little relief. Learning about the virtues of mullein from her minister, she gathered some from a river bank and made a tea out of it. This she did by steeping a handful of coarsely cut leaves and flowers in 1 quart boiling water for half an hour, then drinking two cups of the warm brew sweetened with some honey each and every day. In no time at all, her asthma was brought under control.

Medicine for the Heart

The French herbalist, Maurice Messegue, recommends mullein for palpitations, irregular heartbeat, angina and other coronary distress. Simmer two handfuls of coarsely cut leaves and flowers in 1-1/2 quarts of boiling water for an hour, covered, until about 1 pint remains. Strain and add 3 tbsps. blackstrap molasses and 1/2 tsp. glycerin to give it longer shelf life. Take 1 tbsp. of this syrup twice daily in between meals, once in the morning and again in the evening, or more if pressure builds up in the heart.

Enema for Intestinal Infection

Mullein leaves were collected and tested by the Michigan State College of Agriculture and Applied Science in 1943-44 for possible antibacterial properties. Experiments showed that mullein extract inhibited growth of *Staphylococcus aureus* and *E. coli*. The former bacteria cause boils, abscesses and wounds filled with purulent matter, while the latter genus of unfriendly microbes produces intestinal inflammation, peritonitis and inflammation of the urinary bladder.

To make an enema solution, steep one handful *each* of fresh cut leaves and flowers together in 1-1/2 quarts of boiling water for 40 minutes, covered. Then strain and use half of this amount, while still lukewarm, for an enema.

Treating Childhood Diseases

Mullein is one of the very best herbs that I know of to successfully treat a wide variety of childhood ailments, including tonsillitis, chickenpox, measles and mumps—especially when it's used in conjunction with catnip. Both herbs work well for pancreatitis, too.

A relatively delicious tea that can be made for sick children to drink calls for 1/2 handful *each* of dried or cut fresh mullein leaves and flowers, and dried or cut fresh herb to be steeped in 1 qt. of boiling water, covered, and then set away from the heat for approximately 35 minutes or so. After this the solution is strained twice, once through a fine sieve and again through a piece of clean cloth. Then while still quite warm 2 tbsps. of dark honey, 1 tsp. of pure maple syrup and a couple of drops of pure vanilla should be mixed in to improve the flavor considerably. Give a sick child 1/2 cup of this *warm* throughout the day or every 3-4 hrs. *NO* dairy products, eggs, bread, meat, greasy foods, candy, soft drinks and so forth should be given to the child during his or her recuperation period.

A small enema may also be given as well at least once a day until the fever breaks and glandular inflammation begins to subside. In 1 pint of boiling water, steep 1/4 handful of dried or cut fresh mullein leaves, 1/4 handful of dried or cut catnip herb and 1 peeled, finely chopped garlic clove, covered, for 40 minutes or until lukewarm. Administer the enema to the child according to the previous instructions. Remember to tell the child to try to hold as much of the solution inside of the bowels as possible *before* seeking relief on the toilet. Be sure to give the enema in very short spurts so the child can better retain the solution for a couple of minutes.

Remedy for Skin Problems and Earache

Soak two handfuls of cut dried or fresh mullein flowers and leaves in 2 cups of olive oil or sweet almond oil for 8 days. Strain, bottle and store in cool place. Makes a very useful dressing for skin ulcers, wounds, sunburn, general burns and hemorrhoids. A few drops of this oil, slightly warmed and placed inside the ear canal, helps to relieve painful earache, when the ear is covered with a warm flannel afterwards.

Another variation to this same theme is to use a mix of St. Johnswort oil and mullein oil together. Just a couple of drops of each put into a teaspoon and heated over a cigarette lighter or gas stove burner for about 45 seconds, or until lukewarm, is sufficient. Use an eyedropper to take up the liquid for inserting into the external ear canal. However, be sure there are no perforations of the eardrum before doing this. Then stuff the ear with cotton. Use a hot-water bottle or a cut half of an oven-roasted Bermuda onion to keep the ear warm. Unless there is intense pain and the drum itself is in danger of rupture, using these simple remedies is cheaper, safer and more practical than relying on antibiotics.

MUSTARD
(SINAPSIS ALBA, BRASSICA NIGRA)

Brief Description

Mustard is a collective name for several cruciferous (cross-shaped) plants, some of which are related to the cabbages. (See my other book, *Heinerman's New Encyclopedia of Fruits and Vegetables* (New Jersey: Prentice Hall, 1995) under CABBAGE and MUSTARD for more information on both.) Most important are the two species mentioned in the parenthetical heading. The terms "white" (or yellow) and "black" (or brown) mustard are often applied to these two, respectively.

As a rule, the prepared mustard we buy in stores—like the "English" mustard powder we make our own variants with—consists of white mustard, perhaps yellowed by an additive such as turmeric (a key ingredient in curry powders). The product's taste can be improved by adding (besides water) apple cider vinegar or red wine vinegar, sugar, and salt. It can even be seasoned with honey, garlic, tarragon and much else. Black mustard is the most common in local "peasant" varieties of mustard, more notably in France and Sweden than anywhere else.

Mustard is a peculiar spice, in that its taste develops only after the seeds are crushed and their powder is mixed with water. Two substances from different types of cells then come into contact: sinigrin and myosin. The resultant "mustard oil'" has the slightly sour, but primarily pungent, taste that we expect of mustard. About 15 minutes is needed for the mixture to reach its full aroma.

The television ads for Grey Poupon Mustard are some of the most memorable and humorous in advertising history. Various ads will always depict two fancy chauffer-driven limousines pulling alongside each other and their wealthy backseat owners rolling down their windows to speak with each other. The one stately gentleman then asks his equally rich neighbor if he can borrow some of his Grey Poupon Mustard to put on a sandwich he is fixing for himself; the other always obliges this request with the same grace and dignity expected of those in high circles of wealth and power.

Oriental Treatment for Knee Pain

Kato Ti, a Hong Kong herb doctor, has a sensible solution for treating knee pain. I've watched him in his small clinic treat knee injuries quite success-fully using mustard. He takes one cup of yellow mustard powder and mixes it with an amount of some type of alcohol adequate to form a paste which he then applies to the knee by smearing it on with a rubber spatula or flat wooden stick. A new application is made when the old one has dried. Treatment is continued until the blisters start to appear. He used this method on 11 different patients, ranging in age from 7 to 71 years old. Everyone responded well to his treatment during the several days I spent with him.

Relieving Lower Backache and Joint Pain

My informant from Hong Kong showed me how he has his patients treat their own lower backaches and joint pains. He filled an ordinary tub bath one-quarter full of fairly hot water, but not hot enough to damage the skin. Next he sprinkled over the water about 1-1/2 cups yellow mustard pow-der, then bent down and stirred both together with his hand. A young ath-lete suffering from a pulled muscle in his lower back after throwing some javelins was told to climb into the tub and lie down. He was kept in the tub for 15 minutes. After this, he stood up and rinsed off with a shower hose using cold water. He reported that all his discomforts were gone and he felt much better.

Cure for Chest Cold and Deep Cough

Dr. Yi treats chest colds and deep, rattling coughs with a mustard/ginger powder plaster. He told me it was "quite marvelous," but always cautions his patients when using this. He noted that sometimes a skin irritation may arise from the mustard, producing a burning sensation that lasts about ten minutes. He said that washing the mustard off won't alleviate the redness and only chills the patient. He assures his patients that the redness will sub-side in a matter of minutes and will disappear in two days.

He shows each patient how to make his or her own plaster. He has each one mix one teaspoon of mustard powder with one teaspoon of ginger root powder, and then combine both with 2-1/2 tablespoons of sesame seed oil or olive oil. The patient then rubs this over the chest and has someone else rub it on the back.

He advises wearing an old T-shirt or tank top instead of a good shirt or blouse, since the article of clothing will become easily stained. The next morning the individual is supposed to take a shower to wash it all off. He guarantees that his plaster is very effective in clearing up the worst kind of chest cold or deep cough.

An Easy Mustard Sauce

This sweet and sour sauce can be used as a savory gravy for garlic or spinach or beet noodles, or over rice, potatoes, or mushrooms.

> *Needed:* 1 tbsp. Kingsford cornstarch; 1 cup vegetable broth; 1 tbsp. apple cider vinegar; 3 tbsps. Grey Poupon Dijon mustard; 2 tbsps. honey; and 1/2 tsp. tarragon.

> In a small bowl, combine the cornstarch with 1/4 cup cold stock, stirring until smooth. In a small saucepan over medium heat, combine the remaining stock with vinegar, mustard, honey and tarragon. Whisk in the cornstarch mixture. Bring to a slow, rolling boil and simmer for a couple of minutes, being sure to stir constantly until thickened to your satisfaction. Yield: Makes 1-1/3 cups.

MYRRH
(COMMIPHORA MYRRHA)

Brief Description

Shrubs yielding myrrh gum grow upwards to 30 feet in height and are native to northeastern Africa and southwestern Asia, especially in and around the Red Sea. The part used is the exudation from natural cracks in the bark or from manmade incisions. The exudation is a pale yellow liquid which soon hardens to form yellowish-red or reddish-brown tears or masses which are then collected.

Cures Breath, Gum Problems

In 1 pint boiling water, steep 2 sprigs coarsely chopped parsley, 3 whole spice cloves, 1 tsp. of powdered myrrh and 1/4 tsp. powdered goldenseal.

Stir occasionally while cooling, and then pour the clear liquid part through a strainer and use as a mouthwash to help get rid of bad breath, or gargle to get rid of a sore throat.

Raymond Saunders of Detroit, Michigan wrote to me several years ago about his own experience with myrrh for canker sores. They were caused by a certain food he was allergic to. One day, while reading through the Bible, he came upon a verse mentioning myrrh. A thought immediately flashed into his mind, "This will help you with your mouth problems."

He bought a box of cotton swabs, then some Nature's Way brand myrrh gum at a local health food store. He emptied the contents of 2 capsules of the powdered gum onto the surface of a clean plate. The he wet 2 cotton swabs under the tap before dipping them into the powder, and applied them directly to the cold sores in his mouth.

Using this treatment twice each day, his condition completely cleared up in less than a week. This same remedy also works well for fever blisters that form on the lips. For curing gingivitis or inflammation of the gums, just dip your wet toothbrush in a little powdered myrrh and brush the gums every day until the problem disappears.

Because of its decided antibiotic effects, myrrh gum appears in certain formulas (Sinese, Herpese, Resist-All, and Ginger-Up) used to treat allergies and infections. These are available from Great American Natural Products of Florida (see Appendix).

Sore Gums Relieved

Kenneth Murray of Cleveland, Ohio submitted the following true experience he had with finding quick relief for an annoying problem through natural means.

"I suffered from sore and bleeding gums, even though I brushed and flossed daily. I began taking 1,000 mg. of vitamin C three times a day. After just two weeks, the bleeding stopped. I also started rinsing my mouth twice a day with a combination of warm water and myrrh tincture after brushing. My gums are now completely healthy."

Kenneth made himself a simple tincture by combining 4 oz. of powdered myrrh gum with 10 oz. of vodka. (You can dilute this to a 50% alcohol solution by adding some distilled water.) He let the solution stand for two weeks, shaking it vigorously each day. The solution was then strained into another bottle suitable for storage. He used 15 drops of the 100% alcohol tincture in 3 fluid ounces of tap water for an effective oral rinse.

N

NASTURTIUM
(TROPAEOLUM MAJUS)

Brief Description

The common nasturtium is cultivated in the United States, along with several other species, as ornamentals for their yellow or red flowers. Some nasturtium plants are occasionally used for food: the tuberous rooted T. tuberosum or anu of the high Andes Mountains, the seeds (pickled as capers), and the tart flowers and leaves (used in salads). Properly used, Nasturtium is the botanical name for the water cresses, which isn't related to the genus Tropaeolum at all, but instead is an entirely different genus belonging to the mustard family.

Nasturtium Is a Marvelous Expectorant

This winding ornamental really helps break up the mucus congestion in the breathing passages and the lungs during colds and flus. A warm tea made of the flowers and leaves also acts as a disinfectant helping to kill unfriendly bacteria on contact, besides promoting the development of more white blood cells which fight infection inside the body.

The tea to be taken *isn't* made like your regular herb teas. Put a level double-handful of snipped nasturtium leaves and flowers into a food blender or processor. Then add enough hot *tap water* (*not* boiling) and liquefy to make a drink of smooth, somewhat runny consistency. Drink half of it and take the balance 3 hours later on an empty stomach, making sure both amounts are warm.

Festive Side Dish

NASTURTIUM RICE SALAD

This colorful, exotic rice dish can be served as part of a festive menu or at a picnic or barbecue. Or it can be eaten by itself as a meal.

Needed: 1 clove garlic, crushed; 3 tbsps. olive oil; 3 tbsps. nasturtium vinegar; 3 tbsps. apple juice; 1 cup cooked brown rice, cold; 1 medium onion, chopped; 1 medium green pepper, seeded and sliced; 4 slices fresh pineapple cut into chunks; 3 tbsps. cooked sweet corn; 1/2 cucumber, diced; nasturtiums to garnish.

In a small bowl, whisk the garlic oil, nasturtium vinegar, and juice together until smooth. In a large mixing bowl, toss the rice and onion with this dressing. Then stir in the pepper, pineapple, corn, and cucumbers. Arrange on a glass serving dish with flowers. Yield: Serves 5-6.

To make the nasturtium vinegar, cut into small pieces enough nasturtium leaves and flowers to make one-half cup. Put this amount into an empty quart glass jar and pour over it 2 1/2 cups apple cider vinegar. Screw on the lid and store in cool, dry place for 5 days, shaking the contents vigorously several times each day. Strain and store the liquid in another bottle for use later on.

NEEM
(Azadiracha indica)

Brief Description

The neem tree grows tall with masses of honey-scented white flowers throughout Pakistan, India and Sri Lanka. It yields fruit which looks a lot like olives. Flourishing along roadsides and clustered in market places and millions of city and village backyards, neem trees provide badly needed shade from the blistering Indian sun.

Neem grows vigorously in its arid environment and has been introduced to other parts of the world, where it is helping to reforest nations in West Africa and the Caribbean. Mature neem trees are capable of withstanding mild freezes and can grow in the United States as far north as central Florida and along coastal California to San Francisco.

A Preventive Aid Against Scabies, Fungus, and Mosquitoes

A pilot study in India involved 814 people treated for scabies (a contagious skin disease occurring in sheep, cattle and man, caused by parasitic mites that burrow under the skin) and resulted in a 97% cure rate within 3 to 15 days of treatment. The researchers found that neem paste was an inexpensive, easily available, effective mode of treatment for the villagers.

German researchers investigated neem preparations, including oils and extracts, and their effects on fungal parasites, yeasts and molds. Some of the neem extracts showed modest antifungal activity, probably due to the presence of a flavonoid known as quercetin.

A 2% neem oil mixture, smeared on uncovered body parts like the face, neck, forearms, hands, calves and legs, provided Indian volunteers complete protection from the bites of Anopheles mosquitoes for up to 12 hours. The application of neem was, therefore, deemed safe when used as a protection from malaria in endemic countries.

Neem oil preparations are available at many health food stores, herb shops, and nutrition centers, or through mail order companies like Great American Natural Products or Old-Amish Herbs, both located in St. Petersburg, FL (see Product Appendix for more information).

NETTLE
(see STINGING NETTLE)

NUTMEG
(MYRISTICA FRAGRANS)
(also see MACE)

Brief Description

Nutmeg is the seed of the nutmeg tree, which is an evergreen with spreading branches and very dense foliage, reaching to a height of 66 feet or so. A native of the Molucca Islands of Indonesia, nutmeg is now cultivated in many tropical regions, but is produced commercially mainly in Indonesia and the island of Granada in the West Indies.

The fruit of the nutmeg tree is fleshy like an apricot and about 2-4 inches in length. Upon ripening, it splits in half, exposing a bright-red, net-like aril wrapped around a dark reddish-brown and brittle shell within which lies a single seed. The net-like aril is mace, which on drying turns from red to yellowish or orange brown. The dried brown seed, after the shell is broken and discarded, is nutmeg.

Wonderful Stomach Tonic

Nutmeg and mace have been used for centuries to treat gas, indigestion, nausea, vomiting and other stomach as well as kidney problems. Mix thoroughly 1-1/2 tsps. of powdered slippery elm bark and dashes of powdered nutmeg and mace together with a little cold water in order to form a smooth paste that's not lumpy. Then bring a pint of half-and-half to the boiling point, removing immediately from the heat and quickly adding the powdered herb and spice paste. Keep stirring with a wooden ladle for about half a minute until the paste is thoroughly mixed in. Let it cool until lukewarm before drinking 1/2 cup. Repeat this procedure three times daily, always drinking the mixture warm to help heal stomach problems.

Marijuana Substitute for Mental Disorders

In our present society, more and more people are turning to drugs and alcohol in order to escape reality and enter into a world of mental bliss and trance-like happiness. Especially is this so with high-school and college-age youth. Unfortunately for them, most of the psycho-active substances which they turn to are not only illegal to use, but also very bad for their personal health as well. In most cases, they become addicted in time to such things as marijuana, cocaine, "crack," LSD, heroin and alcohol.

Some medical doctors and psychiatrists who work with young people under such addictions have explored alternative possibilities for those of their patients who apparently still need some kind of mind-altering substance from time to time in order to help them better cope with reality, but which isn't addictive. Catnip is one of these, which is mentioned elsewhere in this book (see CATNIP for details). Another, even more effective agent, is the food spice, nutmeg.

Both the *Journal of Neuropsychiatry* (March-April 1961) and the *New England Journal of Medicine* (August 22, 1963) have mentioned only 1 tbsp. of powdered nutmeg as being necessary to achieve somewhat "dream-like, floating and slightly euphoric" sensations. Such sensations of narcotic bliss have been equated with similar experiences produced by LSD, hashish, marijuana and alcohol.

One psychiatrist with the Department of Psychiatry at the University of Maryland School of Medicine in Baltimore subjected himself to an intake of nutmeg before recommending it to some of his own patients, in order to learn more about its hallucinogenic effects on the body. At 9 a.m. he took 1 tbsp. of the spice and drove to the university for his morning lectures. A particularly irritating problem had put him in a very angry mood. But "by 10:30 a.m.," he said, "the anger was dispelled and I felt at peace with the world. I wandered out to a leisurely lunch with some friends and felt quite unconcerned about my work. This is unusual for me." Other feelings of detachment and isolation from reality reached a peak that ranged from between 6 to 24 hours and didn't completely disappear until some 36 hours later.

Prison convicts have often benefited from the use of nutmeg when other forms of illegal drugs were absolutely impossible to obtain. As with LSD, they usually lose all sense and meaning of time. Their guilt tends to disappear as they learn to be more forgiving and loving of themselves. Feelings of sensuality likewise increase, and it is not unusual for many male prisoners to experience near-constant erections for most of the 24 to 36 hours while under the influence of this incredible spice.

Another feature preferred by some psychiatrists who might recommend nutmeg to some of their patients on a very limited and controlled basis is that the user can wrench himself or herself back to reality anytime it is so wished; this isn't the case with either LSD, "crack," cocaine, heroin or marijuana. Also the spice doesn't have any serious lingering side effects once it wears off like the others seem to have. And nutmeg isn't addictive like the rest are.

Dramatically increased mental awareness, a closer communion with Nature and Infinity, a sense of drifting through time and space, deeper feelings of humility and peace, and an attitude of being in control of what one wishes to experience, are some of the sensations reported by college students, some nurses and a few doctors who have voluntarily tried nutmeg under carefully controlled conditions.

Certain physical discomforts are to be expected when under the influence of nutmeg, but nothing, it seems, that would be life-threatening. Bones and muscles in the body tend to ache, the eyes tend to hurt a little, the sinuses drain, and limited diarrhea result from taking this spice. But some therapists and some of their patients suffering from certain mental disorders seem to believe that these few inconveniences are worth enduring in lieu of the greater therapeutic benefits to be derived from nutmeg.

Besides eggnog, there are other creative dishes which call for the use of nutmeg and may be yet another way of obtaining this spice for mental pleasure without always having to ingest it straight.

NUTMEG-BAKED GOLDENS

Pare and core 8 Golden Delicious apples 1/3 of the way down from the top. Place in a 13 x 9 x 2-inch baking pan. Combine 1 cup dark honey, 2/3 cup water, 1/4 cup lemon juice, 1/2 tsp. each grated lemon and lime peels, 1 tsp. nutmeg and 1 tsp. mace. Bring everything to a boil, then pour over and around the apples.

Bake, uncovered, at 350°F. 50-60 minutes or until apples are tender. Frequently baste with the liquid mixture in the pan every 10 minutes. Cool in the pan. When ready to serve, remove apples to serving dish. Add 1/4 cup boiling water to the pan to dilute mixture, or simply use the nutmeg syrup in its full strength after heating up on the stove. Drizzle the mixture over the apples before topping with genuine vanilla ice cream. If desired, add rum or your favorite liqueur to softened ice cream and freeze for several hours or until sufficiently firm. Makes 8 delicious and invigorating servings.

NUX VOMICA
(Strychnos nux vomica)

Brief Description

The strychnos tree has been exploited by numerous cultures for many centuries for its dried, ripe seeds, which are potentially very toxic. The tree itself is deciduous, grows well throughout Pakistan, India and Sri Lanka. It has a thin gray bark (similar to the ash tree in appearance) and shiny elliptical leaves with greenish-white flowers arranged in terminal cymes.

The fruit is about the size of a large apple, having a smooth hard rind or shell, which when fully mature turns an orange hue. The inside is filled with a soft white jelly-like pulp containing five seeds covered with a soft woolly-like substance that is white and horny internally. The seeds are removed when ripe, thoroughly washed, dried in the sun, and then sorted before being shipped to various parts of the world.

The seeds are often used in Ayurvedic medicine (an ancient healing system indigenous to India) but only after first being treated to detoxify them. The process is known in Hindi as *shodhana* and consists of soaking them in fresh cow's milk for a week and then peeling off their softened outer coats.

Many alkaloids are obtained from the strychnos tree, but none has been more thoroughly studied than strychnine, which is contained in the bark and leaves of the tree. Strychnine is an extremely poisonous substance used for destroying rodents and predatory animals and for trapping fur-bearing animals.

Cures Opium and Heroin Addictions

So what is such a toxic plant material doing in an herb book like this? Well, believe it or not, in skilled hands and under *strict medical supervision* the seeds have some wonderful healing benefits.

The Ayurvedic physicians of India routinely boil the seeds in milk (as previously mentioned) and then pound them into a paste using a mortar and pestle. Very small doses (usually no more than 1/8 teaspoon) are given each day on the tongues of heroin and opium addicts to cure them of their addictions. The success rate ranges anywhere from 63 to 77%, depending on length of treatment (up to two months in some cases) and severity of the addiction itself.

Potent Homeopathic Remedy for Hangover, Drug Overdose, and Cardiac Arrest

A fairly recent work by Dr. Michael Weiner, *The Complete Book of Homeopathy* (NY: Avery Publishing Group, Inc., 1989; p. 180) declared that nux vomica is a very useful antidote for "the effects of overdrugging from allopathic medications, coffee, tea and alcohol." Furthermore, the author insisted, nux vomica should be "the first remedy for patients who have been dosed heavily with allopathic drugs" in order to clear the system and thereby restore these individuals to full health.

In various states where homeopathic physicians are properly licensed and legally allowed to practice their craft and prescribe their unique drugs, nux vomica has been frequently used *in very minute and carefully mea-sured dosages* for the treatment of surgical shock and cardiac arrest. A homeopathic extract of nux vomica is usually given in 1/4 to 1/2 grain amounts, while a tincture of the same thing is given in 10 minims. These are medical terms that only a skilled homeopathic practitioner would understand.

Those who suffer from such problems and wish to explore further the natural alternatives offered by homeopathy may do so by checking tele-phone Yellow Pages or alternative medicine directories, or by inquiring at local health food stores, herb shops or chiropractors for the homeopathic practitioner closest to them.

WARNING: Nux vomica is a violent poison! It can induce terrible mental and emotional hallucinations and may even prove fatal in unskilled hands. Only a competent and qualified homeopathic doctor with the necessary training should be administering nux vomica to you.

In the event that symptoms of poisoning become evident, syrup of ipecac (see IPECACUANHA) from a local drugstore should be taken as directed on the package in order to evacuate the stomach promptly!

For a listing of certified homeopathic physicians in your city or state, write to the following center and request its *Directory of Homeopathic Practitioners*. Be sure to enclose $5.00 to cover costs.

The National Center for Homeopathy

1500 Massachusetts Ave. N.W.

Washington DC 20005

Two old and established companies which supply nux vomica and other homeopathic remedies are:

Boericke & Tafel, Inc.

1011 Arch Street

Philadelphia, PA 19107

and

John A. Borneman & Sons

1208 Armosland Road

Norwood, PA 19074

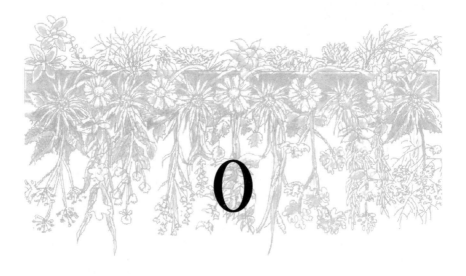

O

OAK
(QUERCUS SPECIES)

Brief Description

The genus Quercus, with many species of deciduous and evergreen trees and shrubs, is the most important aggregation of hardwoods found on the North American continent, if not the Northern Hemisphere. The oaks are widely distributed throughout temperate regions of the Northern Hemisphere, and extend southward to the mountains of Colombia in South America, and to the Indian Ocean Archipelago in the Eastern Hemisphere. There are 70 species native to the United States, and about 58 of these reach tree size. There are also about 70 recognized hybrids. The uses of oak include almost everything the human race has ever derived from trees: timber, food for people and animals, fuel, water-shed protection, shade and beauty, tannin and extractives, and cork. Consequently, the oaks are widely planted for many purposes.

Antidote for Medication Poisoning

Boil 1-1/2 pints water, then add 1 tablespoon each crushed acorn and white oak bark. Cover and simmer for 12 minutes, then set aside and steep for another 20 minutes. Strain and add one-half cup to an equal amount of milk and take internally to help neutralize the effects of medication poisoning.

Reduce the Swelling of Varicose Veins

The same tea will also help to reduce swollen varicose veins. Drink one cup of the tea every evening. At the same time soak a cotton washcloth in some of the *hot* tea, wring out excess liquid and apply over swollen veins. Cover with a dry, folded hand towel and leave until the first cloth becomes cool. Then soak another washcloth in some *cold* tea, wring out and apply as before. Leave on until it becomes warm. Alternate between hot and cold packs for 25 minutes, after drinking a cup of the *warm* tea. Continue this procedure for up to ten days.

A Remedy for Other Problems

This tea is also of service for other health problems. (Whether to take the tea hot or cold depends a lot on the type of problem for which it is being used.)

bloody stool/urine (cold)	mouth sores (cold)
fever (hot)	skin irritations (hot)
hemorrhoids (cold)	sores (hot)
menstruation (excess) (cold)	sore throat (hot)

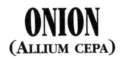

ONION
(ALLIUM CEPA)

Brief Description

Not too many people may be aware of the fact that the elegant lily family (which includes the beautiful Easter lilies) contains a branch of aromatically opinionated cousins that includes onions, garlics, leeks, chives, scallions, shallots, and asparagus. Although each has a strong and distinct personality, there is a strong family resemblance. All are rich in the trace element compound sulphur, which brings out their potent flavor and also makes them stink when they rot.

Some of these things were consumed with obvious relish in ancient Egypt not only by the Hebrews but by their Egyptian taskmasters as well. For we find that after leaving the land of their captivity under the capable leadership of Moses, the Hebrews began missing such items and complained to him on more than one occasion: "We remember the fish, which we did eat in Egypt freely; the cucumbers, and the melons, and the leeks, and the *onions*, and the garlick..." (Numbers 11:5). Pliny, the great Roman historian, wrote that the Egyptians also invoked the onion when taking oaths, much as people do today in court on the Bible.

There are hundreds of varieties of onions on the market today. California ranks first in the country for dry onion production, providing virtually all of the fresh-market dry onions, and about 60% of the dehydrated onions. To buy good onions, select only those that are firm bulbs with clean papery skins, avoiding any that are soft, wet, or sprouting. They should be stored in a dry, cool, well-ventilated place. When sliced, wrap them in plastic and refrigerate. Whole onions should keep for almost a month. There is nothing more foul-smelling than rotting onions!

Green onions (also called spring onions or scallions) are often used in Asian cooking. Wilder than many dry onions, they are also served raw in relish plates and salads.

Shallots are shaped somewhat like garlic, with tissue-wrapped cloves, but they taste like a delicate dry onion. Shallots are frequently used in French cooking and considered more of a gourmet herb than regular dry onion.

An Onion a Day Keeps Old Age Away

The late Belle Boone Beard, a sociologist who once worked for the National Institute of Aging, had files on 8,500 centenarians whom she had interviewed in her lifetime. One interesting thing Beard kept noticing in the thousands of surveys she filled out on their eating habits: nearly everyone who reached 100 years of age enjoyed eating *lots* of onions! In fact, many of them admitted to her that they had onions just about *every day* with a meal. Knowing that onions are strong antioxidants and can control free radicals, which are implicated in the aging process, Beard assumed that this played a *major* role in these centenarians living so long in remarkably good health. Certainly a little "onion a day" will go far in helping to "keep old age away."

Terrific Burn Medicine

The February, 1944 *Bulletin of the History of Medicine* (15:143-49) contained a most informative article by medical historian Henry E. Sigerist entitled "Ambroise Pare's Onion Treatment of Burns." Pare was a famous French surgeon (1510-1590), who was looking for a simpler, easier, and more effective remedy for burns than the standard cooling ointments of his day. He discovered it in a most remarkable way in Piedmont around 1537. At that time he was a young surgeon of 27 and was attached to the army of the Marshal de Montejan in the third war between Francis I and Charles V. One of the kitchen boys employed by this Marshal "fell by chance into a Caldron of Oyle being even almost boyling hot," Pare later recounted in his memoirs. The good doctor was immediately called on to attend to the poor lad's injuries. He quickly went to the local apothecaries "to fetch refrigerating medicines commonly used in this case," when he met "by chance a certaine old countrey woman, who...perswaded mee...that I should lay to raw Onions beaten with a little salt" on the boy's injured skin. "Wherefore," he continued, "I thought good to try the force of her Medicine upon this greasy scullion. I the next day found those places of his body whereeto the Onions lay, to be free from blisters, but the other parts which they had not touched, to be all blistered."

And so came about Pare's famous onion dressing for all degrees of minor or serious burns. He soon had occasion to use it on some soldiers who were unfortunate enough to have some gunpowder explode in front of them, severely burning their hands and faces. In a mortar and pestle, Pare crushed slices of onion with a little salt and applied this dressing to part of their injuries and regular ointments to the other part. He recorded: "I observed the part dressed with the Onions quite free from blisters and excoriation, the other [covered only with ointments] being troubled by both...."

On more than one occasion have I recommended that freshly expressed onion juice be mixed with a pinch of salt and applied directly to even the worst burns and left overnight, with fantastic results the next day. This may be a folk remedy from the Middle Ages, but it was constantly tested by a competent doctor of the times and always proven to be effective. My own experience with the same thing through the years has only confirmed what Pare himself discovered and proved as valid therapy for burns.

Syndicated Columnist Recommends Onion for Insect Bites and Stings

Ann Landers is one of America's most beloved and well-read columnists. For almost three decades now, her daily syndicated column has appeared in over 1,000 newspapers nationwide, including those of several foreign countries. The helpful advice offered has been of definite assistance to many of her readers.

Her column for Monday, December 15, 1986 appeared in the *Salt Lake Tribune* (p. A-14) and contained a brief account by a beekeeper on the West Coast, who had followed some of her advice in a previous column. "I read in your column," he wrote, "that rubbing a bee sting with half a juicy onion would not only stop the pain, but also cause the swelling to go down. It sounded improbable and I forgot about it until a few days ago when I was stung by one of my 'ladies.' I applied the onion and lo and behold, as if by magic, the pain stopped within minutes and the swelling went down." Her short response was to this effect: "Dozens of readers have written to say they, too, had instant results. (It works for wasp stings, too.) It's a great feeling to know I've helped."

How Chicago Got Its Name

Here's a little tidbit of history I bet you didn't know about. The French explorer Père Jacques Marquette happened to be around a point on the southern shore of Lake Michigan in 1624 with some trusted Indian guides, when they showed him an unbelievable abundance of wild onions grow-ing on thousands of acres of wilderness land. With their faces and noses wrinkled in disgust, these Indian scouts pointed in the direction of the onion fields and spoke a word which they gave to the highly offensive odor coming from that direction. "*Chicago!*" they muttered, "bad *Chicago!*" And that is how Marquette came to call the spot by which it would be for-ever known thereafter as "Chicago," thanks to the Illinois Indians who were with him on that momentous occasion.

An Excellent Room Disinfectant

During the Civil War, so strong was General Ulysses S. Grant's belief that onions could prevent dysentery and other ills of warm climates that he wired the War Department, "I will not move my army without onions." The next day, three trainloads were promptly dispatched to the front lines.

Mary Thorne Quelch, a British herbalist of some years ago, mentioned that if "at least one sliced onion" were placed "in every room" during "any epidemic in the neighborhood" and then replaced the next morning with fresh ones, the disease germs that caused smallpox, diphtheria, measles, mumps, chickenpox, scarlet fever and tuberculosis, would be absorbed into the onions themselves, thereby preventing the contagion from spreading to other members of the household. She claimed that the onions "acted as traps" for these airborne bacteria, but warned that " the cut onions should be burned daily" and never, never eaten!

An Asthma Treatment That Works

Some years ago I read about an unusual experiment conducted with guinea pigs, in which they were sensitized to ovalbumin, the major protein con-stituent of egg white from hens' eggs. This sensitization brought on bela-bored breathing in all the test animals, mimicking the asthma or bronchitis attacks that humans routinely suffer from. Thirty minutes *before* bronchial obstruction was induced, however, half of the guinea pigs were *pretreated* orally with an alcoholic extract of onions or just with alcohol alone. The simulated asthma or bronchial attacks in guinea pigs pretreated with onion extract were substantially reduced.

Based on this information, which appeared in the journal *Agents Actions* (14:626-29, May-June 1984), I developed a very simple remedy of my own to test on asthma or bronchitis sufferers. Using a Vita-Mix Whole Food Machine, I pureed one large peeled and quartered red onion and scooped it out with a rubber cake spatula into the center of a clean white cotton handkerchief. I then drew the four ends together in the middle and tied them with a piece of string. I then placed this inside a medium-sized *crockware* mixing bowl and poured enough brandy over to cover it entirely. (Glassware may be used instead, but avoid using metal.) I covered the top of the bowl with a clean dish towel and set it in the corner for about 5 days. Wearing rubber gloves so that the onion juice wouldn't irritate my skin, I took the bound handkerchief in both hands and slowly twisted the top and bottom in opposite directions in order to squeeze out every drop of juice I could. I emptied the handkerchief of its onion contents and later washed it by hand. I then strained the onion-brandy mixture through a paper coffee filter, bottled it, and stored it in the cupboard.

I divided this liquid into equal shares for several asthma and bronchitis cases I personally knew and had them take two tablespoons of this liquid about 20 minutes *before* they thought an inhalation challenge might occur. They reported back to me later that *none* of them suffered their usual asthma or bronchitis attacks and were able to sleep at night without any further disturbances to their breathing.

Delicious Recipe

This delicious blend of onions and fresh, pungent parsley is sure to be a favorite with yourself, your family or invited guests.

CREAMY ONION SOUP WITH FLOWERS

Needed: 2 large onions, thinly sliced; 1 tbsp. sage or thyme flower oil; 2-1/2 cups nonfat milk; 1-1/2 cups water; pinch of granulated kelp for flavor; 5 tsps. whole wheat flour; 5 tbsps. nonfat yogurt mixed with 1 tsp. lime juice; and sprigs of parsley and flowers to garnish.

In a saucepan, sautee the onions in oil on medium heat for 2 minutes. (If herb oil isn't readily available, then just use extra virgin olive oil instead.) Reduce the heat to low, add the milk, 1 cup water, and kelp. Cover and simmer for about half an hour or until the onion is tender.

In a small bowl, blend the flour with the remaining water, and stir into the pan. Increase the heat to medium high, bring to a rapid boil and cook, stirring constantly, until slightly thickened. Remove from the heat

and add the yogurt and lime juice. Reheat but without boiling this time.
Serve garnished with parsley and flowers.

Yield: Serves 4.

OREGANO
(see MARJORAM & OREGANO)

OSHA
(LIGUSTICUM PORTERI)

Brief Description

Osha is a typical member of the parsley family. It has finely divided, hollow stems, flat-topped umbels of seeds and flowers springing from a simple juncture like an umbrella. It may also be distinguished by its strong celery or parsley aroma. The root is large, dark brown, and hairy, with a yellow, soapy inner pith and a strong, distinctive celery-butterscotch scent. It
is common to the West and Southwest and readily obtainable in the wild.

A Legion of Medicinal Uses

Osha is one of only a very few roots that I know of which should *not* be
made into a tea, because heat of *any* kind will render it worthless. It's most
effective taken as a tincture or chewed or in capsules. I recommend the
first; here's how to make it.

Take two full osha roots and wash them thoroughly under running
water. Pat them dry with an old towel. Grate them on a hand-held vegetable grater just as you would with carrots. Then place into a medium-
sized stainless steel pot and cover them about one-half inch above with
three-quarters blackstrap molasses and one-quarter brandy. Cover, set over
low heat, and simmer for an hour, checking every so often to make sure
nothing is burning in the pan. When partially cooled, strain through a
muslin cloth bag and squeeze to get out all of the liquid. Then store in a
pint fruit jar.

This tincture is ideal for viral infections, especially a sore throat. It is
also quite effective with allergies, asthma, bronchitis, and indigestion. Take
one tablespoon of the liquid tincture on an empty stomach every few hours
for these complaints.

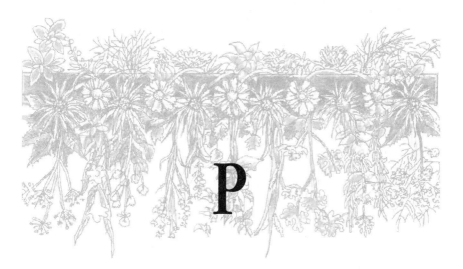

P

PANSY

(see VIOLET)

PAPRIKA

(see CAYENNE)

PARSLEY
(PETROSELINUM CRISPUM)

Brief Description

Parsley is a non-hairy biennial or short-lived perennial with a much-branched stem. A thin, white, spindle-shaped root produces the erect, grooved, glabrous, angular stem that can reach a height of slightly over 2 feet. The plant is often cultivated as an annual for its foliage, especially in California, Germany, France, Belgium and Hungary. There are numerous varieties. Parts used are the ripe fruits (seeds), the above-ground herb and the leaves.

White or greenish-yellow flowers appear in compound umbels from June to August. Curiously enough, parsley is poisonous to most birds but is very good for animals, curing maladies such as foot-rot in sheep and

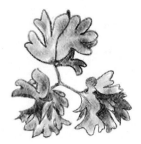

goats. The wild parsleys found throughout the British isles are closely allied to the celeries and were used by the Anglo-Saxons in ancient times to mend skulls broken in combat.

Removing "Dragon Breath"

Ever smell a dog's breath, or someone with acute halitosis? They're bad enough to gag you. But now there's a simple cure for both conditions. The next time you feed your dog, mix several sprigs of parsley in with a little raw chopped or ground beef, then combine that with the animal's regular dry chow. You'll be surprised how well this works! And as for human breath problems, simply dip a couple of sprigs in vinegar and thoroughly chew them slowly before swallowing. The purifying effect should remove offensive odors for at least 3-4 hours.

CleanLife Products of Stanton, California introduced in the summer of 1995 a new breath spray that neutralizes the odor of alcoholic beverages and other substances. BreathAmint's "all-natural formula is able to eliminate the presence of such odors as alcohol, tobacco or garlic instead of simply masking them with a different odor," a company spokesperson told me. Beyond this, however, it can neutralize sulphur compounds in the mouth, act as a natural antibacterial agent to help prevent tooth decay, and can increase natural saliva flow.

One of the principal ingredients is parsley; another is rosemary and a third is peppermint. A few other minor herbs are included as well as vitamin C, lecithin and xylitol from birch bark. According to Donna Carlson, the company's marketing director, "Once someone applies our product, the odor will not be detected because it will be gone for good."

An Ignored Cancer Preventative

Most people don't know that a few sprigs of parsley pack a wallop so far as cancer goes. For one thing, they contain about as much vitamin A as 1/4 tsp. of cod-liver oil. For another, they yield about two-thirds of the vitamin C that an *entire* orange does! Furthermore, parsley ranks higher than most vegetables in an important amino acid, histidine, which strongly inhibits tumor development within the body, according to *Mutation Research* (77: 245-50). And vitamins A and C are now recognized as significant nutrients in the fight against cancer. Therefore, it seems we'd all be better off eating more parsley than just leaving it on our plates.

Yucatan Remedy for Kidney Problems

Throughout the Yucatan Peninsula of southeastern Mexico, a tea is made out of fresh parsley herb to treat kidney inflammation, inability to urinate, painful urination, kidney stones and edema. Bring 1 qt. water to a boil. Remove from heat and add 1 cup of coarsely chopped parsley. Cover and let steep 40 mins., then strain before drinking. Take 1 cup of warm tea 4 times daily with meals.

Overcomes Sexual Frigidity

This same parsley tea also manifests mildly aphrodisiac properties for couples experiencing sexual frigidity of any kind in their relationships. The same directions would be followed, except that 2 cups of chopped parsley are used with 1 qt. of water, steeping time is an hour and 2 cups of *very warm* tea are consumed by each partner at least 20 minutes before sexual activities begin.

Interestingly enough, parsley has been fed to sheep in Spain to bring them into heat in any season of the year. Some couples with whom I've spoken after they've tried the above remedy have reported to me somewhat increased stimulations in their sexual desires, although several wished that this herb worked more powerfully in this respect.

Clears Up Bruises

An old Romanian gypsy remedy called for several sprigs of parsley leaves to be crushed, then applied directly to any bruise on the skin and left there for a while. Repeated applications would usually clear up any black-and-blue marks within a day or so.

Exciting Recipe

The following dish is part of a traditional Iranian New Year's feast that's both delicious as well as very tempting.

PARSLEY-GREEN ONION RICE WITH FISH

Needed: 3 cups uncooked rice; warm water; kelp; 2 bunches chopped green onions; 2 bunches chopped parsley; 3 lbs. fish fillets; sea salt as needed; pinch of turmeric; 2 tbsps. butter.

Rinse rice several times until water is clear; soak in warm water with salt added. Bring a large pot of water to boil (about 8 cups water). Drain water from soaked rice and add rice to boiling water. Boil about 10-15 mins. until rice is not crunchy but still quite firm. Store occasionally to prevent grains from sticking together.

Drain rice in a strainer; add chopped onions and parsley. Pour some cold water over rice, parsley and onions. Cover the bottom of the pot with butter and some water. Sprinkle rice and these two vegetables into the pot, a spoonful at a time, keeping them in the center of the pot so as not to touch the sides of the pot. Cover pot lid with paper or dish towel and place lid tightly on pot. Cook approximately 10 mins. over medium heat, then reduce heat to low. Allow rice to steam 30-40 mins.

Cut fish into serving pieces; sprinkle with sea salt, kelp and a bit of turmeric. In a skillet, brown fish, cooking until done on both sides in butter. Serve with rice.

PASQUE FLOWER
(see ANEMONE)

PASSION FLOWER
(Passiflora incarnata)

Brief Description

Passion flower is common to the Deep South and the Midwest. It is also commercially grown for culinary and medicinal purposes in cooler environs. The plant itself is a rather hairy, woody vine that likes to climb trees and walls. The stems can be anywhere from 12 to 26 feet in length and climb by means of axillary tendrils. The flowers bloom from May to July, are milky white and with purple, blue or pink calyx crowns.

State Flower Also Potent Medicine for Hyperactive and Drug-Addicted People

"T.W." (as everyone calls him) Edwards is an old friend of mine residing in Memphis, Tennessee. He has treated folks for miles around over the years using nothing but herbs from the woods and meadows of his state.

But more than that, he swore, it was *the* perfect medicine to give hyperactive kids or adults as well as senior citizens suffering from tranquilizer addictions. He claimed it worked well for insomnia and nervous tensions, too. He preferred it in the form of a tea.

Both the vine tendrils and flower are employed. His method for making the tea is this: Boil 1 pint of water. Clip with scissors into small pieces enough vine and flowers to equal two-thirds cup. Add this to the water, cover and simmer on low heat for ten minutes. Then set aside and steep for 40 minutes. Strain and refrigerate. Reheat to lukewarm and drink one cup every 5 hours on an empty stomach.

PAU D'ARCO
(TABEBUIA SPECIES)

Brief Description

In the ever dwindling rain forests of South America may be found huge trees reaching upwards of 100 feet in height and frequently with a trunk circumference exceeding *four feet!* The leaves are deciduous, opposite, on yellow-green stems; they have five elliptic leaves of unequal size that can be either lanceolate or ovate shaped. These leaves are uniquely placed in whorls comparable to the fingers of someone's hand. They reside on stems that are dark green on top and yellowish-green below.

The flowers vary in color depending on the species. They can range from blue and yellow to magenta and purple. They have yellow throats and are either bell-or funnel-shaped.

The Elimination of Pain from Almost Any Disease

Pau d'arco has been around in the American health food industry for sometime now, as an especially popular folk treatment for a variety of *cancers.* It is taken in tea, tincture or capsule forms. My friend, Michael Tierra (a practicing herbalist residing in Santa Cruz, California) has wisely cautioned customers to be careful of their source for the bark; he said that some companies have tried to harvest the pouter bark from immature trees, when the real potency lays within the inner bark of older trees.

Mike especially likes pau d'arco in tea form, believing it is more efficacious when taken this way. And while herbalists like himself have recommended it for a wide variety of problems, ranging from *osteomyelitis, ringworm,* and *bronchitis* to *gastritis, colitis, cystitis, prostatitis, lupus* and *Hodgkin's disease,* he prefers to keep things simpler than this. Having had considerable experience with the herb tea himself, he has categorized its use this way: "Pau d'arco's chief purpose seems to be in the elimination of *pain* caused by almost *any* disease you can think of."

Boil one quart of water. Add two cups of crudely cut inner bark. Cover and simmer for 20 minutes. Set aside and steep 1-1/2 hours. Strain and refrigerate. Drink one cup 5 times daily on an empty stomach.

He claims it is also very effective in eliminating *parasitic* penetration through the skin; in cases like Schistosomiasis (snail fever) it would be very good.

Consumer Beware

Consumers purchasing pau d'arco products in health food stores or from direct marketing companies may not always be getting what they expect or pay for. A review of a dozen such pau d'arco products from different Ottawa, Canada health food stores revealed that all but two of them lacked adequate amounts of lapachol (an important naphthoquinone) to make them medically effective. The study, which appeared in the *Journal of Herbs, Spices & Medicinal Plants* (2(4):37, 1994) shows that most pau d'arco products sold today aren't very potent or effective.

PENNYROYAL
(HEDEOMA PULEGIOIDES)

Brief Description

Pennyroyal is an annual herb found in forests and fields from the Midwest to the Northeast. The plant's erect, square, branching stem grows from 10 to 20 inches tall and bears small, opposite, thin, ovate leaves which are sparingly toothed. Axillary clusters of small, tubular flowers, lavender or somewhat purplish in hue, appear from the early summer to the middle of autumn. The entire plant yields a nice, aromatic odor.

Relieves the Itching of Skin Eruptions

One of the best uses for this herb is in the form of a tea used as an external wash for scabies, psoriasis, hives, shingles, and childhood diseases like measles, mumps and chickenpox. It also works well in cases of rash due to wet diapers and contact with poison ivy or poison oak plants.

Boil two pints of water; add one cup fresh or dried cut herb. Cover and set aside to steep for an hour. Strain and refrigerate. Gently wash the afflicted skin surface frequently, about every two hours. Using a sponge to do this is preferable to using a washcloth. Some of the cool tea may also be sprayed on to the skin through an empty plastic spray bottle.

PEONY
(PAEONIA OFFICINALIS)

Brief Description

Peony is a perennial plant which occurs in the wild as well as being cultivated in a number of gardens. It has distinguishing large, solitary, red or purplish-red flowers somewhat resembling roses, a green and juicy stem between two and three feet high, and a thick, knobby rootstock.

A peony common to the West Coast is the California peony (P. californica). It has inch-wide, hanging, maroon and red flowers atop fleshy 6-to-18-inch-high stems. The foliage is an attractive blue-green during the spring growing season.

Useful Remedy for Gout and Asthma

A useful extract for treating gout and asthma can be made from the root. Bring 1-1/2 pints of red wine to a slow rolling boil. Add 1/4 cup chopped peony root, cover and simmer on low heat for 15 minutes. Set aside, steep for 30 minutes, strain and refrigerate. Drink one-half cup twice daily on an empty stomach. CAUTION: The flowers and leaves of peony can make you sick; therefore, they should not be used internally.

Peony root is very popular in Chinese medicine. It is used to alleviate the pain and swelling of traumatic injuries, and to clear away congealed blood resulting from serious bumps or bruises. It is useful in the early stages of abscesses, boils and carbuncles.

PEPPER
(see BLACK PEPPER and CAYENNE PEPPER)

PEPPERMINT
(see MINTS)

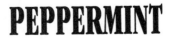

PERUVIAN BARK
(see CINCHONA)

PINE
(PINUS SPECIES)

Brief Description

The genus Pinus is one of the largest and most important of the coniferous genera. It comprises about 95 species and numerous varieties and hybrids. Pines are widely distributed, mostly in the Northern Hemisphere, from sea level to timberline. They range from Alaska to Nicaragua, from Scandinavia to North Africa, and from Siberia to Sumatra. Some species, such as Scotch pine, are widely distributed from Scotland to Siberia, while others have very restricted ranges. Canary Island pine is found growing naturally only in the Canary Islands, and Torrey pine numbers only a few thousand individuals in two California localities.

There are 42 species of Pinus native to America. Artificial planting has extended the range of several of these.

The pines are evergreen trees of various heights, often tall but occasionally shrubby. Some species such as sugar pine, western and eastern white pine, and ponderosa pine, grow to more than 210 feet tall. On the other hand, the Mexican pinyon and Japanese stone pine may not exceed 33 feet in height.

Famous French Explorer Discovers Powerful Antioxidant in Pine

Since about 1992 an extract obtained from the outer covering of conifer trees has been making headlines nationwide and has virtually revolutionized the whole antioxidant movement within the health food industry. The substance is called pycnogenol (pronounced pick-naw-jen-all) and comes mostly from the pine bark which coats the maritime pine found in the Canadian province of Quebec and along the Atlantic seacoast of southern France.

Dr. Jack Bordeaux (now at the University of Bordeaux), while working at the University of Quebec some years ago, rediscovered this remarkable antioxidant. He invented and developed a patented extraction process for removing it from pine bark and putting it into a form which the human body could more easily assimilate. An average of 2 to 4 capsules a day, (or 60 to 120 milligrams) in divided doses of 1 or 2 in the morning and the same again at night, is recommended for a number of things. These include but are not limited to: acne, blood clot, bronchitis, cholesterol (elevated), diabetes, emphysema, gout, fatigue, fever, free radical activity, fungal infection, hypertension, influenza, leukemia, lupus, migraines, morning and motion sicknesses, paralysis, Parkinson's disease, rheumatoid arthritis, scurvy, skin ulcers, sinusitis, stroke and varicose veins. In every instance, where people who have suffered from one or several of these disorders have started taking this pine derivative in the amounts previously suggested, there have been noticeable improvements in their health. Mind you, *this is not a cure*; but pycnogenol has produced enough incredible results to astound doctors and amaze even the most ardent skeptics!

But where did it all begin? To understand this we must travel back in time to the spring of 1534 when the famous french explorer Jacques Cartier landed with three ships and 110 men inside the Strait of Belle Isle near the mouth of the St. Lawrence River in present-day Quebec Province. Driven by greed and the hope of finding gold, these men pressed relentlessly forward into the Canadian wilderness. They subsisted that entire winter on nothing but ship's provisions, which was mostly hardtack (hard flour biscuit) and salted meat. No fresh fruits or vegetables of any kind were ever consumed. It wasn't long before scurvy set in, claiming large numbers of their party. They grew progressively ill with these various disease symptoms becoming all too apparent in many of them: weight loss, bone/joint aches and pains, bleeding gums, loosened teeth, loose bowels, internal hemorrhages, large black-and-blue areas painful to the touch appearing on various parts of the anatomy, eventual pathology of the heart, lungs, and bone marrow, blood loss occasioned by hemorrhages leading to anemia, and then total utter fatigue and hideous death.

It might have been curtains for the lot of them had not an old wizened Indian shared with the Frenchmen a life-saving secret. He showed them how to make a tea brewed from the bark and needles taken from the Anneda tree, a plant-relative of the maritime pine. Once they started drinking copious amounts of this, they quickly recovered from their multiple miseries and weren't long in regaining their health.

So poignant an experience is this that I decided to include the full excerpt dealing with it in this book. I took as my historical source for this *The Voyages of Jacques Cartier* by H.P. Biggar (Ottawa, Quebec: Publications of the Archives of Canada No. 11, 1924; pp.213-15).

"The captain [Cartier] seeing the aforementioned Dom Agaya healthy and deliberate, was joyous, hoping to learn from him, how he was cured, so that his men could be given aid and help. So when they had arrived near the fort, the captain asked him how he was cured of his sickness [scurvy]. Dom Agaya replied that it was with the juice of the leaves of a tree and the water the leaves were boiled in, that he was cured and that this was the special remedy for the sickness. Then the captain asked him if there were any such trees around there, and asked him to show him one so that he could cure his servant, who had caught the aforesaid sickness in the house of seigneur Donnacona [at Quebec] not wanting to let him know the number of his companions who were sick.

"Then Agaya [the old Indian chief] sent two women with our captain, to cure him, they brought nine or ten branches; and showed us how the bark must be pulled off and the leaves [needles] of these branches, and all put into water to boil; then the water drunk once in two days; and the juices of the leaves and bark pressed out and the water put on the swollen and sick limbs; and he said that the tree will cure all manner of sickness. They call the said tree in their language, *anneda.*

"Immediately afterwards, the captain had the drink made, so the sick could drink, of these however no one wanted to try it, only one or two, who decided to try it [on account of its intense bitterness]. As soon as they had drunk, they felt much better, which they found a true and evident miracle; for of all the sicknesses they had suffered from, after having drunk two or three times, they recovered their health and were cured, so that some of the company who had syphilis for more than five or six years before getting this sickness [scurvy], by this medicine were they completely cured. After having seen this, there was such a great demand made for this medicine that a tree, as large and as tall as I have ever seen was used in less than eight days, which made such a cure that if all the doctors of Louvain and Montpellier [in France] had tried, with all the drugs of Alexandria [Egypt], they could not have done as much in one year as this tree did in eight days; For it profiteth us so much, that all those who wanted to try it, recovered health and were cured, by the Grace of God."

Rash Brought on by Indian Witchcraft Cured with Pine Ashes

One of the most fascinating uses for pine that I've ever come across concerned the burning of pine boughs and the use of their ashes to remove a rash brought on through Indian witchcraft. It is related by Edna B. Patterson in her very entertaining book *Sagebrush Doctors* (Springville,UT: Art City Publishing Co., 1972; p.37). She referred to the use of peyote by members of the Native American Church. She noted that the peyote cult had even spread to the northeast part of her own state (Nevada) from the Wind River (Wyoming) and Fort Hall (Idaho) Indian Reservations by the 1930s, affecting "some members of the northern Paiute tribe of Miller Creek, Duck Valley Reservation. One negative aspect connected with the use of this natural hallucinogen from the mushroomlike crown (or peyote) of the spineless cactus, was its association with witchcraft.

"One example of this fear," she wrote, "concerns two Lee Indian Reservation ranchers, one a user of the drug and the other an abstainer. In 1965 both men irrigated acres from the same water ditch and this led to trouble between the two with the argument reaching a crescendo as the peyote man made threats and called on Friend Peyote to bring evil down upon his neighbor and his family. The man against whom the menace had been directed returned home only to find his twelve-year-old daughter broken out in a violent skin rash and was convinced peyote 'voo-doo' had taken place. To counter the evil magic he resorted to oldtime Shoshone medicine. Building a fire of pine boughs he let it burn to ashes and taking the residue, rubbed the girl's body with the waste. After one application of the ashes the rash receded and in twenty-four hours completely disappeared."

Some years ago, while conducting interviews on the Navajo Indian Reservation with a number of medicine men, I learned from one particular shaman named George Running Mule Begay that he had sometimes sprinkled the ashes of burnt pine boughs over the skin of young children afflicted with measles, mumps and chickenpox with good results. He claimed that the itching soon ceased and the rash promptly cleared up of its own accord.

PLANTAIN
(PLANTAGO MAJOR)

Brief Description

Common plantain is a very common weed found in lawns, backyards, gardens, and roadsides all over America. It is a hardy perennial and, like the dandelion, must be taken out by the roots if it once gets firmly established in a yard.

Its leaves are broadly ovate, entire or toothed, and characterized by a thick, channeled footstalk. The flower stalks grow for 7-20 inches high and are tipped with long, slender spikes of greenish-white flowers whose color is again overshadowed by brownish sepals and bracts.

A Useful Weed for What Ails You

For many years the late Edwen Rollin Spencer, Ph.D. taught biology at McKendree College in Lebanon, Illinois. From his writings and numerous lectures, it was obvious that the good professor loved plants which he considered to be useful or attractive, but despised others which he relegated to the lower class of nuisance weeds. In his classic work *Just Weeds* (New York: Charles Scribner's Sons, 1940; pp. 1; 237-38), his prejudice became very apparent.

He believed that such bothersome plants were endowed with "the traits of a Bonaparte or a Hitler," stating that if they were "given an inch [they] will take a mile." He claimed that nature had endowed weeds "with supervitality" that made them outlast ordinary plants. He especially hated plantain: "There is no beauty in the flowers either, and so it has not a single redeeming feature." In fact, he termed plantain as a downright "ugly plant," which should be eradicated at all costs from a person's lawn or backyard.

But don't tell that to a skilled herbalist or plant expert like me, unless you're prepared for a vigorous debate on the subject. For, you see, I have worked with this wonderful plant for many years and can testify to its many healing virtues. Let me share with you a few of these personal experiences.

Some thirteen years ago I, along with a distinguished biologist named Max Barlow, were invited to give a three-day herbal seminar at the Dow Conference Center on the campus of Hillsdale College in Hillsdale, Michigan from June 26th to June 28th. Delores Spence of the local Holistic Study Group was the person in charge who had organized this large event for us.

In referring to my journal notes of the time, I read about a woman who had accidentally cut her foot quite badly on a broken piece of glass while walking barefoot on the campus lawn. Max and I were summoned to her aid, and we proceeded to treat her on the spot with what was readily available. I showed one of the other attendees where to push firmly on some vital acupuncture pressure points in order to slow down the bleeding. Max found a good clump of plantain growing along one wall of a campus dormitory and picked a number of its leaves. He brought them over to me and I put them in an old pillow slip borrowed from one of the beds inside. I took a brick lying nearby and proceeded to crush the leaves inside until they were pretty well macerated. Max then removed this pulpy affair and gently laid it over the woman's laceration and held it in place for a while. Within less than seven minutes (I know it was so because I timed it with my watch), *all bleeding ceased!* Everyone was amazed by this rapid recovery. The woman was taken to a local hospital to have the wound cleaned out and properly dressed; she was given a tetanus shot just for good measure to prevent blood poisoning from possibly occurring.

The evening meal of the first day for the several hundred conference participants was taken in the campus cafeteria. Some rather spicy food was served. A man in his mid-fifties began complaining of severe gastrointestinal discomforts. Alarmed by his growing agony, his wife rushed over to our table and asked for help. Again, Max and I turned to our trusty plantain for help. We procured some more leaves from outside and took them into the back kitchen where we made up a nice brew. We boiled about one quart of water while at the same time cutting up the leaves into irregular pieces that were about two-inches-square until there was enough to equal two full cups. These were added to the water, the pot covered and set aside to steep for 30 minutes. We strained a large glass of the tea later on when it was lukewarm and gave it to the poor fellow to sip. Within a matter of minutes his condition began improving and in no time at all, he said his peptic ulcer had stopped acting up on account of the spicy food he had previously consumed.

A woman's ten-year-old son started complaining of a toothache on the lower right side of his jaw. Again we turned to plantain for help. We crushed part of a leaf and inserted the squishy matter between his gumline and inner cheek and had him press his hand against the outside of his face for a while to hold it in place. Soon the throbbing pain was gone and he was happy again.

These are some of the marvelous things plantain can do for you. Max Barlow and I found it to be "a weed with useful dignity and helpful grace" in what ails us.

PLEURISY ROOT
(see MILKWEED)

POKEROOT/POKEWEED
(PHYTOLACCA AMERICANA)

Brief Description

Pokeroot is usually found in moist, disturbed soils along field borders, fence rows and wood edges, from New England to Minnesota and southward to Florida and Texas. The plant grows anywhere from a yard to nine feet tall. It has thick, fleshy stems that are reddish-tinged as they get older, which are adorned with large, soft, oval leaves and greenish-white flowers arranged in drooping spikes. In late summer they give way to drooping clusters of distinctive rich, purple berries containing a beautiful, magenta-colored juice. (See *Heinerman's Encyclopedia of Nuts, Berries and Seeds* Englewood Cliffs, NJ: Prentice Hall, 1995) for more information on poke-berries.)

Good Medicine for Chronic Skin Diseases and Glandular Swelling

In her popular book *Indian Herbalogy of North America* author Alma R. Hutchens (Windsor, Ontario: Merco, 1973; p.223) praised the herb this way: "Very few, if any of the alternatives have superior power to Poke if prop-erly gathered and prepared for medicinal uses; both the berries and root have high recognition [for healing]..."

As an external medicine, pokeroot makes a dandy wash or ointment for a wide variety of skin afflictions. In 1-1/2 pints boiling water put 3/4 cup chopped *green* pokeroot, cover and let simmer on low heat for about 15 minutes. Set aside and steep for another 25 minutes, then strain and refrigerate. Wash diseased areas of the skin several times a day with some of this tea solution, using a natural sponge for this purpose. To make an ointment, just simmer two cups of finely chopped *green* pokeroot in about six cups of olive oil for approximately two hours at a temperature slightly below the point where the oil would otherwise start bubbling. Keep a lid on the pot while doing this. Pour the oil through a fine-mesh wire strainer into another pot. To this add about 6-8 tablespoons of *melted* beeswax to obtain the desired consistency of firmness you wish. Finally, add a small amount of gum benzoin or tincture of benzoin to help preserve your oint-ment (usually about one teaspoon per quart of salve).

Use both the herbal wash and ointment as a dual approach in treat-ing the following skin conditions: chickenpox, measles, mumps, herpes, shingles, psoriasis, eczema, leg ulcers, scabies, ringworm, fungal infection, boils, carbuncles, bedsores, rash, itch, and so forth.

The other use for which pokeroot is renowned is in the reduction of glandular swellings. In this instance, a tea works best. Make it according to the directions previously given for the herbal skin wash. Small amounts (about one-half cup) can be taken *with meals* several times daily. And a clean washcloth can be soaked in some of the *hot* tea, the excess liquid wrung out; it is folded several times and then applied directly to the swelling itself. A dry hand towel should be placed over this in order to retain the heat and delay cooling as long as possible. Hutchens claims in her book that pokeroot " is very useful in the removal of" chemical poisons from the body and in the treatment of sexually transmitted diseases. She praises the root for its ability to reduce any kind of glandular inflammation. This makes it especially valuable in treating tonsillitis, swollen lymph nodes, mastitis, and even breast cancer.

POPLAR
(POPULUS CANDICANS)

Brief Description

The poplar tree is medium-to large-sized with simple, deciduous leaves of dull, whitish, dark green color with white veins, attached alternately to the twigs. In several species, the leaf stalk, or petiole, is laterally compressed and the leaves "tremble" or "quake" in the slightest breeze (hence, its other common name of "quaking aspen").

A Drugstore Tree

I like to think of poplar as a type of "forest pharmacy." For where else could you find medicines for cancers, skin ulcers, gangrenous wounds, eczema, burns, and strong perspiration all derived from just a single source?

Bring one pint of water to a rolling boil. Then add one-half cup of poplar leaves, finely chopped buds, and shredded bark. Cover and let simmer for 20 minutes. Set aside to steep for 40 minutes, strain and refrigerate. Bathe areas of the skin afflicted with malignant growths, sores, rash, burns, or foul odor frequently (as many as five times a day, if necessary). You'll be absolutely amazed at the changes occurring in each of these conditions. One-half cup of poplar buds slowly cooked in two cups of olive oil for an hour and then made into an ointment (see preceding POKEROOT for directions) is equally useful for many skin problems, including acne.

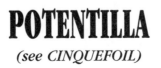

POTENTILLA
(see CINQUEFOIL)

PRICKLY ASH
(ZANTHOXYLUM AMERICANUM)

Brief Description

This tall shrub, or rarely a small tree, can reach heights of over 20 feet. It is characterized by thorny stems and branches and leaves that are hairy when young, smooth when older with resinous dots on them and emitting the smell of lemon when crushed. The greenish flowers, in clusters on last year's wood, appear before the leaves. They are followed by reddish-brown, rough capsules containing black seed or seeds, the taste of which is spicy. Prickly ash is found from Canada to Virginia and Nebraska.

Great Relief from Paralysis and Pain

The 19th century plant authority, Charles F. Millspaugh, had a great deal to say about the wonderful virtues of prickly ash bark and berries in his book on *American Medicinal Plants*. For instance, while walking in the woods one day doing botanical research, his tooth began to ache. "But upon chewing the bark of prickly ash for relief," he recounted, "speedy mitigation of the pain followed!" A little dried bark ground into a powder and then sprinkled on an inch-square piece of white bread coated with a little peanut butter to hold in place inside the mouth, or a wad of cotton soaked with some tincture and firmly held against the tooth, will relieve any kind of pain within minutes.

Millspaugh also praised its remarkable action upon inactive saliva glands, where the bark can promote full saliva flow within a very short time. Dr. Mary R. Leason, an herbalist practitioner from Federal Way, Washington, wrote to me once how she effectively cured a friend named Fern Roemer, who had lost all salivary and taste functions due to the strong antibiotics given her while in the hospital. "I just fixed her up with some powdered prickly ash bark," Dr. Leason said, "which I had her put on her tongue every few hours. Pretty soon she was drooling all over the place and got back her taste buds again."

In his book, Millspaugh recited the success of various Cincinnati, Ohio physicians in the mid-19th century when they used tincture of prickly ash on their patients suffering peritonitis, distention of the bowels, severe abdominal inflammation and swelling, intense fevers like cholera, typhus and typhoid—and pneumonia.

Generally 1 tsp. of the tincture in 3/4 cup of water sweetened with a little honey was administered every hour and about 12 times these amounts (minus the honey) were given in the form of an enema too. "The action was prompt and permanent," Millspaugh wrote. "Prickly ash acted like electricity, so sudden and diffusive was its influence over the entire system. I consider the tincture of prickly ash berries and bark to be superior to any form of medication I know of."

Certain Native American tribes relied on prickly ash for curing rheumatism, joint stiffness, muscle paralysis, lower back pain and other arthritic-like symptoms. The Algonquins, for example, made a tea by combining two cups of the fresh or dried bark with 2 qts. of hot water and simmering the same in a kettle or black iron pot over a low fire for an a hour or so, uncovered, until the liquid had been reduced to half this amount. They would then drink freely of this brew in order to work up a good sweat, after which they would go and bathe in a nearby river or stream. This method never failed to bring them several hours of lasting relief from pain.

The Chippewa made the same kind of tea, which was used to bathe the legs and feet of sickly, weak children or the elderly in order to give them additional strength to walk and move about more freely. The fresh or dried cut bark was also steeped for several hours in hot bear grease (substitute lard for this) before rubbing on painful muscles and joints for incredible relief from pain.

Remedy for Sickle Cell Anemia

Sickle cell anemia is a disease occurring most frequently among Blacks throughout the world. Symptoms include those of anemia, leg ulcers, arthritic manifestations and acute attacks of pain, with the hemoglobin being quite abnormal. In his scientific reference work, *Medicinal Plants* and *Traditional Medicine in Africa*, Abayomi Sofowora, who is Professor of Pharmacognosy at the University of Ife in Ile-Ife, Nigeria, indicates that a water extract of the active principle from the powdered root of prickly ash "will revert sickle-cell anaemia." "Studies show that the extract of the root is not toxic orally," he adds. "It has reduced significantly the painful crisis of sickle-cell patients in a clinical trial carried out in Ibadan." Besides the root, however, the young leaves of the prickly ash are also a very rich source of the anti-sickling acids, which stop the progress of this terrible disease.

Nigerian folk herbalists have consequently used strong tea extracts made of these young leaves of an African species of prickly ash for curing their patients who've been afflicted with sickle cell anemia. Usually a generous handful of leaves is added to a quart of boiling water and permitted to steep away from heat, covered, for 1-1/2 hours. The dosage generally administered to those in their care is approximately 3 cups daily in between meals as a rule.

Nature's Own Toothbrush

During my several trips to the African continent in the past, I've had the opportunity of observing and using the African version of a toothbrush. The root or slim stem of species of prickly ash is thoroughly chewed until it acquires brush-like ends. The fibrous end is then used to brush the teeth thoroughly. These chewing sticks, as they're called, are used frequently during the day.

When I tried them, they imparted a tingling, peppery taste to my tongue and left it and my gums kind of numb for a while. But they sure helped to remove food particles from between my teeth and from those hard-to-get-to crevices. They worked better, I thought, than regular toothpaste, brushing and flossing did. My teeth and gums never felt stronger, cleaner or better than when I used these chewing sticks from prickly ash! If you have access to a prickly ash in your immediate vicinity, then I heartily encourage you to utilize its twigs for this very purpose. You may never want to go back to brushing with Crest or rinsing with Listerine after you've tried this method for a while,

PSYLLIUM
(PLANTAGO OVATA)

Brief Description

Psyllium is a stemless or short-stemmed annual herb. Its leaves are in a rosette or alternate, clasping the stem strap-like, and average 3 to 10 inches in length and 1/4 to 1/2 inch in width. The flowers are white, minute, four-parted, in erect, ovoid, or cylindrical spikes. The fruit is ovate with the top half separating when ripe, releasing smooth, dull ovate seeds that are either pinkish-gray-brown or pinkish-white with brown streaks on them. Each seed is encased in a thin, white, translucent husk which is odorless and tasteless. When soaked in water, all the seeds expand considerably in size.

Obesity and Constipation Cured

Certain bulk laxatives such as Metamucil, Effersyllium and Syllamalt are all composed of the ground husks or seeds of psyllium in combination with sugar to make them taste pleasant. Clinical studies have shown that psyllium by itself is superior in its action to other known laxatives such as mineral oil, milk of magnesia, cascara sagrada, methylcellulose or phenolphthalein.

And various clinical experiments conducted in Italy have demonstrated the value of psyllium seed in obese and diabetic patients. In obese subjects, there was a noticeable decrease in serum cholesterol and a reduction of food intake as well. Diabetic patients benefitted from a drop in their blood sugar levels. A Southern California group of medical doctors observed that psyllium helped relieve irritable bowel syndrome in many of their patients. An average of 3 capsules daily of a unique product called Fiber Cleanse is suggested for the above problems. The product may be obtained from any local health food store.

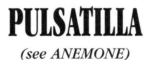

PULSATILLA
(see ANEMONE)

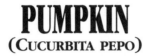

PUMPKIN
(Cucurbita pepo)

Brief Description

Pumpkin is the fabled jack-o-lantern of Halloween tradition, and that very same object that the headless horseman threw at a frightened and fleeing Ichabod Crane with great fury and deadly accuracy, in the immortal tale by Washington Irving. Pumpkin is a variety of winter squash recognized by its smooth round shape and hard-ribbed, orange-colored rind. For cooking purposes, the small sugar pumpkins averaging 7 lbs. or so are best. But for scaring the wits out of young kids, varieties like the Big Max weighing 100 lbs. or more are hard to beat.

The name "pumpkin" goes back to the Greek word "pepon," meaning ripe or mellow. In time the early French had it down to "poupon" and, having been nasalized into "poumpon," entered the King's English as "pompion," to which was later added the diminutive "-kin" ending.

An Effective Cure for Tapeworms

Speaking from personal experience, I can attest to the wonderful benefits of either pumpkin or squash seeds for getting rid of tapeworm. Even now I can recall having to chew very thoroughly each day for 5-1/2 days a cup of dried pumpkin seeds from the health food store when I was just 13 years old.

For several years prior to this, I had been eating voraciously, but never gained a single pound of weight. At first everyone thought it was just the "growing boy" syndrome, which every tall, lanky kid goes through during his teenage years. In time, however, several naturopathic doctors who examined me (my folks never believed in regular M.D.s as such) confirmed that it was a severe case of tapeworm, which was robbing me of the proper nourishment I should have been getting from the tons of food I was shoveling down.

They recommended the pumpkin seeds, which apparently worked quite effectively within just a short period of time. A succession of different bowel movements on my part discharged chunks and sections of what had been a pretty long parasitic worm attached to the walls of my intestine. Various estimates were made as to its overall length, ranging from 20 feet to well over 45 feet. For myself, however, I never bothered keeping track of these statistics. I was just glad to get the ordeal over with and back to a more normal diet. In the course of time I filled out very nicely. I would recommend grinding the seeds up into a powder and serving them 1/2 cup of powder at a time in 1-1/2 cups of apple sauce, or mixed in with some carrot juice in a food blender as a vegetable shake in order to make them more palatable. Some have even suggested making a tea of the seeds, but I have never found this to work as effectively as taking the seeds straight.

A folk healer friend of mine from Merida on the Yucatan Peninsula shared with me some years back an old Mayan remedy for expelling intestinal worms of any kind that he had found never failed once in those of his patients to whom he had prescribed it in times past.

On an empty stomach 2 tbsps. of castor oil were first ingested. The next day 1/2 cup of shelled and powdered seeds of pumpkin or squash mixed with a little water were taken, followed by 1 cup of goat's milk. Then some two hours later, another 2 tbsps. of castor oil were ingested.

PURSLANE
(PORTULACA OLERACEA)

Brief Description

The plant can be either an annual or biennial. It has fleshy, prostrate or decumbent stems, leaves that are opposite, fleshy, spatulate and sessile with a slight pinkish tinge, and bears small single yellow flowers or in groups of 2 or 3. These appear in late summer; the petals soon fall away, revealing a small seed capsule. Purslane is widely distributed from Greece to mainland China and has been introduced elsewhere. It prefers dry, sandy, nitrogen-rich weedy soils in full sunlight.

Excellent Food for Vitamin-Mineral Deficiencies

People in other countries such as Britain, France, Italy and India do not have ready access to the vitamin and mineral supplements that we have here in America or that are available in Canada. If we want a vitamin A or C, iron, or potassium supplement, we can just visit any local health food store or nutrition center in our city and buy what we need. Such a convenience isn't found so easily elsewhere. Consequently, people must rely upon the foods they eat to obtain the nutrients their systems require.

Purslane has long been used as a foodstuff in Asia and the Middle East. It is incredibly rich in vitamin C (700 mg. per 100 grams fresh plant) and vitamin A; has considerable potassium salts (about 2% in fresh or 75% in the dry plant); enough iron to equal any serving of raw or cooked spinach; and lesser amounts of calcium, magnesium, phosphorus, and sodium. Purslane also has a nice cross-section of several important trace elements, including boron, molybdenum, tin, and zinc.

The herb, when made into a tea, is good for all respiratory disorders and skin afflictions. It also induces more vigorous contractions of the heart in cases of low blood pressure (hypotension). For urinary tract disorders, it has often proven very useful. Bring a pint of water to a boil and then add one-half cup of cut purslane herb. Cover and set aside to steep for 30 minutes. Strain and drink one cup twice daily with meals.

PUSSY WILLOW

(see CATTAIL)

PYRETHRUM
(Pyrethrum roseum)
(Also see CHRYSANTHEMUM)

Brief Description

The genus *Chrysanthemum* includes pyrethrum, feverfew, marguerite and daisy. But only those in the section *Pyrethrum* are known to possess distinctly insecticidal properties. In former times this earned the several pyrethrum species the appropriate nickname of "insect flowers."

In some ways, the pyrethrum flowers resemble those of chamomile, with their very small and numerous flowers that are often yellowish or brownish-white in appearance. The plants are mechanically harvested from fields and the heads separated by what would pass for a combing machine. After being dried, they are ground into a fine powder that usually has a greenish-yellow color and an odor somewhat reminiscent of black or green tea.

Marvelous Fly Control

Anyone who has ever kept or been around livestock will know just how easily pesky flies — the buzzing and biting kinds — can accumulate. Warm weather, unburied trash, piled manure, and domesticated animals such as horses will surely bring every winged insect imaginable within flying distance.

But by using pyrethrum flower products (which are perfectly safe for man and beast alike, I might add), you can control horse flies, common house flies, horn flies, face flies, biting stable and deer flies, not to mention gnats and mosquitoes.

Pyrethrum powder can be liberally sprinkled around the kitchen and other parts of the house, as well as in barns and stables to help eradicate such insects of nuisance. The usual method of application is to just sprinkle the powder in such places as are frequented by them and, in the case of humans and animals, to apply it to the surface of the body. There are also a few lotions that can be applied around the face of a person or animal, where powders or sprays aren't desired. This natural fly control artillery also includes sprays that are either water- or alcohol-based; both have their advantages and disadvantages, however.

Before purchasing any product, review its label. If the label shows the active ingredient as pyrethrin, you know it automatically contains the extract from pyrethrum flowers that has an immediate kill effect. But pyrethrins don't provide a long-lasting residual effect. There is, however, the synthetic ingredient permythrin, which is based on the natural pyrethrin molecule, that does have a residual kill effect, lasting from 3 to 5 days as a rule. Just because it's synthetic, though, doesn't mean it's harmful and should be avoided.

Permythrins are most apt to be found in alcohol-based products. Alcohol provides a faster speed of kill because it does some damage to the cuticles of flies. Alcohol delivers the active ingredient better and disperses it better. But don't overlook a definite advantage to using water-based products containing either pyrethrin or permythrin. With a water base you don't have any alcohol odor. If a human or animal has any kind of skin sores or abrasions, a water-based spray is far less likely to cause problems or irritations.

This is one herbal-based product that you *will never* find in an herb shop or health food store. You must visit a tack shop, equine (horse supply) store, or local veterinarian for pyrethrum-containing products. Be sure to read their labels carefully so that you fully understand how to use them.

If not readily available in your immediate area, then I suggest that you contact the following company that makes *natural* pyrethrum insecticides:

Chem-i-matic, Inc.
P.O.Box 920706
Houston, TX 77292
(1-800-231-2966)

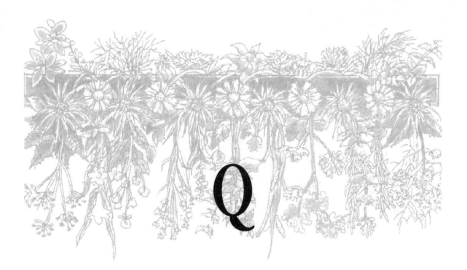

Q

QUAKING ASPEN
(see POPLAR)

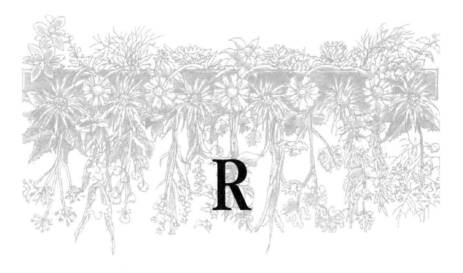

R

RAMPS

(ALLIUM TRICOCCUM)

Brief Description

As far as I know this is about the only herb and spice book in which you will find any information on ramps. All other consumer books on herbs (and I checked through forty of them at last count) *do not* have a single mention of ramps at all. But they are extremely popular and grow wild throughout the appalachian Mountains. In fact, there are annual celebrations held in some small West Virginia and Pennsylvania towns which attract tens of thousands of spectators and revolve entirely around ramps.

So just what are they? They are native leeks with leaves resembling those of lily-of-the-valley and bulbs looking a lot like scallions, while their earthy flavor is a curious mixture of garlic, leek, and dandelion greens. The best time to harvest ramps is between the end of March to the middle of May; after that the leeks grow so strong in flavor that they can, quite literally, overwhelm the taste buds and knock the brain into a momentary stupor!

If you've ever eaten raw garlic or onions, then you know all about the odor that remains on your breath. And even if you eat these spices cooked in meals, some evidence of their presence in your gut will stay with you for a while. But ramps are notorious for their odor, which lingers in the mouth, and in the air where they have been cooked. And cooked they need to be if they are to be tolerably enjoyed. I've written down plenty of ramp recipes from my informants who reside in the quaint Swiss settlement of Helvetia, West Virginia (1-1/2 hours by car from Clarksburg or two hours from Morganstown). There is ramp Bloody Mary (a whiff of this will kill Dracula for sure!), ramp chili (even Hispanics who like their food extra spicy will have a hard time downing this), ramp home fries (these will *never* be served at MacDonald's), ramp vinegar (which is guaranteed to take some of the finish off a new car in less than 24 hours!), ramp oil, ramps and eggs, ramp meat loaf, ramp-flavored bourbon (an excellent cure for the failing alcoholic), and ramp pie (guests won't ask for seconds when this dessert comes around).

Every April, ramp suppers are held statewide in West Virginia — in community halls, Elks' Clubs, elementary schools, and even some churches. The Helvetia Ramp Supper is especially popular (it is held on the last Saturday of every April). When I was there one year, I saw long lines of people patiently waiting for hours to savor both the food and the spirit of the event, which is like a warm gathering of some giant family. Bowls and platters are passed down the long tables as kids of all ages run back and forth from the kitchen to replenish them while their folks and grandparents man the huge black stoves. For roughly $6.25 (it has since gone up to about $7.15) I was able to get my fill of country ham, fried spuds, corn bread, cole slaw, beans, applesauce, and fried ramps. My oh my, but was that ever a heavenly combination that churned around in my gut for hours afterwards!

A Community Effort

Everyone pitches in to make the Helvetia Ramp Supper a community success. The most difficult chore is cleaning approximately 65 bushels of ramps still clumped with dirt. Cement trowels, garden hoes, screwdrivers and even small crowbars are used to excavate the bulbs intact. They are dug up within a month's time by a few local families, who leave before the crack of dawn to go to their secret ramp sources deep in the woods.

The town turned out the year I was there to clean the ramps, peeling the bulbs of their outer skins, removing the roots, and rinsing them a number of times. In the basement of the community hall, volunteers, paring knives in hand, faced each other as they straddled hardwood benches, engaging themselves in local gossip with piles of dirty ramps between them. Behind the hall, several men tended a wood fire under two gigantic iron kettles suspended from booms. The ramps were parboiled in batches, stirred with a pitchfork, drained through an oilcloth punched with holes, and then chopped with an axe. They were then frozen until the day of the supper, when they were fired in rendered bacon fat.

Ramps Have Kept These Octogenarians Fit and Trim

When I visited Helvetia's most famous trio — three sisters named Anna, Freda and Gertrude Balli — a while back, they were then in their late seventies and still doing quite well working their remote 215-acre farm on which they were born. Known locally as the Balli Girls, they spoke to me in thick Swiss-German accents. But we really hit it off together when I switched to German (in which I'm pretty fluent). They told me the reasons they felt so good physically: "We work hard, pray to God, love each other and our fellowmen, and frequently eat ramps in some form with our meals."

When I checked in with them again during the summer of 1995, they were still going strong in spite of the fact that they were then *pushing towards ninety* (Freda and Gertrude are twins, by the way). One of them was just recovering from a broken hip, but all were still doing the same chores I had witnesses when I was there some time ago: they milked their cows, made their famous cheese, handcut their hay, and split their own wood to fuel their ancient Monarch coal-and-wood stove in the large kitchen. Freda took a turn to speak, reminding me again that " without our ramps, we'd probably all be in nursing homes by now or in our graves!"

In the likely event you can't readily get access to ramps, there is a more reasonable alternative. The late sociologist Belle Boone Beard worked for a number of years for the National Institute of Aging, where she managed to compile data on some 8,500 centenarians. In doing hundreds and hundreds of dietary surveys on many of them through the years, she discovered one very remarkable similarity with all: they ate lots and lots of onions, either every day or else several times a week! Since ramps and onions are known antioxidants, they can stop the ravages of scavenger molecules within the body called free radicals, which have been blamed for aging. Once they are successfully held in check, then the body stops aging so fast. Also, ramps and onions are incredibly rich in sulphur, which helps to boost immune defenses and protect the system from viral and bacterial infections. No wonder the Balli Girls are doing so great!

Smelly Medicine That's Good for What Ails You

Granted that ramps or the alternative onions may not be the best smelling or most flavorful medicine around, but they sure can work health wonders when you're ill. My Helvetia informants explained to me some of the different ways in which they've used ramps (you can substitute onions instead). Some of the bulbs are washed, peeled and pounded to extract a juice, a little of which is warmed in a metal spoon over a lit candle or the top of a kerosene lamp, and then slowly dropped into the ear to relieve the worst earache. Some of the warm oil is also put in a teaspoon and given internally to children suffering from croup or cold.

Some of the juice is mixed with several tablespoonfuls of warm water and a pinch of salt, and then gargled in the mouth to relieve sore throat. Cold sores are rubbed with ramp juice several times each day until they go away. A tiny piece of crushed ramp no bigger than a thumbnail is inserted into the mouth and placed next to the gumline to relieve a throbbing toothache. One-fourth ramp juice and three-quarters warm water taken internally once a day on an empty stomach gets rid of intestinal parasites and worms. A tea made from one-half ramp or onion bulb makes an excellent " spring tonic" for getting rid of "bad blood."

RED CLOVER
(TRIFOLIUM PRATENSE)

Brief Description

Red clover is a biennial or short-lived perennial herb reaching almost a yard in height. It grows in clumps consisting of several smooth or hairy stems. The green leaves are stalked and each one has three oval leaflets. Every one of these usually carries a distinctive whitish V-shaped marking. The characteristic rose-to-pink flowerheads are round and close to an inch wide; the blossoms appear from May to October.

Whooping Cough and Sore Throat Cured

A registered nurse in Buffalo, New York wrote to me sometime ago and mentioned an herbal cure her grandmother used all the time to cure members of her extended family of whooping cough and sore throat. The grandma made a tea of red clover blossoms by putting nearly a cupful in a quart of boiling water, covering and setting aside to steep for 20 minutes. The nurse remembers the aged lady telling her to "never, never cook the flowers, just simmer them gently for a spell." My anonymous informant insisted that the remedy worked every time and wondered "why modern medicine isn't using some of these old granny remedies again that are cheaper and safer" instead of relying so much on synthetic antibiotics that can leave harmful side-effects. The usual dose was to take 1 or 2 cups of the warm tea on an empty stomach as well as gargling with it.

Natural Blood Thinner

Some years ago, Georgia Wohl of Seattle, Washington sent me a testimonial of how she had used red clover blossoms. "I make a tea of them," she wrote, "and drink 3 cups a day for 3 days. Or until it becomes so revolting to me that I then know I've had enough...at least for the time being. I find it wonderful for relieving heart pain. And blood clots just disappear from my legs when I drink it. It's helped to relieve my phlebitis of ten years or better, after all the stuff the medics gave me failed to work as good as this has done. Someone should be growing this stuff by the acres and harvesting the blossoms. I bet you they could make a mint out of that."

A Very Remarkable Case of Cured Cancer

Without a doubt the most controversial application for the internal use of red clover has been as an alternative cancer treatment. It was originally included in the famous Hoxsey formula and more recently in Essiac, another popular herbal cancer remedy. Scientists who've evaluated the herb extensively now believe it is the flavonoids present in the plant which account for its dramatic anti-cancer activity. One study published in *Cancer Research* (48 (22): 6257-61, 1988) found that the total flavonoids from the blossoms inhibited by 40% the activity of a common laboratory carcinogen called benzopyrene, a compound always found in charcoal-broiled foods. An even earlier study in the same journal (30:1922-25, July 1970) observed that one of these flavonoids, in particular quercetin, kept this same benzopyrene from becoming active in the liver and small intestines, where liver and colo-rectal cancers frequently occur.

However, the *real* proof for red clover's effectiveness in fighting off cancer comes from a letter that appeared in the *New York Evening Post* sometime in the last century, but was originally printed in the *Phrenological Journal* of December 1867. It is reproduced here in its entirety and was submitted by the recovered cancer patient himself, one Truman Woodford of West Hartford, Connecticut:

"When about fifty years of age (A.D.1836), there appeared near the outer corner of my left eye a small scab, which slowly enlarged and soon became painful, attended with a constant itching, or rather a twitching sensation.

"Feeling anxious about it, I applied to a physician in Hartford, Conn., who said it was a cancerous affection, but advised me to let it alone and give it no medical treatment. As the affected place continued to enlarge and the irritation increased, I applied to another physician, who attempted to cure it by applying caustic, which treatment proved an injury instead of a benefit."

"The sore increased in size, spreading over the temple, eating off both lids of the eye, discharging matter constantly, destroying the sight of the eye, and causing almost insufferable pain. Thus matters stood at the end of twenty years' affliction, and I had reached the age of seventy. I had up to that time consulted six physicians, from none of whom did I receive any relief. The cancer now assailed the substance of the eyeball, eating it out entirely. The sore spread over the temple to the size of the palm of my hand, and below the eye about three-quarters of an inch.

"I then applied to an eminent physician in New York (Dr. Blake), and remained under his treatment one year without any benefit, but rather grew worse. I now gave up all hope of recovery, ceased taking medicines, and merely washed the affected part often in cold water. During the summer of 1865, it had become so painful that I slept but little, was very weak and nervous, was confined to my bed most of the time, and expected soon to die; my friends thinking I could not live till the following spring.

"In the month of August, 1865, I heard of a remarkable cure of cancer by the use of a tea made from common red field clover. Thinking it was at least harmless, I used it as a common beverage, making it very strong, and also washed the eye with the same. In less than two months, to my utter astonishment, the pain entirely ceased, and the sore began to heal at the inner corner of the eye. The healing process went on rapidly until the eye socket was healed over, forming a skin as smooth as that on my cheek, and the redness is now gone.

"There is not over my eye even the semblance of a scar, and but a few scars remain on the temple. My sleep is now sweet, my appetite good, am more fleshy than ever before, my general health was never better, and I think I have as few infirmities, and am as hale and hearty as any man of my age, which is now eighty years."

The *New York Evening Post* introduced the old gentleman's letter with this brief testimonial gathered by one of its correspondents:

"Mr. Joel Reed, son-in-law of Mr. Truman Woodford, has a cousin residing in Great Barrington, Mass., the wife of a hotel-keeper, who had cancer in one breast, which became so serious that the whole gland was removed by a surgeon and the wound healed.

"About a year after the cancerous tumor broke out in the other breast and was beginning to be serious. Mr. Reed, seeing the good effects of the clover tea and wash on his father-in-law, Mr. Truman Woodford, wrote to his cousin informing her of the fact, and urging her to try the remedy. She adopted it at once, and in a few months was entirely healed, and at the time of receiving this information, which was a year or more afterwards, no reappearance of the tumor had occurred."

The sum and substance of everything presented conclusively points to just one thing: so long as red clover blossoms are available for making into a tea, there should *never* be any reason why cancer victims need to go to medical doctors to have their bodies poisoned by chemotherapy drugs and/or to have their entire immune systems nuked into oblivion with lethal doses of cobalt radiation.

And in the event that the cancer is too well advanced for even this herb to do any good, then may I suggest that the individual make his or her peace with God and spend whatever time remains *at home* instead of the hospital. By doing so, one passes on with his or her dignity and respect intact, rather than enduring the horrible pain of barbaric medical practices. At least this way it is natural and more humane than the other.

RED EYEBRIGHT
(see EYEBRIGHT)

RED LILY
(see LILY)

RED RASPBERRY
(RUBUS IDAEUS)

Brief Description

Of all the raspberries, the red raspberry is the best known and most beloved. This cherished plant has arching canes that can extend as long as six feet, and sometimes they have a slight whitish tinge. An obliging shrub, the red raspberry doesn't even have as many prickles as other Rubus species, such as the blackberry. In the wild, it can be found growing on rocky hillsides and also in clearings. Even its leaves point to its sweet nature: they are heart-shaped at the base and have a whitened, downy underside. Raspberry leaves were brewed as a tea by American colonists; the drink was known as Hyperion tea, named for the Grecian father of the sun god, for raspberries thrive on sunlight.

The red raspberry's flowers are a lovely white and blossom from May to July. The fruits, growing in fragrant bouquets, ripen from July through

September. In North America, the hardy red raspberry may be found growing from Newfoundland to British Columbia, down through the Midwest, and south to North Carolina. It is especially prolific in California, where it boldly fruits into November, daunted only by the first frost. In the eastern states, "Latham," an early-to-midseason mainstay, is the grandfather of cultivated red raspberries. In the West, berry connoisseurs are more likely to encounter the dependable, sturdy midseason "Williamette" and the two-crop "Heritage," although the latter grows nicely in the East as well. The red raspberry is equally hardy in northern Europe because it thrives in cool climates. Red raspberry varieties often seen in the British kitchen garden are "Malling Jewel," "Glen Clova," and "Malling Admiral" — easily harvested and resistant to blight.

Most cultivated red raspberries are the result of crosses between the Eurasian species *R. idaeus* and the American native *R. strigosus* and are so finely melded that they are usually grouped under the European nomenclature. Even botanists are perplexed by the red raspberry's comings and goings. Cultivated European raspberries escaped from New England gardens centuries ago: they mingled with native red raspberries and produced their own transatlantic lineage.

Three other types of raspberries worth mentioning are the purple-flowering, the black, and the rare golden kinds. The first lacks the hooked prickles of red raspberry, and its fruits aren't as sweet as other raspberries. The second is often mistaken for a blackberry; when unripe, it can also masquerade as a red or even a yellow raspberry. Mountain folk of Appalachia harvest this ebony berry for preserves, wine, and liqueurs. The rare golden is, botanically speaking, really the same species as the red raspberry. A result of crosses between reds and native yellow Asian raspberries, it has merely lost its pigmentation. But it makes up for its lack of ruby color with a flavor that is infinitely sweeter than that of the red type.

Fight the Flu and Common Cold

Dr. Jaroslva Kresanek practiced medicine for many years in the former Czechoslovakia. While using some Western drugs and surgery for the more difficult cases he encountered, he was also very much a strong advocate of natural remedies. He believed that for common complaints, turning to herbs and food was better for the body than simply writing a prescription.

For many years he has been using the fruits and leaves of red raspberry in decoction form to treat the common cold and flu in many of his patients. He discovered early on in his research that this combination worked best when it was sipped while still quite warm. The addition of a small dose of rum helped to strip accumulated mucus from the bronchial tubes and sinus cavities, so it could be expectorated from the body.

Dr. Kresanek's recipe for making this incredible antibiotic tea is very simple. He shared it with me some years ago when we briefly met during a tour I made of the former Iron Curtain countries. Boil 1 quart of water. Remove from the heat. Add two tablespoons each fresh or dried berries and cut leaves. Mix well, cover, and let the brew steep for 25 minutes. Uncover, strain, and pour one eight-ounce glass. Add 1 teaspoon of brandy, stir, and slowly sip so as not to burn the mouth or tongue. Repeat every couple of hours until recovery is imminent.

By doing it this way, the loss of vitamin C is minimized. And by adding the alcohol just before drinking, it prevents its evaporation.

Childbirth Made Easy

The following anecdote in an abbreviated form appeared in *Heinerman's Encyclopedia of Fruits, Vegetables and Herbs* (West Nyack, NY: Parker Publishing Co., Inc., 1988, p. 38). I believe it deserves to be repeated here in its original expanded form the way I received it.

A Mormon mother of nine children residing in West Jordan, Utah (who asked that I never divulge her name) had her virtually *pain-free* deliveries after her second child when she started drinking red raspberry leaf tea on a regular basis.

She made the tea by boiling a quart of water, turning off the heat, adding 6 tablespoons of dried raspberry leaves, covering the pot with a lid, and letting it steep for 40 minutes. She would drink a cup each day for the first eight months of her pregnancy. And when the nausea of morning sickness would set in, she would double her intake.

In the last month or a couple of weeks prior to the estimated delivery time, she would drink *four* cups of strong hot tea, always in between meals. Due to lack of space in my first *Encyclopedia*, I wasn't able to mention that her husband even brought her several thermos bottles full of the hot tea when she was admitted to the hospital a couple of days ahead of each delivery.

Other women with whom she shared rooms each time she was in to have another delivery always complained to her about how much suffering they endured during their labor periods. "But as for me," she stated with a smile, " it was always a moment of joy, always a pleasant experience without hardship." That's what hot red raspberry leaf tea did for her multiple pregnancies.

RHODODENDRON
(RHODODENDRON GENUS)
(Also see AZALEA)

Brief Description

These shrubs belong to the heath family and are found mostly in the mountainous areas of the arctic and north temperate regions and also in the
mountainous tropics. They are especially abundant throughout Asia, where
many of the popular cultivated species and hybrids derive. They ordinarily have large, shiny, leathery, evergreen leaves and clusters of large pink,
white, or purplish flowers. Native American species include the great laurel, or rose bay (this is the common eastern species and is the state flower
of Virginia); the mountain rose bay of the southern mountains; and the
western rhododendron (which is the state flower of Washington). Azaleas
and rhododendrons look very similar but can be distinguished by their
deciduous leaves.

Alleviates Chronic Cystitis

Judging from the well-landscaped yards of many middle-and-upper income
homes I've been to visit, it seems pretty obvious to me that people love
rhododendrons. Their handsome evergreen foliage and lavish floral displays are unmatched by any other temperate ornamental shrub.

But what most folks don't know is that a tea made from the leaves
helps to alleviate the painful miseries accompanying chronic cystitis. Boil
two pints of water. Then add one-third cup of cut rhododendron leaves.
Cover, simmer on low heat for ten minutes; set aside to cool. Strain and
refrigerate. Drink one-half cup of the *warm* tea on an empty stomach every
4 hours, or as needed.

Flushes Out Mucus Like Crazy

Many of us periodically suffer from excess mucus. It accumulates in our
sinuses, the backs of our throats, in our lungs, and elsewhere. One-half cup
of the *warm* tea made from the shrub leaves and slowly sipped will strip
out this unwanted phlegm in no time at all.

Useful for Kidney Disease and Kidneystones

The same *cool* tea is helpful for resolving kidney complaints. Drink one-quarter cup every five hours on an empty stomach for this. Don't worry about the color of your urine changing; that's normal for a tea like this.

CAUTION: Rhododendron tea is meant only for short-term use and medical situations. It is *not* advisable to be drinking it for very long. In the event of stomach distress, eat a piece of bread for relief.

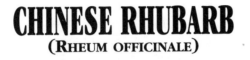

CHINESE RHUBARB
(RHEUM OFFICINALE)

GARDEN RHUBARB
(RHEUM RHAPONTICUM)

Brief Description

Species of rhubarb are denoted by their large and sturdy sizes and large leaves borne on thick petioles. These hardy perennials grow between 7 and 10 feet high, are native to southern Siberia, China and India, and widely cultivated elsewhere.

Chinese rhubarb is used more for medicinal purposes, while the garden variety is grown more for its edible stalks (petioles) and ornamental beauty.

Strengthens Tooth Enamel

Rhubarb is high in potassium and calcium with a lesser amount of phosphorus. These mineral salts, according to a Rochester, N.Y. dentist, occur in rhubarb juice and seem to coat tooth enamel with a thin protective film. Dr. Basil G. Bibby of the Eastman Dental Center believes that more frequent consumption of cooked rhubarb might be of some positive benefit in helping to reduce extensive decay.

Better still, a little bit of the expressed juice from fresh rhubarb stalks brushed on the teeth with a soft bristle brush or else rubbed on with some cotton balls every other day, should coat the enamel with these protective materials.

Shows Anti-Tumor Value

Rhubarb has demonstrated some excellent tumor-blocking abilities. For instance, the first supplement of vol. 20 of *Pharmacology* related that two of the laxative compounds in rhubarb, rhein and emodin, also blocked Ehrlich and mammary tumors in mice by 75% at the relatively high dose of 50 mg. per kilogram of body weight per day.

A 1984 issue of *Journal of Ethnopharmacology* reported that rhein and emodin inhibited the growth of malignant melanoma at a daily dosage of 50 mg. per kilogram of body weight. The percentages of inhibition were 76% for rhein and 73% for emodin. In certain parts of mainland China, rhubarb juice and rhubarb tea are used in the treatment of some forms of cancer with good success. About 1/2 cup of the juice twice daily obtained by putting fresh stalks through a mechanical juicer, are administered to patients. More often, though, tea is made by simmering 2 cups of finely chopped stalks in 1 quart of boiling water, covered, for up to an hour. Afterwards, the liquid is strained off and given to cancer victims in 1-cup amounts two to three times a day.

Relief for Psoriasis and Arthritis

The anthraquinones in rhubarb, besides exerting wonderful laxative action, also help to relieve the itchiness and pain accompanying psoriasis and arthritis. Combine 1 cup of chopped, slightly mashed rhubarb root, 1/2 cup of chopped, slightly mashed rhubarb stalk, 10 tbsps. of powdered wide Oregon grape root, and 8 crushed zinc tablets (50 mg. size) in 3 cups of quality gin or rum. Put in a tightly sealed bottle and shake twice daily for 15 days.

Then strain the tincture through clean muslin cloth and add 1-1/4 cups of cool cabbage juice. Thoroughly stir or shake up until both liquids are well mixed. The vegetable juice may be obtained by simmering half a head of chopped or shredded green cabbage in 1 qt. of boiling water until only half the amount (or 1 pt.) remains. Strain and cool before mixing with the alcoholic tincture. Then put in a bottle with a tight lid.

One level teaspoon of this tincture should be taken five times a day on an empty stomach. Not only will this help bring relief to psoriasis and arthritis, but also it will work equally as well for eczema, herpes, acne vulgaris and hepatitis.

Great Laxative and Anti-Diarrheal

Two important compounds in Chinese rhubarb root, called sennosides E and F, exhibit the identical properties on the bowels as do sennosides A and B, which occur in another well-known laxative herb, senna. And when used in large doses, it will quickly remedy even the most obstinate form of constipation. But strange to say, it's also an astringent and will stop diarrhea when used in small amounts.

As many as 4-6 capsules of powdered Chinese rhubarb root may be necessary for chronic constipation, but a mere 2-3 capsules should be all that is necessary for clearing up diarrhea. Or a tea can be made by bringing a pint of water to a boil, and adding 1-1/2 tbsps. of cut, dried rootstock for constipation or just 1-2/3 tsps. of rootstock for diarrhea.

Reduce heat and simmer for 3 mins. before removing to steep, covered, for an additional half hour. One cup at a time may be taken for constipation, but only 1/4 -1/2 cup for diarrhea.

Heals Digestive Tract Diseases

Some interesting clinical studies conducted with Chinese rhubarb emerged from the Central Hospital of Luwan District in Shanghai in the early 1980s. In the first study, some 890 cases (79% male) of upper digestive tract bleeding (57% were duodenal ulcers complicated by hemorrhaging) were treated with rhubarb either in powder, tablets or syrup. These were administered in 1 tsp. equivalents three times a day until the bleeding ceased, usually averaging only two days with most. A 97% success rate was achieved.

A random comparison between this single use of rhubarb and the combined treatment of Western medicine and Chinese herbs was made in other patients experiencing the same type of difficulties. Furthermore, six different combinations of rhubarb were also tested. In all tests made, the single use of rhubarb took the shortest time to stop bleeding, reduce fevers and help patients toward quicker recovery than the others did. This action exhibited by rhubarb may be due to the presence of tannic acid, which constricts blood vessels.

In the next set of studies, 100 cases of acute inflammation of the pancreas (pancreatitis) and 10 cases of acute inflammation of the gall bladder (cholecystitis) were successfully treated with the equivalent of 4 tbsps. of a decoction of rhubarb between 5 and 10 times a day until full recovery was noticed in most of them. Related symptoms like abdominal pain, high fever and jaundice usually cleared up within 5 days or less. To make a decoction for any of these problems, simmer 2-1/2 tbsps. of cut, dried Chinese rhubarb root in 1-1/2 qts. or 6 cups of boiling water, covered, for 40 mins. or until about half (3 cups) of the liquid remains. Strain this and take as previously directed for any of the foregoing maladies.

Lowers Dangerous Cholesterol

A liquid solution of rhubarb root was fed orally to normal and hyperlipi-demic rabbits. Those with the elevated levels of cholesterol, triglycerides and lipoprotein experienced a significant *decrease* in all of these. This sug-gests that a meal heavy in fats should be accompanied by a simple dessert of delicious cooked rhubarb to help control cholesterol.

To make this dessert, wash and cut into inch pieces about 7 cups (approximately 2 lbs.) of rhubarb. Cook in a double boiler with a little water and 1/4 tsp. sea salt until nearly tender. Then add 1-1/4 cups of dark honey and continue cooking another 40 mins, or until done. It may also be cooked in a covered casserole in the oven using 1/2 cup water, but with the same amounts of salt and honey. Bake at 350° F. for 50 mins. A thera-peutic dessert served with greasy or fatty foods should be about 1-1/2 cups of cooked rhubarb. Adding a little cardamom, 1/2 tsp. pure maple syrup and a touch of pure vanilla improves the flavor more for those who don't especially care for its puckering tartness.

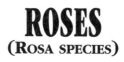

ROSES
(ROSA SPECIES)

Brief Description

For many centuries, gardeners have adored the gorgeous aromatic flowers of the rose, but they have also prized the hips. These are the oval or round-ed fruits of the rose that appear in late summer or fall. A rose hip is actu-ally a receptacle that encloses the true fruits of the plant, called the *ach-enes*, or "seeds." Some linguists contend that the original English word for rose was *hip*.

Rosehips were once regarded as sacred. In fact, during the Middle Ages, the Catholic rosary was so named because rosehips were once used to count the prayers as they were being said. Come to think of it, the beads of the rosary do, indeed, resemble smooth, elongated rosehips, similar to the graceful fruits adorning many species of roses.

In general, species roses are easier to care for than hybrids, and they also tend to produce more succulent hips for eating. So if your intention is culinary as well as ornamental, you might wish to cultivate plants from this group. If you plant climbing roses and want them to fruit, remember to *not prune* them directly after their summer flowering.

Rosehips will usually remain on the plant throughout the early part of the winter or until birds, rabbits and field mice have eaten or stored them. The hips have a zesty acidic but fruity taste, due to the rich amount of ascorbic acid present. Fresh rose hips contain 60 times as much vitamin C as oranges, and rugosa roses, with their large round fruits, are considered to have one of the highest contents. I've had the pleasure of eating some of them raw in the dead of winter in the high Uintah Mountains here in Utah. I ate only the walls of the hips and spit out the seeds. I found them to have quite an exciting taste in the cold weather.

Preventing Infection

Treating infectious diseases when you have them is one thing, but trying to prevent them before they occur is even better. In parts of Europe rosehip syrup has long been a popular tradition for keeping the immune system strong enough so infections don't start. A French horticulturist, while admiring his lovely rose hedge, commented one time, "When I was very young, my mother would give me a tablespoonful of rosehip syrup every day to keep me well. I never got sick that I can recall."

If you want to remain free from sickness, here is a time-honored recipe from a resident of Der Hague in the Netherlands. He writes (translated from the Dutch): "Use about 1-1/2 pounds of rosehips for every 5 pints of distilled water. Mince the hips after removing the stalks and calyces. Cover with water and boil, then strain through a jelly bag. Reduce the liquid to approximately half of what it was before, add 2 cups of honey, and boil for 5 minutes to sterilize. Pour this mixture into sterilized bottles and seal up right away with sterilized screw top lids."

Rosehip tea is excellent for treating present infections. In a pint of hot water, steep 2 tablespoons of dried rosehips, covered, for 20 minutes. But DO NOT COOK or else the vitamin C, which is heat-sensitive, will be substantially reduced. Strain and drink 4 cups daily on an empty stomach.

Roses for Enhanced Skin Beauty

Maurice Messegue is a world renowned folk healer residing in Provence in France. He is the son of a farm worker and much of his own botanical knowledge has been handed down in his family from father to son for several generations. He has had a reputation throughout Europe as being a very skilled healer, numbering among his patients famous deceased figures of the past, such as King Farouk of Egypt and Pope John XXIII of the Roman Catholic Church.

Over the course of time he has put many of his healing secrets into different books. One of these was *Mon Herbeir de Santé* (Paris: Laffont/Tchou, 1975) in which he discussed the merits of roses for skin treatment. The parts quoted here have been translated from the original French edition. "There is nothing better than rose water for the daily care of the skin," he began. "Nothing compares to it for cleansing the face, for preventing and getting rid of wrinkles. Nothing is more effective against acne and blackheads. Why make use of chemicals that burn the skin," he asked, " when rose water will do all that is needed?"

"But that is not all," he adds. "Rose water is also excellent for minor cuts, bruises, sprains, and pulled muscle ligaments. And there is nothing that makes a better eye-bath for sore or running eyes than rose water. Not to mention gargles for inflammation of the mouth and throat, too."

Messegue prefers using dried roses, believing that they are more potent than fresh ones. "Pick the petals on a dry day," he admonishes, "when the flowers are in bud, remove the stamens, and cut off the claws at the base of the petals. Dry the petals quickly so that they retain their bright color and keep their smell sweet. Keep them in a tin box or a tinted hermetically sealed jar. Their scent should improve every day, but do not forget that these plants lose the best part of their medicinal properties in three or four months."

To make his famous rose water, he suggests this: "Put a handful of dried rose petals into a litre (1-3/4 pints) of boiling water. Cover and let steep until cool. Drink two cupfuls a day." Or use externally as a wash or wet pack for any of the aforementioned conditions.

Good for Stomach Ulcers, Nervousness, Liver Problems, and Rheumatism

Messegue tells of a certain "rich industrialist who was in the habit of putting several handfuls of rose petals in his bath, and one day he found that his rheumatism had disappeared." He said that several cups of his rose water each day will do well for the stomach, the nerves and the liver.

An Exotic Luncheon Treat

ROSE PETAL SANDWICHES

Needed: 4 ounces light cream cheese or goat cheese; 1/2 to 1 cup fresh rose petals; granulated kelp (a seaweed available from health food stores) for flavor; 8 thinly cut slices of seven-grain, whole wheat, honey-wheat, pumpernickel, or dark rye bread (crust removed).

In a small bowl, combine the cheese with 1/2 of the rose petals. Wrap well and refrigerate overnight. Spread the cheese on 4 pieces of bread and press in the remaining rose petals. Place the second piece of bread on the top and cut into quarters diagonally. Makes great finger sandwiches for healthy hors d'oeuvres. Serve with warm chamomile tea.

ROSEMARY
(Rosmarinus officinalis)

Brief Description

This evergreen shrub originated in the Mediterranean area and is now widely cultivated elsewhere for its aromatic leaves. The many branches have an ash-colored, scaly bark and bear opposite, leathery thick leaves which are lustrous and dark green above and downy white underneath. They have a prominent vein in the middle and margins which are rolled down.

Effective Mouth Wash

Rosemary tea makes a wonderfully refreshing mouth wash for getting rid of bad breath. In 1 pint of boiling water removed from the heat, steep 3 tsp. of the dried flowering tops or leaves for half an hour, covered. Strain and refrigerate. Gargle and rinse mouth each morning or several times a day.

Remarkable Water Purifier

Certain of the aromatic spices like peppermint, rosemary, sage, savory and thyme, are believed to hold tremendous value in sterilizing water contaminated with unfriendly bacteria. Rob McCaleb, editor of the *HerbalGram*, speculates that if one were to boil suspected water and put in a little of

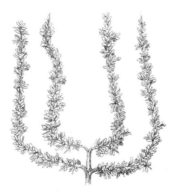

any of these aromatics, a person would have something pretty safe to drink without fear of coming down with diarrhea, cramps and fever due to a harmful microbe with a long Latin name to it. Any of these spices is especially handy to carry with you when traveling in Third World countries such as Mexico, where the conditions of cleanliness leave much to be desired.

Youthful Elixir

The famous French herbalist, Maurice Messegue, calls rosemary "the miracle herb that restores youth" to the physically decrepit and elderly. Some time in the 14th century Queen Elizabeth of Hungary fell in love with it when she was well into her 70s. She had been crippled with rheumatism and gout for a number of years, but rosemary gave her back her youth to such an extent that the King of Poland asked her to marry him!

The herb's tremendous diuretic action explains its effectiveness against rheumatism and gout, as well as kidney stones and the inability to urinate. Moreover, it's a nice digestive, helping the liver to do its work by increasing the flow of bile into the intestines.

To make an elixir similar to that used by the Queen of Hungary for restoring some of your lost youth, lightly crush 2 handfuls of the flowering branches of fresh rosemary, then soak for 10 days in 2 cups of expensive brandy. Repeat the same process and measurements with fresh lavender. Place each solution of herbs in separate bottles with tight-fitting lids. Be sure to shake each one twice daily.

Strain each and store in a cool place until needed. The next part to making this elixir involves mixing together 3 parts tincture of rosemary with 1 part tincture of lavender. An older person should take 1 level tsp. of this a couple times each day on an empty stomach.

Soothing Liniment for Sore Muscles

An oil of rosemary can be made at home to rub on sore, aching muscles or sprained areas for soothing relief. Coarsely chop a double handful of fresh rosemary tops and leaves before soaking in 1 pint of olive oil in a well-sealed jar for a week. Strain and store oil in a cool, dry place. Since rosemary is a natural antioxidant and has been previously used to preserve cereal, luncheon meat and pizza in place of synthetic BHA and BHT, it should keep the oil from turning rancid.

Natural Skin Softening Agent

Most cooks may not realize, when they're using rosemary to flavor their favorite dishes, that this culinary spice makes a wonderful skin softening agent when combined with special water and other herbal extracts. But the irony to this is that the product in which these things appear is normally used in the care of *horses!* You read it correctly. I said *horses!* Coat-So-Soft (as it is called) is a botanical spray intended to soothe the coat of horses and leave their skin feeling soft, healthy and refreshed.

The transition to human skin care came about in a gradual way. Horse owners around the country who were using Coat-So-Soft on their animals began noticing that their own hands, which regularly came into contact with this natural spray, started feeling softer and smoother, too. Some of them switched from their own hand lotions and creams to this product and soon discovered the wonderful benefits it gave to their face, arms, hands and legs. It wasn't long before Rio Vista, the Santa Barbara, California company which markets this and other equine products, began receiving more numerous requests for its Coat-So-Soft than it was usually accustomed to getting.

Besides an extract of rosemary oil, the product also contains an extract of chamomile flowers, deionized water, an herbal woodland fragrance, and other natural ingredients. I've even had a few Avon distributors tell me confidentially that they switched from their own company's Skin So Soft to Rio Vista's Coat-So-Soft, simply because they liked it better.

Quit Horsing Around with Your Regular Shampoo and Use This

Even more incredible is the fact that Rio Vista's Tail & Mane Detangler/Conditioner works *better* on gnarly and unmanageable human hair than ordinary shampoos and conditioners. That's what more than one horse owner has told me in the past. They claim that the rosemary-based Tail & Mane has helped to repair their damaged hair, preventing individual follicles from becoming brittle, made combing or brushing easier and given their hair a more luxuriant shine than they had before. Apparently what seemed to have worked well for their horses has also done an equally splendid job on their own scalps as well.

To find out more about these rosemary-containing products, just call or write: 1-800-248-6428 / Rio Vista, Inc., PO Box 60806, Santa Barbara, CA 93160.

Tasty Spuds

ROSEMARY POTATOES

Needed: 12 russet potatoes; 4 tbsps. extra virgin olive oil; 1/4 cup rosemary sprigs; and granulated kelp (a seaweed available from health food stores).

Peel and wash the spuds. Dry well, cut in half lengthwise, and place in a roasting pan. (Or you can roast the spuds in the same pan that you might roast beef, lamb or venison.) Drizzle olive oil over the spuds, add the rosemary, and sprinkle liberally with kelp. Place in a preheated 350°F. oven 1 hr. before serving. Yield: Serves 8.

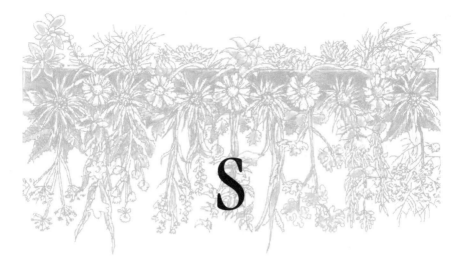

SAFFLOWER
(CARTHAMUS TINCTORIUS)

Brief Description

Safflower is commonly found in Mediterranean regions, but cultivated extensively in Europe and America. It is an annual with a glabrous, branching stem that can be anywhere from a foot to a yard tall. The plant bears alternate, sessile leaves that are either oblong or ovate-lanceolate-shaped and marked with small, spiny teeth. The orange-yellow flowers give the appearance of saffron, which has earned for the plant the moniker of false saffron.

Hysteria and Seizures Brought Under Control

I attended the 1994 annual convention of the American Association of Naturopathic Physicians which was held in San Diego, California. The following item was communicated to me by one naturopathic doctor who, although wishing anonymity, granted me the liberty of reproducing what he told me for this book.

"In my private practice I sometimes see cases of hysteria and seizures in different stages of progress. The single most useful thing I have ever found in controlling these conditions is safflower. I prescribe it in the capsule form (4 daily) as well as in the oil (1-1/2 tbsps. every day).

"But the very best form I like my patients to take it in is as a *warm* tea. I instruct them to steep 2 tbsps. of dried safflower blossoms in 1-1/2

407

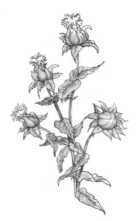

pints hot water, covered, and set aside for 25 minutes. They are told to strain and drink 3 cups morning, noon and night on an empty stomach. It works better than anything else I know of."

SAFFRON
(Crocus sativus)

Brief Description

The saffron we can buy from food stores or spice shops today consists of the dried stigmas from the flower of the saffron crocus, which is indigenous to the Near East and Mediterranean countries.

Saffron is, without doubt, *the* most expensive spice around. It takes 150,000 flowers just to produce one kilogram of the stuff. A planted bulb takes a couple of years even to begin flowering. And once exploited for a few years, the plants must be dug up, cleaned and replanted. Such effort and delay make it easy to understand why it is so costly to use.

The Ultimate Aphrodisiac?

Forget what you've read about ginseng, yohimbine or a number of other herbs with purported aphrodisiac powers. I have been reliably informed by colleagues of mine in other countries where saffron crocus fields bloom by the thousands of acres, that *this is the ultimate* love-making agent! Over half a dozen authorities on medicinal plants and spices from around the Near East, in places such as Syria, Turkey, Iraq, Egypt, and Greece, have been unanimous in lavishing their praise on this very costly food and dye item.

I was reminded that in the *Song of Solomon* (one of the books of the Old Testament) a new bride was compared to a garden that did not lack for saffron. A world-famous scholar, who specialized in the ancient Assyrian language, wrote a monograph seven decades ago about some of the plants used by the Babylonians back in 2500 to 2000 B.C. The gentleman's name was R. Campbell Thompson and he got his data by translating hundreds of cuneiform clay tablets found deep in the sands of Iraq and Iran many years ago. His classic work, *The Assyrian Herbal* (London: Luzac and Co., 1924), was published in a very limited number and is probably one of the rarest botanical works around. Fortunately, I have a copy that I purchased some years ago at a bookstall in London, England. This very learned man stated that the ancient Assyrians used saffron quite frequently "to create" or "set the mood" for an intimate lovemaking experience. Based on the scanty data he gleaned from ancient writings, it seems that saffron acted more on the mental and emotional psyche than it did on any physical organ of the body.

My scholar friends in the Middle East reminded me that the ancient Phoenicians, for instance, spent their wedding night on sheets colored yellow with saffron. A distinguished expert on spices from Cairo University called to my attention that saffron is more than just a spice: it is also *a perfume* and widely used dyestuff to make colorful clothing. Good saffron that is less than a year old and of brilliant orange color, yields a *strong perfume* aroma and a pungent, medicinal, honey-like taste. The ancient pharaohs, my informant said, would mix a tiny pinch of golden saffron with a few drops of wild rose petal water (see under ROSE). This paste they would then judiciously anoint on very selected parts of their bodies which, when touched, would effect a sexual arousal in their genitals. Male body parts most apt for this were the upper lip, both chest nipples, and around close to their armpits. Their wives or concubines would similarly rub small dabs of the same saffron paste on their throats, on the ends of both ear lobes and breast nipples, and on their belly buttons.

The idea or at least theory behind this ancient practice was that as the couple were together in bed, caressing and kissing each other in these particular areas of the body, the *aroma* of the saffron would effect an arousal in each of them, thereby definitely enhancing their moments of love-making.

I wondered if something so ancient would work equally well in modern times. So I asked a young friend of mine in Hartford, Connecticut, who has a rather debonair way with the ladies, to try this out on some of his girlfriends. I supplied the saffron and the *exact* instructions on how the pharaohs of old used it. He reluctantly agreed to the experiment, but found it even more difficult to persuade several of his girlfriends to go along with this. But about six or eight weeks later, he reported back by phone some very pleasant experiences with this saffron paste. He remarked: "I thought you were joking at first. My girlfriends thought I was crazy for something they viewed as being kinky. But I got to tell you in all honesty, John, that my interludes with a couple of them using this saffron stuff like you said, actually made for some very *special* love-making on both our parts. My girl-friends complimented me and used words like ' soft and gentle' or 'tender-hearted' to describe how I was with them. It seems the scent of the saffron brought out *the best* in me instead of the typical 'animal' instincts I've been somewhat notorious for."

A Recipe with Saffron

BOUILLABAISSE

This fish soup originates in Provence, France.

Needed: Appr. 7 lbs. of various fish; 1 fresh lobster, crab or scampi; 40 mussels; 3 medium-large yellow onions, finely diced; 2 fresh fennel flowerheads and leaves, chopped; 6 whole tomatoes (fresh or canned); 2-4 crushed garlic cloves; 1/2 pint extra virgin olive oil; 1/2 pint white wine; 4 tbsp. chopped parsley; 1 sprig of thyme; 2 bay leaves; 1 large piece of dried orange peel; salt and white pepper for taste; saffron; 8-16 slices of French bread and butter to fry them in.

Clean and gut the fish. Cut lengthwise and across the crustaceans and crush their claw shells. Remove mussels from their shells. Next, dump the vegetables into the oil in a large stainless steel pot, cover them with a layer of the firmer fish, pour in the wine, and add water enough to cover the fish. Then season with salt, pepper and saffron.

Boil with the lid on for about 8 minutes, then add the less firm fish and boil for another 8 minutes. Strain out the fish and crustaceans, laying them on a dish; sprinkle parsley over them and into the soup. Meanwhile, the bread slices should have been fried. Pour the soup into bowls and put a bread slice in each. The rest of the fish can be put on a large platter on the table and some of it cut up and laid into the soup by individual diners. Yield: Serves 6.

SAGE
(SALVIA OFFICINALIS)

Brief Description

This perennial shrub grows wild in southern Europe and the Mediterranean area of the world, but is cultivated in many other places as a valued culinary spice. A strongly branched root system produces square, finely hairy stems which are woody at the base and bear oblong leaves. The floral

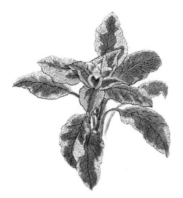

leaves are ovate to ovate-lanceolate. The purple, blue or white flowers are two-lipped and grown in whorls.

Aid for Insect Bites

A quick little remedy for relief of itching and swelling accompanying insect bites is to pick a few fresh sage leaves, then crush or chew them up a bit. Mix them with a little saliva to make a crude, wet poultice and apply directly to the afflicted area and secure in place with a strip or two of adhesive tape.

Relief for Throat Problems

A tea made of the leaves of sage provides soothing, healing relief for sore throat, loss of voice and tonsillitis, as well as helping to remove mucus from congested lungs. Steep 2 tsp. dried or fresh leaves in 1-1/4 cups of boiling water for 35 mins. Strain, sweeten with honey if desired and take 1/2 every few hours as needed. Add 1/4 tsp. of fresh lime juice and gargle well before swallowing for raw, irritated throat.

Stops Milk Flow

More and more mothers seem to be returning to the natural art of breast-feeding their newborn infants, because they feel it is much better for their babies' overall health. When the nursing stage comes to an end, however, many aren't aware of how to properly stop their flow of extra, unneeded milk.

Two cups of warm sage tea daily for up to a week generally dries up the milk supply quite nicely. Bring 1 qt. of water to a boil and steep 8 tsp. dried or fresh sage leaves in it for 45 mins. covered. Strain, add honey and drink.

Intense Itching Disappears

Any kind of intense itching, whether it be due to an allergic reaction to some unknown substance, general nervousness, psoriasis and eczema or coming in contact with poison ivy or sumac, may be effectively relieved *and* healed with an old folk remedy from Nassau in the Bahamas.

A kindly old cook by the name of "Mistress Marshall," who lived to the decent age of 102, was known far and wide for her practice of "bush medicine" (as it was called in those parts) with a touch of black magic thrown in for good measure.

One of her favorite remedies for itching was to steep a handful of cut, fresh sage leaves, that had been lightly crushed first, in 1 pint of boiling water for about an hour. After this, the strained liquid was used to bathe the afflicted parts. Then while the skin was still wet with this solution, she would generously sprinkle *whole wheat* flour (*never* white) over the entire area and leave to dry. Relief came within 10 minutes as a rule and never failed once that I'm aware of.

Darkening Gray Hair

You can make your own home-version of Grecian Formula for taking away gray hair that's a lot safer to use because it's free of chemicals and only contains natural ingredients.

In a heavy ceramic mixing bowl put 2 heaping tbsps. of dried sage and the same amount again of either orange pekoe or black tea. Then fill the bowl or jar half full of boiling water. Cover with a small dinner plate or aluminum foil and place in a moderately warm (275°F.) oven or in a large pan of boiling water on top of the stove on a low setting for at least a couple of hours. Then remove, allow to cool, stir well and strain.

Now a small quantity of this infusion is to be rubbed into the roots of the hair 4-5 times a week. Pretty soon the grayness will start fading away as the hair becomes darker in color once more. Thereafter, this infusion ought to be used just once or twice weekly for maintenance purposes only. Many of those who've tried this for themselves have experienced moderate hair growth in bald places or at the very least, an overall improvement in the tone and texture of their hair. This infusion will keep longer if 3 tbsps. of either gin or rum are added to it.

Inhibits Clots and Prevents Heart Problems

Recently published studies by a team of scientists from the Department of Microbiology and Chemotherapy at the Nippon Roche Research Center in Kamakura, Japan, indicates that powdered sage or sage tea helps to prevent blood clots from forming and is quite useful in the prevention and treatment of myocardial infarction and general coronary pains.

How to Make a Really Good Sage Tea

Ordinarily I haven't given any special heading to making great tea any-where in this book. My emphasis, for the most part, has always been on highlighting effective remedies for unique health situations. But I can't resist the urge to do so here, since I value sage so highly. In his book *Medicinal Plants of The Mountain West* (Santa Fe: Museum of New Mexico Press, 1979; p. 142), author Michael Moore declared that " the Sages *own* the lower mountains of southern California, and often form pure stands of several mixed species," so sage is readily available if you live there or in Arizona, New Mexico or western Texas.

For a bold brisk tea that "slaps you down on the outside and wakes you up on the inside," here are the easy-to-follow directions:

1. Boil 1 1/2 pints of water.
2. Add 2 1/2 tbsps. cut fresh or dried sage.
3. Cover, lower heat and simmer 25 minutes.
4. Set aside and steep 15 minutes.
5. Strain and refrigerate.
6. Reheat the amount needed (usually 1 coffee mug full), adding 1 tsp. *pure* maple syrup for flavoring.
7. Drink and enjoy!

Sage for Physical and Spiritual Purification

I spent America's national holiday, the Fourth of July, 1995, in a most unusual way. I worked in my research center in Salt Lake City, finishing up this manuscript for my publisher. But not before having a 1-1/2 *hour*-long telephone chat with a dear friend of mine, Adrienne Simidian of Carmel, New York. The theme which dominated much of what we talked about was *freedom*. Not necessarily the kind of patriotic freedom which millions of Americans were then commemorating on this special holiday, but rather the type which comes with knowing the truth—the truth about life and our own individual searches for personal identity of *who* we are, *why* we're here, and *where* we intend going.

Because of our long friendship spanning many years, Adrienne felt comfortable enough to share with me a recent experience that she had with sixteen other women high in the hills above San Diego. From Tuesday, June 20th to Sunday, June 25th, l995, these women from all over the coun-try came together under the collective name of the Fireweed Eagle Clan for the sole purpose of holding a sacred sweating ceremony in a sweat lodge constructed by themselves. This was one of six ceremonies held annually, but had added significance because it was to be held during the summer solstice.

The women were from all backgrounds and occupations imaginable. Adrienne works as an executive secretary for a company representing the business interests of a large, Swiss-based manufacturer of heavy equipment. She also plays the piano part time for the advanced adult Ballet A classes held throughout the week at the Northern Westchester Center for the Arts in downtown Mount Kisco, Westchester County, in downstate New York. The woman previously designated as the "spiritual elder" of this clan and going by the adopted name of Grandmother Dragonfly, is British by birth and a retired psychologist in her early seventies. Other members of this exclusive all-female clan hold occupations ranging from nursing and accounting to lawyering and real estate selling. "There is a healthy diversity of personalities and life patterns within the group," Adrienne stated. "Some are outspoken, others more subdued; some are heterosexual, while a few others are gay. But we come together with one purpose in mind, and that is to purify ourselves mentally, emotionally and spiritually. Who we are, what we do, or how we live is unimportant; the central motivation that draws us all together is to become *whole* again and give something back to the planet which has nurtured us for so long."

Sage is an integral part of the sweating ceremony with many early Native Americans. In the construction of the lodge itself, willow was often used. Adrienne's clan was fortunate enough to have had the shell of an existing lodge already in place when they arrived at their designated site. They proceeded to gather willow boughs to cover the exterior. But at a much earlier date in California's history, different Indian tribes incorporated wild sage in the building of their sweat houses. Sometimes the sage would be worked into the willow boughs themselves or at other times intermingled with clay earth and daubed over the wood to make a tighter enclosure.

There has always been much symbolism attending the stones to be used in any sweat lodge ceremony, be it true Native American or a considerably modified version in keeping with modern lifestyles in the late 20th century. The Indians often referred to such stones as "our elders." Adrienne mentioned to me that within her own group, the two largest stones were addressed respectively as "Grandfather" and "Grandmother." The stones are viewed by both groups as being "alive," just like the earth is, and so must be reverently treated. The best stones for sweats have always been igneous, since they retain heat the longest and don't crumble when water is poured on them.

My friend explained how a pit was dug in the center of the lodge and a small latticework of wood laid across the bottom. A few lava rocks were placed on top and then a fire was made beneath the wood. Although no sage was used in this instance, I interrupted her engrossing narrative long enough to point out that some California tribes placed pieces of wild sage in between the firewood in the belief that the plant would help to "purify" even the fire itself. More wood was laid on top and around the sides, she continued, as extra stones were periodically called for, until a total number of 32 had been heated to the point of nearly turning white.

Just prior to everyone entering the lodge, Adrienne said, the designated "elder" of their clan (in this case, the retired psychologist "Grandmother Dragonfly") entered alone, carrying in one hand a long, beautifully carved peace pipe in the shape of a buffalo head and in her other hand a smoldering bunch of tied sage plants. Like a priest slowly swinging a chained dish of burning incense, this woman stood in specific spots and waved her "smudge bundle" around, while at the same time speaking certain words intended for that special occasion. She then took several puffs on her pipe and proceeded to repeat everything several more times, but facing in different directions each time. The entire ritual took about 20 minutes; when she emerged form the lodge, Adrienne noted, "she manifested an unbounded energy which indicated to the rest of us that there was a really strong spirit present within the lodge."

My friend confessed to not knowing very much about the *true* manner of the sweat ceremony as conducted by Native Americans in the past. But she mentioned that theirs was held in four separate increments, each one lasting about 15 minutes. Everyone entered the lodge about 6:30 p.m. in the early evening of Friday, June 23rd, 1995. The first sessions occupied any personal problems that members of the clan may have had; the second one, a while later, dealt with events in the world. After this followed another brief interlude outside, before returning for a third session in which their unseen "spirit guides" appointed to each of them specific "tasks" to try and perform in the hopes of making the world a little bit better place to live in. Finally, there came a "quiet period" of silence in which each one was encouraged to meditate on what they had just experienced.

In the course of our long-distance conversation, I brought up the fact that some early Indian tribes boiled up wild sage into a tea, and used this to splash on to the heated stones every so often when more steam was required, as well as to splash some on their own bodies, besides periodically drinking it. They did this with the idea in mind that sage is capable of purifying the body as well as the soul. From what we now know concerning the actual chemistry of sage, this concept is quite correct. Adrienne said she had never heard of sage being used in this manner before, but I reassured her as an anthropologist that I knew what I was talking about.

For individuals coming from the modern world as each of these seventeen women did, something so simple and beautiful as an Indian sweatlodge ceremony offered a means by which they could obtain a release from all of their pent-up mental anxieties and emotional hostilities. It was "a deeply satisfying way for each of us to cleanse our souls, purify our bodies and heal our spirits," as Adrienne so eloquently put it. "I found this time spent with the others to be some of the most defining moments of my entire life!"

Obviously, not everyone can have access to a sweatlodge as she frequently does. But soaking in a hot tub of water or sitting in a sauna with a *warm* mug of sage tea in your hand, is going to have enough of an impact on your mind and body to renew you for another day. I personally *guarantee* that will happen. You'll feel like a million bucks afterwards! (An easy-to-read book on the subject that I recommend is *The Native American Sweat Lodge* by Joseph Bruchac, Freedom, CA: The Crossing Press, 1993.)

SAGEBRUSH
(Artemisia tridentata)

Brief Description

In his outstanding book on nature and philosophy, author Douglas Rigby correctly noted in *Desert Happy* (New York: J.B. Lippincott Co., 1957; pp. 119; 108) that "sagebrush is a literary symbol" of the West and Southwest, referring to it as "that glamorous plant."

In the Intermountain West extending from British Columbia and Alberta all the way to Baja California and New Mexico, sagebrush dominates the floor of the high deserts. It spreads in wide valleys and up gentle slopes and into the mountains. The most common shrub in western North America, sagebrush is a tough, squat, gray-green plant which blossoms with tiny yellow flowers in late summer and early fall. It is a woody, evergreen perennial with a pungent fragrance similar to the garden plant herb sage. It belongs to the genus Artemisia of which wormwood is a member, and there are some 20 species of sagebrush on the continent; the most common is big sagebrush.

Ranging in height from 1 to 8 feet, sagebrush can be used to determine potential uses for land because it becomes progressively smaller as water availability and soil quality decrease. If the plant averages 3 feet or more, the soil is considered arable. On our family ranch in the southern Utah wilderness just below Bryce Canyon National Park, the sagebrush averages about a yard in height. This indicated to my father Jacob, my brother Joseph (in whose name we put the land many years ago) and I that the soil was good enough to grow potatoes and watermelons.

Throughout the West, sagebrush is used to revegetate land stripped bare from overgrazing by cattle and sheep, forest fires, road construction, and mining. At least 22 animals eat sagebrush; these include everything from pronghorn antelope and mule deer to jack rabbits and gophers.

I recall E. Durant McArthur, formerly a plant geneticist at the U.S. Forest Service Shrub Sciences Lab in Provo, Utah, telling me way back in 1981: "Sagebrush and the West were inseparable; in fact, sagebrush characterizes the whole West. In the years ahead, the much-maligned sagebrush will be regarded with increasing favor. When mixed with grasses and other shrubs, sagebrush adds beauty to the range, food and cover for animals and stability to the soil."

He also mentioned to me a rather interesting piece of scientific data. Chromosome and chemical studies have linked the North American sagebrush with the wormwoods that proliferate in the Central European steppes.

Why I Like Sagebrush So Much

Some readers are apt to wonder why I devote so much space to sagebrush and yet give so little attention to sarsaparilla, sassafras and savory mentioned a few pages hereafter. The reasons for this are quite simple: (1) Sagebrush covers over 130 *million* acres in the West, making it more abundant and more readily available than the others; (2) It is much more versatile in terms of healing than the other three are; (3) It is much more adaptable and tougher to harsh environs than are the preceding trio of herbs.

Diarrhea Stopped Instantly

A friend and his wife came one time from a large metropolitan city some distance away to visit our family ranch south of Cannonville, Utah. Shortly before they had been on vacation to Mexico. While staying in one of our several cabins or bunkhouses, they frequented the outhouse more times in one day than is normal for guests to do.

I bluntly joked: "Got the runs or something?" Whereupon, the husband took me aside and whispered their gastrointestinal problem into my ear. They had contracted what every Yankee who goes south over the border usually gets: an old-fashioned case of "Montezuma's Revenge."

So I got a pair of hand-held pruning scissors and snipped enough sagebrush twigs to make 1-1/2 cups. This I added to 1-1/2 pints of boiling water, covered, turned down the heat and let it simmer for 20 minutes. After it set a while to cool, I strained a cup for each of them, added some honey to allay the bitter taste, and instructed them to drink it.

They screwed up their faces at the still somewhat unpleasant taste, but bravely swallowed the contents of their cups. Within less than an hour, they happily reported to me that all evidence of loose bowels had apparently ceased. And imagine their joy later that same night when they were able to excrete solid "logs" of fecal material instead of more watery waste material.

What an Indian Taught Me About Preventing Dehydration

In May 1995 I employed a Native American named Ed Hunter, whom I met in company with another fellow; both were then sleeping on the ground beside some railroad tracks near the train yard in Salt Lake City. I took them down to our family ranch where they proved to be pretty good "grunt" or common laborers. Everytime I would go down to check up on them, however, I noticed that Ed would always be chewing a little piece of sagebrush. After seeing him do this several different times, I became curious enough to inquire as to the purpose for this. He told me that it kept him from dehydrating. He said his father taught him, and his dad had been taught the same thing by his grandfather. He said that the hot sun beating down on them every day and the afternoon wind blowing constantly made for a constant thirst.

Now Steve Gable, the Anglo companion of Ed's, would always be drinking water or soft drinks throughout the day; it seemed like he could never get enough liquids to quench his great thirst. But I saw Ed only take a couple of swigs of water throughout the whole day; the rest of the time he chewed on sagebrush twigs. I decided to give it a try for myself, and must confess that I wasn't so thirsty thereafter. I've learned to keep an open mind to things like this, for we never know the source from which helpful knowledge may come.

Sunstroke and Eye Inflammation Alleviated

Some 25 miles north on top of the mesa is the entrance to Bryce Canyon National Park. Over a million tourists from all around the world come there each year to admire its scenic wonders and spectacular rock formations. Some years ago a French tourist and his wife visited the place and then decided to head on out into the wilderness south of the town of Cannonville, Utah, They camped for several nights in a little state park called Kodachrome, about 4 miles from our place.

At that time we didn't have our well and plumbing hooked up in a bath house as we presently do. So the hired help and I would drive over to this state park several times a week and take our showers in their public facilities. This is how I met this couple. Upon learning of my scientific background in folk medicine, they asked me what they could do for sunstroke and eye inflammation (due to the lack of wearing dark glasses around so much intense sun exposure).

A clump of sagebrush was within walking distance of their tent. I borrowed a knife and cut off an amount to equal about 2 cups. I filled their empty coffeepot with water from a nearby pipe spigot, boiled it up on their Coleman stove and then added the sagebrush, letting it simmer for 15 minutes. I set it aside to cool for 30 minutes. I then borrowed a couple of their clean wash cloths and soaked them in this sagebrush tea solution, wringing out the excess liquid. I had the woman lie down and placed these over her forehead to stop the migraine and reduce the heat sensation. I borrowed the man's clean white handkerchief, moistened it with enough sagebrush tea, and had him lie down. Pushing back the top and bottom eyelids of one eye, I gently squeezed some of this tea into it, and then repeated the same thing with the other eye. After this, I soaked the whole handkerchief in the tea, gently wrung out some of the excess liquid, folded it in half lengthwise and laid this across both eyes.

I stayed around for an hour to see how they were getting along. The woman reported her headache gone and much of the heat by then had been removed from her skin. She felt a lot better. Her husband exclaimed that his eyes didn't hurt as much following the tea treatment. They asked me how much I wanted in payment, but I declined accepting any money for my services. I said, "Render the same kindness to others in need some time in the future, even as you have both received from me this evening. This is all the payment I ask in return." They gave me their word they would do so, and we heartily embraced each other and vigorously shook hands, and parted with much good feeling between us.

Serious Wound Injury Healed

I had another hired man working for us sometime before this. He was part Cherokee and part Anglo, but proved to be such a nuisance that he eventually was forced to quit. I won't mention his name because he has a criminal past and has served time in both state and federal prisons. In fact, at the time I hired him I had to bail him out of Clark County Jail in Las Vegas, Nevada, which should have alerted me early on as to his character; but I chose to remain blind to this fact, believing that everyone in life deserves at least a couple of chances to prove themselves.

In the late winter of 1994, he was out chopping kindling wood late one night in the dark when the razor-sharp hatchet he was using missed the board and went down through his boot and deep into his ankle. Because the nearest hospital was about 45 miles away in Panguitch, he chose to treat it himself. He had his wife (she divorced him soon after this) cut some sagebrush and juniper twigs for him. What I later judged to be about two handfuls was boiled in a quart of water for 20 minutes. She soaked some clean rags in the tea, squeezed out some of the excess liquid, and applied them over the ugly gash in his foot. She kept this treatment up for several hours. Eventually the bleeding ceased and the wound began to heal slowly of its own accord in the weeks that followed.

Hair Tonic and Skin Remedy

Grizzled old prospectors and weathered cowboys have told me in past years of having used sagebrush tea many times to cure themselves of baldness or early hair loss, dandruff, ringworm, eczema, and psoriasis. They also have said that when the skin is frequently bathed with a strong solution of sagebrush tea that it relieves the itch caused by " bedbugs and similar critters." Soaking in some sagebrush tea that part of the skin into which a tick has partly burrowed itself will cause the insect to quickly back out, where it can then be flicked off the skin or else crushed with a gloved hand. Scorpion stings, lizard bites, mosquito and gnat bites, and stings from angry wasps and wild bees can all be effectively treated by first bathing the injured part in sagebrush tea, and then applying a cold pack of more tea over it to reduce swelling and itching.

A Remedy from God for Blood Poisoning

The following anecdote is true. I found it in the Lot Smith Papers currently housed in the Western Americana-Manuscripts section of the Harold B. Lee Library on the campus of BYU in Provo, Utah. It is an excerpt from a letter written by a former Mormon Church Apostle named Wilford Woodruff to an early Mormon frontiersman and colonizer named Lot Smith. The rest of the excerpt is self-explanatory.

Salt Lake City, January 31, 1882

PREST LOT SMITH.

Dear Brother: - Your letter of Jan. 12 arrived all safe and I was truly glad to hear from you, but certainly sorry for your serious afflication [sic]. I did not know how it happened before, and now I do not know what part of the machinery your leg got into, but it certainly is a serious affliction. I do not know how you are doctoring your leg, but I do want to recommend a remedy which I wish you to try, for it saved my life and was given me by revelation [from God]. I was seriously poisoned through my whole system by being cut while skinning an ox that dies with poison. I drew the poison out of my body into my arm with onions until my arm was all inflamed and liable to do go my vitals and kill me, and while I lay in great misery not knowing what to do, the impression came to me like a flash why don't you use charcoal and wild sagebrush. I immediately got a peck of charcoal, pounded fine & sifted it and boiled up a pot of wild sage, sand stirred in the charcoal in the sagebrush water, and made a poultice of it and covered my arm all over with it, and it took all the inflamation [sic] out of my arm in a short time and I was saved. I want you to do likewise & try it. It is a safe medicine and can do no hurt. I would recommend you to wrap up your leg with cloths wet with strong hot sage tea beside the charcoal poultice. Again, if it becomes inflamed, make a smoke of woolen rags on wood & hold your bare leg over that, and I think you will find benefit from these applications....I shall be glad to hear from you at any time.

W. Woodruff

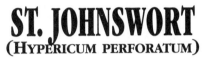

ST. JOHNSWORT
(HYPERICUM PERFORATUM)

Brief Description

This shrubby perennial occurs in dry, gravely soils, fields and sunny places throughout the world. A woody, branched root produced many round stems which put out runners from the base. The opposite, oblong to linear leaves are covered with transparent oil glands that look like holes. The yellow flowers have petals dotted with black along their margins.

Cancer Therapy

Some years ago, while lecturing in Athens, Georgia, I visited an old herb folk healer by the name of Bo "Big Swede" Erikson. He passed along some valuable instructions to make a fairly simple herb oil which he'd formulated for treating certain skin cancers and gangrene. The one skin cancer with which, he said, he always had the most success was basal cell carcinoma—the kind that forms on the forehead, face or nose of light-complexioned people. His key ingredient was St. Johnswort and his main method of preparation was exposing this herb to as much direct sunlight as possible.

"Big Swede" (as he preferred to be called) would first go out and collect some fresh St. Johnswort from nearby fields in his locale. These he would thoroughly macerate with a wooden mallet and then put about 2 handfuls of the crushed plant materials into a gallon jar filled about 1/3 full of olive oil, 1-1/2 pints of good white wine, and 1 cup of gum turpentine. He would seal the jar with a loose-fitting lid and set it in the sun for 10 days.

After this, Big Swede would take a large pot used for canning fruit, and, before filling it 1/3 full of water, would place a large soup bowl *upside down* on the bottom. On top of this inverted bowl he would then put the gallon jar with *the lid left on very loosely*, so as not to build up pressure inside the jar. The pot would be set on the stove on medium heat and the water permitted to boil for an hour.

Following this procedure, the remaining liquid in the jar was then strained several times and put into another clean gallon jar. Into this second jar, an equal amount of more freshly macerated St. Johnswort leaves and flowers were put, but with *no more* oil, wine or turpentine added. This jar was also set in the sun, but only for 5 days instead. After which the entire preparation was set aside in some cool, dry place *without* being strained again until needed.

When treating basal cell carcinoma, he would transform some of this St. Johnswort oil into a simple salve. This was done by heating up 1 cup of the oil inside a pint jar which had been set inside a pot on an inverted dish, with the pot half full of boiling water. When the oil was hot enough he would then add 1-2 tbsps. of melted beeswax and frequently stir until it had been sufficiently dissolved enough to yield a salve-like consistency. A little gum benzoin or tincture of benzoin was also added to help preserve the salve (about 1/2 tsp. of tincture per pint of salve). His patients would then rub this salve on their skin and leave it exposed to the sun. He claimed to have better than a 75% success rate for this. His remedy was also used to treat burns, wounds, sores, bruises, eczema and psoriasis.

Help for Cerebrospinal Problems

St. Johnswort is one of the very few herbs for which there exists some documentation to show its value in treating certain conditions of the brain and spine. One of these is hydrocephalus, a condition marked by an excessive accumulation of fluid enlarging the cerebral ventricles, thinning the brain and causing a separation of cranial bones.

The Feb. 1981 Soviet medical journal, *Vrachebnoe Delo*, cited considerable relief from such intense head pressure in 150 patients who were given an herbal "cocktail" composed of St. Johnswort herb, Siberian ginseng root, peppermint leaves, birch buds and huckleberry or blueberry leaves. A similar brew can be made at home for such a condition. Bring 1 qt. of water to a boil. Add 2 tbsps. each of dried, coarsely cut Siberian ginseng root and 1-1/2 tbsps. of chopped buds from a birch tree. Cover, reduce heat and simmer for 5 mins. If only the powdered Siberian ginseng is present and birch buds are unavailable in your immediate vicinity, then proceed to this method instead. After the water boils, remove it from the heat and add 2-1/2 tbsps. dried St. Johnswort, 2 tbsps. mint leaves, 1 tbsp. blueberry leaves and the equivalent of 1 tsp. of powdered Siberian ginseng root. In place of birch buds, substitute 2-1/4 tsp. fresh, finely minced celery stalk. Stir all of these ingredients together, return the pan to the heat and simmer for 7 minutes. Then remove and steep an additional 25 minutes. Strain through a fine sieve, then strain again through a clean muslin cloth before drinking. Recommended amount is 1 cup three times daily on an empty stomach.

A tincture made from the flowering tops and fresh herb of St. Johnswort has outstanding benefits for various brain disturbances, among which is mental depression. Ten to twenty drops in a 6-oz. glass of spring or distilled water on a daily basis has been highly recommended by some naturopathic and homeopathic physicians in the past. To make your own tincture, combine 10 tbsps. of powdered St. Johnswort herb in 1-1/4 cups of vermouth. Let stand for 15 days, shaking twice each day; then strain through a muslin cloth and bottle. Use as previously directed for mental problems.

For treating any kind of trauma to the nervous system, some of this same tincture may not only be given internally, but just as effectively rubbed on the spinal column, especially in cases of extreme shock or hysteria with reasonably good results. When the drops are given orally, they should be slowly placed beneath the front of the tongue or given sublingually for maximum penetration and benefit to the nerves.

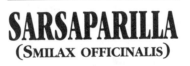

SARSAPARILLA
(SMILAX OFFICINALIS)

Brief Description

This tropical American perennial plant produces a long, tuberous rootstock, from which grows a ground-trailing vine that climbs by means of tendrils coming in pairs from the petioles of the ovate, evergreen leaves. The small, greenish flowers grow in axillary umbels.

Treating Venereal Diseases

For venereal diseases such as syphilis and gonorrhea a sarsaparilla tea has been shown to be effective. Bring 1 qt. of water to a boil, adding 2 tbsps. each of sarsaparilla and yellow dock roots. Reduce heat and simmer, covered, for 5 mins. Remove cover and add 3-1/2 tsp. of dried thyme herb. Cover again and steep an additional hour.

Drink 1-3 cups daily and use as well to douche and/or wash the sexual organs often. Both herbs may be found in any local health food store.

SASSAFRAS
(SASSAFRAS ALBIDUM)

Brief Description

Sassafras is a small- to medium-sized tree, varying in height from 10 to 50 feet. It has furrowed grayish to reddish brown bark that emits a pleasant spicy fragrance.

An Appalachian Medical Standby

Folks residing in the Appalachia Mountains still utilize the root bark of sassafras in the form of a tea for many different things. Boil 1 pint of water; add to it 2 tbsps. sassafras rootbark; cover, simmer 10 minutes, then set aside and steep 30 minutes. Take 2 cups daily for these problems: venereal disease, herpes, eczema, shingles, psoriasis, rash, rheumatism, gout, arthritis, fever, dysentery and lung problems. It is also good to drink for breaking the smoking habit and to slow the flow of milk in nursing mothers.

A quaint idea still subscribed to by many rural folks is that sassafras tea is good to drink in the springtime to "thin and purify bad blood."

SAVORY
(SATUREJA HORTENSIS)

Brief Description

This annual herb grows wild in the Mediterranean area and is widely cultivated elsewhere in the world as a nice culinary spice. Its branching root produces a bushy, hairy stem which grows over a foot high, often taking on a purple hue as it matures. The small, oblong-linear leaves are sessile and usually have hairy margins. The pink or white, two-lipped flowers grow in whorl-like cymes. The entire plant is extremely aromatic.

An Aphrodisiac That Works

Savory has been considered an "herb of love" for centuries! The famous French herbalist, Maurice Messegue, has often used it in place of ginseng to help couples retrieve their married bliss. He advises them to sprinkle powdered savory on all their meat dishes. For impotent men and frigid women he advises them to rub the base of the spine with a decoction of savory and fenugreek.

In 1 qt. boiling water, simmer 3-1/2 tbsps. fenugreek seed for 5 mins., covered. Remove from heat and add 2 handfuls of savory. Steep an additional 50 mins. Drink 2 cups before going to bed and apply to the bottom of the back as well.

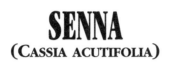

SENNA
(CASSIA ACUTIFOLIA)

Brief Description

This type of senna cones from Egypt and goes by the name of Alexandrian senna. It is a shrub common to North Africa, reaches upward of 3 feet in height and has pale green stems. The brittle and grayish-green leaflets and oblong pod fruit are the parts used for medicinal purposes.

Herbal Dynamite for the Most Stubborn Constipation

The only thing you ever need to remember about senna is this: if your bowels are hopelessly blocked up, and nothing else seems to work, then senna will surely clean you out fast. It is the herbal equivalent of dynamite and will remove even the most impacted feces within a matter of hours, if adequate amounts are taken. But because it can produce abdominal cramping, I always advise that it be used *with* cinnamon. Take 4 capsules of senna and 3 capsules of cinnamon with one full glass of canned milk, goat's milk, or soybean milk. For older people this is the safest and easiest way to go, but expect prompt results within a matter of hours. Another way is to drink the *cold* tea. Boil 1 pint of water. Add to it 1 tbsp. of senna leaves and fruit and 1 tbsp. cinnamon bark. Simmer for 5 minutes, covered, then steep for 20 minutes. Strain and drink two cups.

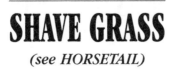

SHAVE GRASS
(see HORSETAIL)

SHEPHERD'S PURSE
(Capsella bursa-pastoris)

Brief Description

Shepherd's purse is a white-flowered, weedy, annual herb. It is a member of the widespread mustard family. Its tiny blossoms grow in the form of a four-armed cross.

Stops All Forms of Bleeding

Here's one for your natural emergency kit: Include some shepherd's purse, because it's outstanding for stopping all forms of bleeding very quickly.

If a persistent nosebleed fails to respond to other conventional treatments, then soak some cotton balls with a little bit of the tea, squeeze out the excess liquid, and insert them into the nostrils to quell further hemorrhaging.

For internal use, drink one-half cup of the tea every hour on the hour, as necessary, but do so on an *empty* stomach for greatest effects. Externally, the cold tea may be applied to *any* wound with saturated cloth compresses or by holding wet cotton balls firmly against the wound until the bleeding eventually ceases. Scratches, skin ulcers and bites are similarly treated.

This is also one of *the very best* teas for a woman to drink following hemorrhaging after childbirth. The tea should be taken cold and several cups at a time. It is also marvelous for bloody urine and stool as well as bleeding from the lungs.

Here's how to make the dynamic tea for theses serious medical problems. Bring a pint of water to a boil. Add two tablespoons dried herb. Cover, remove from heat, and steep for 45 minutes. Strain and refrigerate. Best used when cold.

SIBERIAN GINSENG
(see GINSENG)

SKULLCAP
(Scutellaria lateriflora)

Brief Description

This North American perennial grows in wet places throughout Canada and the northern and eastern U.S. as well as in other parts of the world, such as southeast Asia. The fibrous, yellow rootstock produces a branching stem from 1-3 feet high, with opposite, ovate, serrate leaves that come to a point. The axillary, two-lipped flowers are pale purple or blue.

Soothes Nervous Spasms or Convulsions

Skullcap by itself or in conjunction with valerian root makes an ideal sedative for nervous muscle spasms, twitches and general convulsions. Three capsules of each herb should be taken every 4 hours for the worst cases, less, of course, for minor symptoms. Either 1-1/2 cups of warm tea every couple of hours or 1/2 cup, as the case may be. In 1 pt. of boiling water simmer 1 tbsp. cut, dried valerian root on low heat, covered, for 3 mins. Then add 2 tsp. of cut, dried skullcap herb, cover again, and simmer an additional 1-1/2 mins., before removing from heat entirely and steeping 40 mins. longer.

Lowers Cholesterol, Relieves Arthritis

Not all uses generally ascribed to medicinal herbs come from indigenous folk healers and makeshift herbalists. Nor is the full potential for some herbs to be found in the plethora of herb books currently inundating the health food market. Skullcap is a case in point to be more carefully studied by those who *think* they know something about this herb, but, in reality, may know very, very little.

Various Japanese scientists have been investigating the remarkable capabilities of this herb in regard to the heart and joint inflammation. As reported in various issues of *Chemical & Pharmaceutical Bulletin* (29:2308; 32:2724) skullcap inhibits the increase of serum cholesterol in the blood, increases the production of "good" cholesterol instead (high-density lipoproteins), inhibits fat cells from clumping so as not to cause hardening of the arteries and reduces muscle and joint swelling so common to rheumatoid arthritis.

Two to three capsules of skullcap from your local health food store after a heavy meal rich in fats is recommended, as well as 4 capsules once or twice daily for arthritic relief. Or 1-2 cups of tea may be taken instead, as needed for the same conditions.

SLIPPERY ELM
(ULMUS FULVA)

Brief Description

This deciduous beauty reaches heights of 65-70 feet and may be found planted along streets and growing in forests from Quebec to Florida, the Dakotas and Texas. The tree is covered with a reddish, dark brown, rough, furrowed outer bark, with the inner bark being whitish, slightly sweet and somewhat aromatic. The twigs are hairy, the buds dark brown, blunt and coated at the ends with long, rusty hairs. The leaves are very rough to the touch, thick and stiff, with both surfaces being hairy.

Incredible Hip Joint-and-Socket Replacement

One of the most amazing accounts I've ever read concerning what an herb can do is found in the rare, out-of-print book, *The Women of Mormondom* by Edward W. Tullidge. In there is related in great detail how a woman named Amanda Smith was inspired with a divine cure, which kept her young son from being permanently crippled.

On Tuesday, October 30, 1838, the small Mormon settlement of Haun's Mill in Caldwell County, Missouri was unmercifully attacked by a heavily armed band of religious hooligans. Close to two dozen young boys and teenage-to-adult men were murdered in cold blood and their bodies later dumped down a deep well for concealment.

Amanda Smith's youngest son had his one entire hip joint completely blasted away when one cruel attacker put the muzzle of his gun against the lad's waist and deliberately fired. The mother recovered from her initial shock and prayed to God for inspiration. She was told by an unseen voice to make a lye out of the ashes of shagbark hickory and carefully wash out all dirt and debris from the ugly, gaping wound.

Next she proceeded to get some roots and inner bark from nearby slippery elm trees and pounded them with rocks until they were quite pulpy. This mucilage poultice was then put directly into the wound until it was full and finally dressed with clean line. The boy's mother changed the poultice every few days. In about 5 weeks her son had completely recovered—a flexible gristle having grown in place of the missing joint and socket which amazed physicians for years to come. The family later migrated to Utah where the boy enjoyed a full, active adult life without any physical hindrance whatsoever from his terrible childhood ordeal.

A tea made of the bark is also good for appendicitis.

Ideal Remedy for Sores and Eczema

Certain 19th century Native Americans like the Menoiminee and Potawatomi would mix water with some powdered slippery elm bark and put it on sores and boils with good results.

And a rather remarkable remedy for eczema using slippery elm bark was contributed by a Minnesota couple. The husband's teenage sister had once been severely afflicted with eczema on both arms. The parents had exhausted their funds on the medical profession in trying to find a cure for her miserable condition, but without any success. Someone recommended an application of boiled jimsonweed (a poisonous herb) and slippery elm bark, which cleared it up in no time at all.

I recommend substituting chaparral in place of this dangerous herb. Bring 2 quarts of water to a boil, adding approximately 4 heaping tbsp. cut, dried chaparral. Reduce heat to low and simmer an hour and a half until the liquid has been reduced to just 1 quart or so. Strain liquid into a clean jar and store unused amount in refrigerator until needed. Pour a cup of the warm liquid into a small saucepan. In a cup, combine enough cold water and powdered slippery elm until thoroughly mixed. Turn this into the hot chaparral liquid on the stove and heat up, stirring constantly until a thick type of paste is formed. You'll need to do a little experimenting perhaps in order to achieve the right consistency (close to cooked cream-o'-wheat).

Spread this mixture on several strips of clean surgical gauze with a wooden ladle. A tbsp. of olive oil may be added to the mixture in the pan before spreading to keep it from drying out so fast. Apply this to any rash, eczema, dermatitis, or in smaller amounts to any venereal sores, herpes lesions, leg ulcers, wounds that will not heal and so forth. Leave for several hours at a time. Repeat process a couple of times each day. Healing should be imminent before you realize it.

Recipes to Get Well By

This is the best herb of nourishment to administer to those recuperating from any kind of mild or serious illness, be they infant or elderly.

We are indebted to the late Euell Gibbons for these recipes found in his *Stalking the Healthful Herbs.*

Elm Lemonade for Recuperation

Gibbons calls for us to pour 1 pint of boiling water over 5-1/4 tbsp. (1 oz.) of cut, dried elm bark and let steep until cool. Then add juice of 1/2 lemon and enough honey to sweeten to taste. "This same elm lemonade is highly recommended for feverish patients; allow them to drink all they take, for this drink will quench their thirst and help relieve their illness by giving them strengthening, easily digested food at the same time," he wrote in his chapter on this herb.

Homemade Anti-Smoking Lozenges

Although a great lover of the outdoors and a true believer in Nature, Euell Gibbons wasn't very health-minded in many other ways. He believed in the excessive use of white sugar, and, like the late health food faddist Adelle Davis, he was a compulsive chain-smoker. But he found that slippery elm bark really helped him to cope with the constant craving for another cigarette.

His recipe: Put some finely powdered slippery elm bark into a bowl. Make a little nest in it, pour in some dark honey and carefully work the powder into the honey with the back of a wooden ladle or strong metal tablespoon. Do this until the dough is somewhat stiff. Place on a board and cut into small squares. Roll these squares again in powdered slippery elm, then store in your refrigerator. I recommend adding a dash of nutmeg or cinnamon to the powdered bark the squares are to be rolled in, for added flavor. Said Gibbons: "They make very effective lozenges, soothing my throat, dispelling my hoarseness, and allaying my cough, and I find that sucking on these lozenges satisfies my infantile oral cravings, so that I'm not constantly taking another cigarette that I really don't want."

SMARTWEED
(POLYGONUM HYDROPIPER)

Brief Description

This annual plant is prolific throughout the country except for the southern half of Georgia and its neighbor, Florida. The herb has reddish jointed stems, narrow-shaped leaves, and tiny, greenish-white, often red-lipped blossoms borne on long, slender, drooping spikes It gets its name from the strong peppery taste of the leaves and stems.

Prehistoric Food Condiment and Medicine

Archaeologists excavating ancient paleo-Indian sites in the Ohio and Illinois River valleys have uncovered seeds of smartweed from garbage pits and very old campfire sites. They believe this herb was used in prehistoric times as a common flavoring agent on account of its hot, biting taste, since regular salt and pepper were then virtually unknown to paleo-Indians.

It is further believed by paleobotanists (scientists who study the prehistoric use of plants) that smartweed may have been used for its terrific hemostatic properties in stopping bleeding from wounds suffered in battle or by accident. A cold compress of the tea held against the injured site will hasten blood coagulation in minutes. The tea is also good for hypertension.

To make the tea, add 1-1/2 tbsps. of cut stems and leaves to one pint boiling water; cover and simmer 7 minutes, then set aside for 20 minutes. Strain and drink one cup or soak cloth compresses or cotton balls in the tea for external injuries.

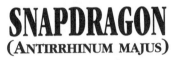

SNAPDRAGON
(Antirrhinum majus)

Brief Description

The name "snapdragon" applies to any showy white, crimson, or yellow bilabiate flowers fancifully likened to the face of a roguish dragon.

Great for Sore Eyes

My Hungarian grandmother, Barbara Leibhardt Heinerman, was an eighth-generation herbalist from the city of Temesvar (now part of Romania). She treated numerous eye disorders ranging from cataracts in the *early stages* and eye inflammations to conjunctivitis, with an eye wash made from snapdragon flowers, leaves and root.

Boil 1 qt. of *distilled* water, adding 1 cup chopped fresh root. Cover and simmer for 15 minutes. Then set aside, uncover and add 1/2 cup cut flowers and 1/4 cup cut leaves. Stir and recover. Steep for 40 minutes. Strain twice and refrigerate. Bathe the eyes frequently with this using an eye cup that can be obtained from any local pharmacy or drugstore.

SOLOMON'S SEAL
(see LILY)

SORREL
(Rumex acetosa)

Brief Description

This perennial can reach nearly 3 feet tall. Sorrel has an erect stem branching at the top into several stalks bearing clusters of small reddish-green to brown blossoms. The plant has rather odd-looking leaves, nearly shaped into the form of arrowheads.

Useful Tea for Stones and Oral Sores

Sorrel leaves can be used in place of spinach, especially in the springtime when a suitable "green tonic" is desired. Boil one pint of water and add 3/4 cup sorrel herb. Cover, set aside and steep 20 minutes. Drink 2 cups daily between meals. This should help in alleviating the pain and the need for eventual removal of gall and kidney stones.

Drink one-half cup *warm* sorrel tea. Swish it around inside your mouth and retain it there for a minute or two before swallowing. Repeat this several times throughout the day. This will get rid of mouth sores. And if the tea is routinely gargled, it will clear up a sore throat or throat ulcers.

SPEARMINT
(see MINTS)

SPRUCE
(Picea excelsa)

Brief Description

Norway spruce is native to Europe, but widely cultivated as an ornamental evergreen in various parts of Canada and the U.S. The trunk is covered with scaly, reddish-brown bark, and can reach a height of 125 feet. The buds in winter are reddish or light brown and produce young shoots at the tips of the branches in May. The dark green, quadrangular needles grow spirally around the branchlets. The catkin-like flowers bloom in May; the male can be either yellow or red, while the female is always bright purple. The light brown cones are cylindric-looking in shape and from 4-6 inches in length.

Indian Headache Remedy

The story is told by Thomas E. Mails in his book *The Mystic Warriors of the Plains* (Garden City, NY: Doubleday & Co., Inc., 1972) about a Sioux warrior in the 19th century named Jaw. He had fought many battles against his enemy, the Crow. He always carried spruce needles with him in his medicine bag. Whenever he got a headache due to anxiety or fatigue from excessive fighting, he would place a few of the needles in his mouth and chew them for a while. His headache would soon disappear.

Native American Medicine for Coughs, Cold, and Flu.

Jaw was quite skilled in stealing horses from the Crow. It is said that he would chew some spruce needles as he went to the windward side of the horses, at which time the animals "pricked up their ears," attracted to his presence on account of the aroma of the chewed needles. This Sioux warrior made a tea of the needles by throwing a handful of them into the equivalent of a pint of water and cooking them over a fire for a while. He would give this tea to other members of his tribe suffering from coughing spells, the common cold or a bad case of the white man's flu.

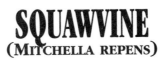

SQUAWVINE
(MITCHELLA REPENS)

Brief Description

This perennial, evergreen herb is found around the bottom of trees and stumps in woodlands from Nova Scotia to Ontario and southward to Florida and Texas. Its creeping or trailing stems grow up to a foot long, rooting at various points, and bear opposite, orbicular-ovate leaves that are dark green and shiny on top and are often streaked with white. The funnel-shaped white flowers grow in pairs and the fruit is a scarlet berry-like drupe up to 1/3 inch in diameter.

The Leading Herb for Pregnancy

A number of America's most famous herbalists concur that this herb is unexcelled in many ways for expectant mothers to take prior to delivery. Both the late Jethro Kloss and John R. Christopher regarded squawvine as the medicine par excellence to take during pregnancy in order to "make childbirth wonderfully easy." Michael Tierra, a practicing herbalist residing in Santa Cruz, California, recommends squawvine "to prevent miscarriages." And the late naturopathic doctor, John Lust, stated that "squawvine makes childbirth faster."

Cut squawvine herb is available from Indiana Botanic Gardens (see Appendix) to make a tea. Steep 2-1/4 tsps. of dried herb in 2 cups of boiling water, covered, for half an hour. A pregnant woman should drink between 1-3 cups a day throughout the length of her pregnancy. A much stronger herbal extract is available from Bio-Botanica of Hauppauge, N.Y. (see Appendix). One tablespoon should be taken every morning on an empty stomach.

When making the tea, equal parts of red raspberry leaves and squawvine herb may be used together with excellent results.

Effective Eyewash for Infants, Elderly

Squawvine makes an excellent eyewash for newborn babies and elderly folks alike, when combined with other herbs. In 1 pint of boiling water, combine equal parts (1/2 handfuls) of cut, dried squawvine herb, raspberry leaves and strawberry leaves. Cover and steep for half an hour. Strain twice through fine sieve and cloth. Wash the eyes of infants and elderly adults frequently with this solution. It also makes an excellent vaginal injection for syphilis, gonorrhea and yeast infection.

Old Indian Remedy for Insomnia

In the 19th century the Menominee Indians of the Upper Great Lakes region made a tea out of the herb and leaves for insomnia. Steep a handful of cut, dried herb in 1-1/2 pints of boiling water, covered, for 45 minutes. Strain about a cup and a half and drink lukewarm before retiring.

STAR OF BETHLEHEM

(see LILY)

STINGING NETTLE
(Urtica dioica)

Brief Description

This is a perennial plant found all over the world. In America it grows in waste places and gardens and along roadsides, fences and walls in the states northward from Colorado, Missouri and South Carolina. The square, bristly stem grows from 2-7 feet high and bears pointed leaves which are downy underneath, and small, greenish flowers that grow in clusters from July to September.

Fantastic Hemostat

Nothing seems to stop profuse bleeding more quickly and effectively than stinging nettle! Because the evidence to be presented is so incredible, the source from which it has been obtained needs to be cited as well in order to make everything more believable.

Francis P. Porcher was a surgeon and physician in the Southern Confederacy. His book, *Resources of the Southern Fields and Forests*, was an important medical text during the Civil War. In it, he related how he and another doctor deliberately cut open and laid bare a major artery of an adult sheep. Then just by soaking some gauzelike material in a strong cold tea made of stinging nettle and applying the same directly to the open wound, he was able to stop all bleeding within just a matter of minutes. More remarkable yet was the fact that when the pressed juice of the plant was added to fresh blood poured out into the palm of the hand, it immediately began coagulating.

To make a strong solution for your own personal needs, bring 1 quart of water to a boil. Remove from the heat and add a generous handful of *freshly* chopped stinging nettle plant. Cover and let steep for an hour before straining. Always best to use when cold. Dried plant materials may be used, but don't work quite as well. Tea may be used internally for bleeding ulcers or externally as a wash or poultice to stop any major hemorrhaging.

Remarkable Hair Tonic for Baldness

Stinging nettle lotion seems to help hair grow again where baldness may now be present. The following two lotions should be used at the same time every morning after washing and rinsing the hair as you would normally do. The alcoholic portion to be used should be diluted by half as much of the infusion prior to rubbing well into the scalp with the fingertips. When doing so, be sure to bend your head down low, massaging the lotion in from the nape of the neck upwards towards the front. Afterwards, allow the scalp to dry naturally without using towel or hair dryer.

In 1 qt. or 4 cups of gin, put 2 handfuls of washed and chopped freshly picked stinging nettle, 3/4 handful of chopped fresh rosemary, 1 handful of chopped or cut fresh chamomile flowers and 2/3 handful of chopped fresh sage. Cover the fruit jar with a tight lid and let stand exposed to *indirect* (shaded) sunlight for 2-1/2 weeks, making sure you shake the contents of the bottle well twice each day. Strain and refrigerate in a clean fruit jar with a lid.

Bring 1-1/2 qts. of Perrier or other bottled mineral water to a boil, adding half each of a small, coarsely chopped rutabaga and unpeeled potato, and 1 diced stalk of celery. Cover, reduce heat and simmer for 25 mins., then strain liquid into another pan, discarding the vegetables. Reheat to boiling point and add 1/2 handful of coarsely chopped, fresh stinging nettle, 1/2 handful of chopped, fresh garden sage, 1/4 tsp. grated horseradish root and juice from half a lemon. Cover and remove from heat, allowing to steep for 50 minutes. When cool, strain and refrigerate in a clean fruit jar with a lid.

When using the alcoholic extract, just remember to dilute one part of it with 1/2 part of the infusion. If used regularly for several months, new hair growth should become fairly evident.

Fun Recipes for a More Slender Image

The late plant forager, Euell Gibbons, once wrote that "stinging nettle is very efficacious in removing unwanted pounds!" Those obese individuals who've written to me in the past desperate for advice on how to reduce and who I've put on a semi-diet of stinging nettle have reported losses up to 32-1/4 lbs. in just three months or less!

Nettles should be collected in the early spring when they are 4-8 inches high. As the plant matures, it becomes pretty tough and quite unpalatable. A pair of good leather gloves is recommended to protect the hands when handling the stuff. Heavy paper bags to carry the nettle are preferable to plastic ones.

After you've gathered enough nettle it should be washed in cold water. A pair of kitchen tongs will be of considerable help when removing the washed greens from the water. Allow them to drain on paper towels for a few minutes before refrigerating. They'll keep for up to a week.

Nettles freeze very well. Place the rinsed nettles in a large kettle. Pour boiling water over them to cover. After 5 mins., drain off the water, pack them into freezer containers and freeze. In the frozen state they'll keep for up to 9 months as a rule.

NETTLE GREENS, GEORGIA STYLE

Needed: 2 qts. stinging nettles; 3/4 cup stock from boiled chicken wings and chopped, cooked meat from those wings; 3 sliced green onions; 2 hard-boiled eggs and 1/4 tsp. lemon juice.

Snip greens into bite-sized pieces. Put in pan with other ingredients except the eggs. Simmer on low heat for 20 minutes.

Remove and serve, topped with sliced hard-boiled eggs. Season to taste with a little kelp, if needed.

CREAM OF NETTLE SOUP

Needed: 1-1/2 qts. nettle greens; 1/3 cup Perrier or other mineral water; 1/4 cup sesame seed oil; 1/4 cup whole wheat flour; 3 cups canned goat's milk.

Cook the nettles with water in covered saucepan over medium heat for 10 mins. Cool 15 mins., then puree in blender or food processor. In a saucepan, warm up the oil and stir in the flour, mixing both well. Then slowly add the goat's milk and cook until the mixture thickens over a low heat. Add the pureed nettles and heat thoroughly. Add some kelp to season. Serves 4.

NOTE: I'm deeply indebted to Darcy Williamson, author of *How to Prepare Common Wild Foods,* for her nettle recipes, which have been somewhat adapted to fit the needs of this book.

Nettles Ease Benign Prostate Enlargement

Prostate enlargement, technically known as benign prostatic hyperplasia or hypertrophy (BPH), tends to affect most men past age 50. Sometimes BPH can cause painful urination. Often, it's just a nuisance or an embarrassment, causing frequent nighttime urination, an unfinished sensation or dribbling.

Naturopathic physicians in Europe, America and Canada for years have recommended stinging nettle and saw palmetto together in the treatment of this problem. French and Italian studies have shown that when these two herbs are used together in low doses for at least a month, remarkable improvement is always made in cases of BPH.

Two capsules of each herb are taken once daily with a full glass of water. Or make a tea by adding one tablespoon each of stinging nettle and saw palmetto to 2-1/4 pints boiling water. Cover, set aside and steep for 40 minutes. Drink 2 cups daily, one in the morning and the other at night.

SUMA
(PFAFFIA PANICULATA)

Brief Description

Suma (also called "Brazilian ginseng" or "Brazilian carrots") is a suffrutescent shrub growing prolifically in the Goias area south of the Amazon Basin in Brazil. Here much of the soil is very red, signifying large amounts of iron oxide and aluminum hydroxides, but very little of other nutrients.

In this rocky, lateric soil, this member of the pig weed (amaranthacene) family grows. Its top part is rather fragile, but the below-ground rhizome is usually quite thick. Even with limited amounts of rainfall, suma has adapted quite nicely.

Women's Tonic

From what we know about the soil of the region in which it grows, we may assume that this herb is relatively high in iron. Additional research data from Japan indicate the presence of a number of natural sugars and several regular ginseng-related compounds.

In cases of anemia, fatigue, and even premenstrual syndrome to some extent, it would appear that suma is very useful for women to take. One of the few companies that I'm aware of obtains its suma from this area of Brazil. Great attention is paid to the purity and integrity of the herb materials imported. An average of 2 capsules daily helps to supplement the diet with iron.

Possible Anti-Cancer Value

Some American herbalists have ascribed virtues to suma which cannot be substantiated in regular scientific literature. In addition to this, the actual ethno-botanical lore surrounding it is quite sparse. That is, there are virtually no officially recorded folk uses for it for any great length of time. One botanist, in fact, has told me in private that the folk uses attributed to it have all been of fairly recent vintage and, in his professional opinion, "were mostly created by a few Brazilian businessmen, to help sell more of the stuff." When I reported on this herb at a recent gathering of health food retailers in Philadelphia, a number of proprietors were quite surprised to hear this.

Recent experiments in Japan with malignant melanoma cells in a culture medium showed that certain naturally occurring constituents in suma manifest anti-tumor properties. These cancer-inhibiting compounds (pfaffic acid and pfaffosides) have been written up in volume 23 of *Phytochemistry* and Volume 102 (191149n) of *Chemical Abstracts*, among others.

Although not specifically recommended here for cancer per se, yet in an overall program of sound nutrition and good herbal supplementation, suma appears to have certain preventative value in regard to cancer. An average of 3 capsules daily is suggested.

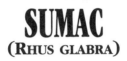

SUMAC
(RHUS GLABRA)

Brief Description

Sumac can be either a shrub or small tree, growing anywhere from 10 to 18 feet high. Its branches have smooth, gray bark and leaves that are green on top and silvery white or whitish gray underneath; in the autumn they turn a brilliant red and add wonderfully to the rich kaleidoscope of colors to be seen at that particular season of the year.

Venereal Disease and Rash Treated

A tea made from parts of the sumac makes an excellent skin wash in cases of venereal disease or poison ivy rash. Add one tablespoon each of sumac bark, leaves and berries to one quart of boiling water. Cover and gently simmer on low heat for 30 minutes. Set aside and steep for another 30 minutes. Strain and refrigerate. Use when cool for external applications.

NOTE: If you intend harvesting these parts from a sumac tree close by, make sure you are well enough acquainted with it to distinguish this species from others which are poisonous!

SWEET CICELY
(OSMORHIZA LONGISTYLIS)

Brief Description

Sweet cicely is a perennial herb found from Alaska, through the Canadian and American Pacific Northwest, and southward through Colorado to Georgia. The thick, bundled roots produce branched stems for 2 to 3 feet in height. The entire plant emits an unmistakable aniselike odor.

An Herbal "Tums for the Tummy"

Believe it or not, Nature often provides us with many of the OTC (over-the-counter) medications that we might otherwise procure from our local pharmacy. Instead of reaching for the Maalox, Rolaids or Tums next time you have a tummyache, try some sweet cicely root tea for a change. You'll be pleasantly surprised at just how effective it is in clearing up heartburn, acid indigestion, abdominal cramps, intestinal gas, and in improving the appetite.

Boil a pint of distilled water. Add 1-1/2 tablespoons of chopped sweet cicely root. Cover, lower heat and simmer 20 minutes. Set aside and steep for 20 more minutes. Strain and drink one cup when lukewarm.

SWEET FLAG
(see CALAMUS)

T

TARRAGON
(Artemisia dracunculus)

Brief Description

Tarragon is a green, glabrous perennial shrub found in sunny, dry areas in the western United States, southern Asia and Siberia. In Europe it is culti-vated for its aromatic leaves that impart a licorice-anise flavor to sauces, sal-ads and vinegary foods. It grows about 2 feet high and has long, narrow leaves which, unlike other members of its genus, are undivided. Tarragon is closely allied to wormwood and has long, fibrous roots spreading every-where by runners and small flowers in round, yellow-black heads that are seldom fully opened.

Tea for Insomnia and Hyperactivity

An old French remedy for insomnia and hyperactivity that's been tried with pretty good success is tarragon tea. And though insomnia for me is extremely rare to say the least, I can testify to those very few times when the tea never failed to put me into dreamland in just a few minutes. Steep 1-1/2 tsp. of the dried, cut herb in 1-3/4 cups boiling water, covered and away from the heat, for 40 minutes. Prepare about an hour before retiring, then strain and drink the tea while it's still lukewarm.

Improves Digestion, Promotes Appetite

The renowned French herbalist, Maurice Messegue, who once treated the likes of people such as Charles DeGaulle, King Farouk of Egypt and Pope

441

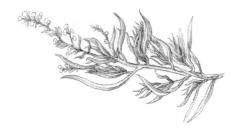

John XXIII, said this about tarragon: "I prescribe the herb basically as a mild stimulant for the bowels and as a stomach aid. It can bring an appetite back to people in a very weak condition, to convalescents, nervous people, those suffering from anxiety and promote recovery from an episode of schizophrenia or nervous exhaustion following mental depression. It fights indigestion, air-swallowing and gassy distension, and is also useful in cases of gout, rheumatism, retention of urine, sluggish kidneys and bladder. It can regulate women's periods, too."

Now the best way to take tarragon for digestive-related problems is in the form of a homemade vinegar, 1 tbsp. before each meal. To make tarragon vinegar, fill a wide-mouthed fruit jar with the freshly gathered leaves, picked just before the herb flowers, on a dry day. Pick the leaves off the stalks and dry a little on a flat cookie sheet lined with foil in a low-set oven (about 225°F.).

Then place in the jar, cover with apple cider vinegar and 1/2 tsp. each freshly squeezed lemon and lime juices. Permit it to stand about 7 hours, then strain through about five layers of cheesecloth or a clean piece of flannel material into another jar with a tight-fitting ring lid. Store in a cool, dry pantry or cupboard.

Culinary Uses

The anise-flavored leaves and flowering tops are used to season salads, sauces, soups, stews, eggs, meat, fish and pickles. Leaves or essential oil are also used in the manufacture of tarragon vinegar, mustard, tartar sauce and liqueurs. Russian tarragon, a separate cultivar, is often confused with and sold as French tarragon. Except for being taller, the Russian variety looks similar to French tarragon but is considered far inferior to the French or true kind as far as taste goes.

TARRAGON CARROT SOUP

Needed: 1 small onion, chopped; 2 tbsps. white rice; 1 tbsp. olive oil; 4 medium carrots, sliced; 2 medium sprigs tarragon, chopped; 2 cups water; granulated kelp (a seaweed) to taste.

In a medium saucepan over medium heat sauté onion and rice in olive oil until clear, about 2-1/2 minutes. Add carrots, tarragon and water.

Bring to a boil, cover, reduce heat and simmer until carrots are tender, about 30 minutes. Remove from heat and cool.

In a Vita-Mix blender puree this mixture until smooth and creamy.

Return to pan, season with kelp, and heat through. Yield: Serves 2.

TEA
(CAMELLIA SINENSIS)

Brief Description

Tea drinking in some Asian countries has evolved into quite a delicate art, much as wine sampling or tasting has done in France. There are connoisseurs of finely brewed tea, who can tell what type of water was used, what kind of utensils were involved and the approximate conditions under which a particular tea is made. In mainland China, some teas are so incredibly strong to the palate that they're served in (literally) thimble-sized cups.

Relieves Migraines

Black and green teas both contain caffeine (1-5%). Since caffeine constricts the blood vessels in the head, it's able to calm the pain caused when they throb and swell. During my 1980 visit to the People's Republic of China, I noticed a number of traditional medical hospitals administer black tea to their patients suffering from migraine headaches.

In the Soochow Chinese Traditional Medical Hospital in Soochow, there was a remarkable 92% recovery rate for migraines. To 1 cup of hot water, simply add 2 teabags of black tea and steep for 20 minutes until very strong. Then drink while still very warm, but not so hot as to burn the tongue or injure the inside of the mouth. "Works every time!" I was told by my hosts in China.

Great Infection Fighter

Throughout mainland China I found black tea being used in numerous hospitals and clinics to successfully treat all kinds of infection and inflammation of the stomach, lower intestines, colon and the liver with recovery rates averaging between 83-100% for the majority of patients treated. A strong cup of warm tea was given four to five times daily for these various infectious diseases.

Reduced Atherosclerosis

University of California scientists have discovered that tea drinkers experience a lot less hardening of the arteries than coffee drinkers do. It seems that the caffeine in coffee is bound with some heavy oils, which tend to elevate serum cholesterol levels quite a bit. But not so with either dark or green teas. In fact, it's believed that the caffeine content in both teas may actually help to cut cholesterol somewhat. Besides this, the tea's polyphenols act in concert with the vitamins C and P present, helping to strengthen the blood vessel walls of the heart.

Tea Removes Dental Plaque

During 1983-84 dental scientists at Washington University in St. Louis conducted a series of experiments proving that black tea definitely inhibits the growth of decay-causing bacteria common to plaque buildup on the teeth. This is probably due to the high natural fluoride content found in both teas.

A 1977 dental study conducted in Taiwan showed that 50 weaning rats given cavity-producing foods like white bread, white sugar and carbonated soft drinks, but also given green or black teas, had anywhere from half to three-fourths fewer cavities than those rodents which didn't receive any tea. Brew a Lipton Brisk Tea bag in a cup of hot water for at least 6 minutes in order to get the maximum removal of fluoride. Also squeezing the tea bag before discarding helps. Use either tea as a good mouth wash and dental rinse after every meal of sweets. The April 1986 issue of *Dentistry* encouraged people to drink more tea in order to reduce cavities and plaque buildup.

Celebrated Food Expert Clears Up Hoarseness with a Cure of Her Own

In the first week of January 1995, the Wilmington [Delaware] *News Journal* carried an interesting story about 83-year-old Julia Child, author of the definitive *Mastering the Art of French Cooking*.

It was a Sunday morning and fog and humidity had taken their toll on her vocal cords. The culinary grande dame's distinctive voice kept breaking up in take after take of the opening shots for "Good Morning America's" visit to the Hotel du Pont in downtown Wilmington. Child was unable to get past her opening line.

She told members of the anxious TV crew that "my hoarseness just isn't normal." After the fourth try, she reluctantly admitted with an apology, "I still have that frog." Shaking her head and narrowing her eyes, she worked desperately to clear her throat, but to no avail.

Finally, turning to hotel manager Jacques Amblard, she ordered some tea. A makeup artist on the set rushed off to fetch some lozenges as a backup measure in case the other failed. The program producer stood with hands on hips, frowning at the hotel lobby's ornate ceiling.

But television's most famous chef wasn't the least bit worried. Once the tea arrived, she added 1/2 teaspoon lemon juice and a teaspoon of honey and slowly sipped the hot liquid. After she had finished, she set the empty cup aside and remarked, "Let's give it a few more tries, shall we?"

By now her voice had assumed the firmness fans have come to expect. And she was correct; in less than six takes, her voice was again clear and distinct and she executed her just-written lines perfectly without any more mistakes.

She told reporter Valerie Helmbreck afterwards that "this remedy will always take care of hoarseness, no matter how bad it gets. I've depended on hot black or green tea with a little lemon and honey for many years to keep my voice in good shape for critical moments like this."

Green Tea May Protect Against Heart Disease and Reduce the Risk of Cancer

An Indian doctor friend of mine, who practices the ancient art of Ayurvedic healing in the city of Madras, called something to my attention not long ago. Dr. Nadu Thiruparamkundram pointed out that it has been the custom of some practitioners like himself to routinely prescribe green tea to protect against heart and liver disease as well as against certain forms of cancer (especially skin, stomach, and colon-rectum). He attributes these helpful benefits to the presence of vitamin-like substances called polyphenols. He recommends to all of his patients that they drink at least two cups of green tea every day. (For additional information on the medical advantages of tea, see one of my other reference works, *Heinerman's Encyclopedia of Juices, Teas and Tonics* (Englewood Cliffs, NJ: Prentice Hall, 1996).)

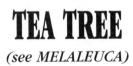

TEA TREE
(see MELALEUCA)

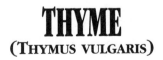

THYME
(THYMUS VULGARIS)

Brief Description

Thyme is the general name for the many herbs of the *Thymus* species, all of which are small, perennial plants native to Europe and Asia. Common or garden thyme is considered the principal type and is utilized commer-

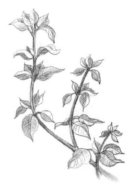

cially for flowering and ornamental purposes. This low-growing, woody shrub has gray-green leaves and white, pink or purple flowers. Thyme is produced and collected in most European countries, including France, Spain, Portugal and Greece, as well as in the western U.S. The three principal varieties of thyme are English, French and German, and they differ in leaf shape, leaf color, and essential oil composition.

A Natural Antibiotic

Europe's most renowned folk healer, the French herbalist Maurice Messegue, had this to say about thyme: "From my long years of experience as an herbalist, I can appreciate thyme because of its antiseptic qualities. It contains thymol and its smell destroys viruses and bacteria in the atmosphere as it destroys infectious germs in the body. I do not know any infection that cannot be mitigated if treated with this precious herb. It is an excellent weapon against epidemics and much cheaper than other means of controlling them. From boils to typhoid and whitlows to tuberculosis, it is excellent beyond compare!" This puts thyme in the same realm as garlic, both being "Nature's antibiotics" and replacements for penicillin and various sulfa drugs.

Messegue devised various preparations for using this wonderful natural antibiotic internally and externally. For gargling (sore throat), mouth wash (bad breath, tooth decay, cold sores) and drinking (common cold, influenza, fever, allergies) purposes, make a tea by steeping a dozen sprigs of fresh thyme in 1-3/4 pints of boiling water, covered and away from the heat for half an hour. Strain and drink 3-4 cups daily.

For external purposes, such as a hot compress on the chest to help break up lung congestion in cases of asthma, bronchitis, cold and flu or as a massage lotion for aching joints and muscles, put 1-1/2 handfuls of fresh thyme in 2 pints boiling water, covered and away from the heat, and steep for 40 minutes. Strain and use.

He also used thyme for footbaths, handbaths, and a douche for promoting better blood circulation, getting rid of nail fungus and athlete's foot, reducing a fever and treating *Candida albicans* or yeast infection of the vagina, respectively. One handful of fresh thyme is added to 1-1/4 pints of boiling water, covered and removed from the heat and permitted to steep about 25 minutes. Strain and soak hands and feet in this solution while still somewhat hot; douche with it when lukewarm.

Any of the above solutions may also be used to bathe wounds and burns, in the form of a compress on bumps and bruises and as a wash for sore eyes when moderately cool. This thyme eyewash is especially good for red eyes which have been irritated by the chlorinated water in public swimming pools. If fresh thyme isn't readily available, then the *cut*, dried herb may be used (2 tbsps. = 1 handful fresh herb).

Even the culinary form of ground thyme has some medicinal application for various skin problems. Mix together 1 tsp. ground thyme, 1/2 tsp. lime juice, 1/2 tsp. onion juice with just enough honey to form a soft, sticky paste. Then apply directly on open, festering sores and boils of any kind and leave for 12 hours or so. Change again or wash away when showering or bathing and apply some new paste. This will help to heal them a lot faster, Messegue discovered.

A health liqueur for tonic and preventative purposes may be made by soaking 6 fresh or dried sprigs of thyme in 1-1/2 cups of fine brandy for 5 days, shaking several times each day. Taking several teaspoonfuls of this throughout the day when you feel a cold or flu coming on will not only help to prevent you from getting the "bug," but will also lessen its seriousness should you come down with it. This same liqueur will tonify the stomach and stimulate the appetite a little, when a person doesn't especially feel like eating but needs to for strength and sustenance.

Another interesting idea that Messegue came up with was prescribing an herbal toothpaste made out of thyme herb for people suffering with tooth and gum diseases. Soak 3 handfuls of fresh thyme, which has been lightly crushed with a rolling pin, in 1 cup of brandy for about 5 hours. A soft-to-medium bristled brush can then be dipped in this solution and the teeth cleaned with it each day. This solution is good for about 4-6 brushings or approximately 2 days use, before some more needs to be made.

Healing Salve for Facial Blemishes

A nice salve can be made at home for helping to heal cuts, bruises, acne, rash and so forth on the skin, especially in the area of the face, neck, throat and forehead. But its use also extends to burns, wounds and sores located elsewhere on the body.

The first part to prepare this salve is to make the base. Ghee is used as an excellent base for many herbal salves and oils in India by Ayurvedic folk healers everywhere. This is nothing more than clarified butter, a delicious and fragrant oil that is semi-solid at room temperature. To make this ghee, melt 2 pounds of butter in a saucepan until it reaches a slow, rolling boil. Remove from the heat and carefully skim off the foam with a spoon. Return the pot to the heat and repeat this procedure twice more, removing as much of the foam as possible and discarding it. Allow the pan to cool a couple of minutes before removing the thin film that forms on top. Let the butter cool down somewhat, and then, while still liquid, pour through a fine-meshed tea strainer, but stop pouring when the heavier solids at the bottom of the pan move to the strainer. Collect the ghee in a glass bottle, cool completely and cover. The entire process takes less than half an hour to accomplish. Two pounds of butter yield about 2 cups of ghee. It can be stored without refrigeration for up to 6 months.

The next step involves reheating the ghee to just below the point where it will bubble without burning and smoking. Add 2 handfuls coarsely chopped and slightly crushed garden thyme to the pot. When the ghee is reheated, and during the gentle cooking of the thyme for an hour, the pot should always *remain covered.* After this, briefly uncover just long enough to strain through a coarse, wire sieve of some kind. Return to the stove and cover again to reheat for about 5 minutes. Then remove the lid and add between 1-2 tbsps. of melted beeswax and stir thoroughly. Also add about 1/2 tsp. of pure vanilla when putting the beeswax in. Finally, pour the entire contents from the pot into clean jars that aren't too deep (empty baby food jars will do). Allow to set up before screwing the lids on. Store in a cool, dry place.

Massage some of this salve into the skin each day after showering, and again in the evening before retiring for the night. I'm grateful to my friend, Michael Tierra, for the data on rendering butter into ghee and making a good, general salve.

Relieving Headaches and Cramps

The antiviral constituent, thymol, occurring in thyme is not only effective in combating unfriendly bacteria, but also helps to relax tense muscles and tight blood vessels. To help relieve migraine headaches or stomach cramps, just make a tea out of fresh or dried thyme, according to any of the previous directions given; and drink 1 cup of warm tea on an empty stomach before lying down for a while. Also, soak a small cloth dish towel in some of the hot tea, wring out the excess liquid, then apply across the forehead and lay another dry hand or small bath towel over that to retain the heat longer. Change several times when it turns cold and continue the process for about an hour before getting up. Having the hot tea on a stool, table or small stand beside your bed or couch will prevent you from having to get up so often to change the compresses if you are alone.

If fresh or dried cut thyme is unavailable, you can effectively substitute some Listerine antiseptic in its place. Just bring a couple of cups of this commercial mouth wash almost to a boil or until quite hot. Remove from the heat to use *only* for compress purposes.

NOTE: *Under no circumstances* are you to drink this!

A milder tea can be made *separately* by putting 1 tsp. ground thyme into 1-1/2 cups boiling water, covering and steeping for half an hour. Then drink slowly while still tolerably warm. The reason Listerine is recommended when thyme herb is not readily available is because this oral mouth wash contains a lot of thymol and eucalyptol from eucalyptus. Both of these constituents really help to relax the muscles when they are exposed to heat and then applied to the surface of the skin. In fact, these are some of the same constituents found in Mentholatum Deep-Heat Rub, which is used to relax sore, aching muscles.

Purifying Contaminated Water

Thyme is one of several aromatic herbs (peppermint, rosemary, sage and savory) which are handy to use in purifying water in countries such as Mexico, Spain, Portugal, Greece, Italy and, believe it or not, parts of the Soviet Union where the drinking waters are in serious question as to purity. Generally, you will find some species of thyme in the public marketplaces, which can then be used when boiling up water for drinking purposes later on. Figure about 1 good handful of cut thyme to 1 quart of water. Cover and boil, then reduce heat and simmer, covered, for 20 minutes. Strain and you now have safe drinking water that won't give you any more diarrhea and fever.

Culinary Virtues

BROWN RICE WITH MUSHROOMS AND THYME

Needed: 1 cup of spring or distilled water; 2 cups chicken stock; 1/2 tsp. sea salt; 1-1/2 cups brown rice; 1/2 cup chopped onions; 1-1/2 cups fresh, coarsely chopped mushrooms; 2 tbsps. butter and 1/2 tsp. thyme.

Bring water, stock and salt to a boil. Add rice slowly and return to boil. Turn down and simmer for 45 mins. Stir occasionally. While rice is cooking, chop onions and wash and chop mushrooms. Melt butter in large, heavy skillet. Sauté onions and mushrooms. Add cooked rice and mix well. Add thyme.

Add a little bit of kelp and some more sea salt to taste. Makes 6-8 servings. I'm indebted to the folks at *Country Journal* (see Appendix) for use of this recipe.

TORMENTILLA
(see CINQUEFOIL)

TURMERIC
(CURCUMA LONGA OR C. DOMESTICA)

Brief Description

This perennial herb of the ginger family has a thick rhizome from which arise large, oblong and long-petioled leaves. Turmeric grows to almost a yard high and is extensively cultivated in India, China, Indonesia, Jamaica, Haiti, Philippines and other tropical countries. The part used is the cured (boiled, cleaned and sun-dried) and polished rhizome. India is the major producer. This spice is the major ingredient of curry powder and is also used in prepared mustard.

Paste for Skin Ailments

In Samoa, natives have used the powdered rhizome to treat skin ulcers, heal the navel of newborn children, get rid of pimples and relieve the pain and itching of dermatitis, eczema and psoriasis. In some cases, such as with diaper rash, the powdered rhizome is just sprinkled into the hand and then rubbed on the baby's skin. In other instances, however, some turmeric is mixed with a little coconut oil and gently applied to more severe inflammations.

In India and China, a little powdered turmeric is mixed with the juice from half a squeezed lime and a little water to make a smooth, even paste, which then is put directly onto herpes lesions, leprosy sores, measles, mumps, chickenpox and so forth with excellent results. Several crushed zinc tablets (50 mg. each) may also be added if desired. The same paste works well for snakebites, insect stings, and ringworm, too.

Curing Ear and Eye Discharges

Among some Ayurvedic practitioners in India, it still is a common custom to use a piece of clean cloth soaked in turmeric solution for wiping away discharges of acute conjunctivitis and ophthalmia. And a little powdered turmeric is sometimes mixed with an equal amount of baking soda and then a tiny portion put into the outer ear to help dry up any fluid discharges.

Stops Bleeding During Pregnancy

According to the *Philippine Journal of Nursing* (50:95), a decoction of turmeric followed by 3 glasses of water is very helpful for alleviating any bleeding experienced during pregnancy. When combined with eggplant, it seems to be even more beneficial for this, and for healing wounds. Early pregnancy bleeding usually denotes threatened abortion and should, therefore, be taken quite seriously.

This remedy may be adapted for American households. In 1 pint of boiling water, simmer 1 cup of diced eggplant on low heat for 45 minutes, covered. Strain into another pan and add 1/2 tsp. of powdered turmeric. Cover again and steep until this liquid becomes lukewarm. Strain through several layers of gauze and drink 1 cup at that time. Repeat this process each day for as long as needed to stop bleeding.

Relieving Sprains, Fractures, and Arthritis

Turmeric has manifested remarkable anti-inflammatory properties by inhibiting induced edema and subacute arthritis in rats and mice. These positive results are comparable to the same effects achieved by popular anti-inflammatory drugs like hydrocortisone acetate and phenylbutazone. Two half teaspoonfuls taken morning and evening in juice can help somewhat.

Additional relief may be obtained for this disease, contusions, sprains and fractures by mixing together 2 tbsps. turmeric with 1 tbsp. lime juice and just enough boiling water to make a nice, smooth, warm paste. This can then be applied directly to the area of swelling and pain, and then covered with some plastic food wrap to retain the heat and moisture longer. The consistency of the paste should be similar to that of creamy peanut butter so that it can be spread on the skin easily.

Counteracts Liver Fat

Turmeric is good at lowering serum cholesterol levels and preventing fatty accumulations in and around the liver. Rats fed on diets containing 10% fat colored with turmeric showed virtually no fat buildup around the liver as did other rodents on the same diet but without the benefit of this spice. It works twice as well when combined with some cooked eggplant. Mix 3/4 tsp. turmeric with 2 tbsps. cooked, mashed eggplant and 1-1/2 tbsps. boiling water until smooth. This can then be spread on a piece of rye or whole wheat bread and eaten following a meal of fatty foods to protect the liver.

Turmeric appears to be of definite value in the treatment of certain forms of cancer. Not so much from a curative aspect as from arresting its further progress *if* it's taken in the early stages of cancer development. For instance, the *Journal of Ethnopharmacology* (7:95-109) for 1983 noted that several constituents in this spice have proven to be very active against cervical cancer, but *only in the early stages.*

These same active components (curcumol and curdione) displayed strong cytotoxic effects against Dalton's lymphoma cells in the beginning stages of development. This research was conducted in India, according to *Cancer Letters* (29: 197-202) for 1985. And *Nutrition & Cancer* for July-Sept. 1986 stated that powdered turmeric is able to prevent cell mutations from occurring when certain types of aggravating food are consumed. Scientists working at the Tata Memorial Cancer Research Institute in Bombay, India discovered that turmeric helps to offset the mutagenicity of hot chili peppers and related dietary mutagens. This seems to suggest that whenever anything this hot or spicy is consumed, some turmeric ought to be taken along with it as a good preventative measure.

Helpful in Diabetes

Dr. Richard Anderson, a researcher at the U.S. Department of Agriculture's Nutrition Research Center in Beltsville, Maryland started experimenting some time ago with several different spices to see what they might be good for besides just flavoring food. He noticed that extracts of turmeric, bay leaf, cloves and cinnamon tripled the performance of insulin in metabolizing blood glucose in the test tube. His next step was to synthesize the spices' active ingredients and dispense them to those with impaired glucose tolerance. To his amazement, they greatly enhanced the production of insulin by the pancreas. He attributed this astonishing activity to possible minute traces of chromium in each of these spices.

Ron Hamilton of Great American Natural Products in St. Petersburg, Florida, made a special product called Spice Caps based on the formulation that Dr. Anderson worked from: a pinch of cinnamon, a couple of cloves, half a bay leaf, and a teaspoon of turmeric. Although he has been very careful to never make any claims for them, those customers who've purchased these Spice Caps from his company reported back that their blood sugar levels all stabilized very nicely. And while those who are diabetics still need *some* insulin every day, they've reported having to use less than before. (See Product Appendix under Great American Natural Products to order Spice Caps.)

Inhibits Gas

In another Indian experiment, some rats were fed a particular diet intended to produce intestinal gas. But when turmeric was added later on, further gas production ceased altogether, due to the yellow-orange pigment present called curcumin. It's advisable to take 1/2 -1 tsp. of turmeric in a cup of warm water to help relieve heartburn and indigestion discomforts.

Increasing Shelf Life of Food

Recent studies from Japan have confirmed that spices can increase shelf life of oils and fats. Turmeric and ginger, among other spices, showed significant antioxidant activity when they were added to olive, soybean or sesame oils. Interesting applications of turmeric have been found in extending the refrigerated storage life of seafoods. Since turmeric is used popularly with most fish preparations, the effect of a dip treatment in turmeric, or turmeric with salt, each at 5% level for 15-30 minutes was studied by one group of scientists.

Control shrimp only had a shelf life of 13 days, developing black spots and fishy decomposition odor. But by dipping the shrimp in a turmeric plus salt dip solution, the shelf life increased another week. And when a combination of spice-salt dip plus irradiation was employed, shelf life increased to 42 days.

Colorful Dishes

Turmeric really adds color to otherwise dull-looking dishes. Plain rice can suddenly take on a nice golden hue when a dash of this spice is added in the final cooking process.

Making Your Own Curry Powder

Needed: 1 tbsp. ground coriander seeds; 1/2 tsp. ground mustard seeds; 1/2 tsp. ground cumin seeds; 1/2 tsp. ground turmeric; 1/4 tsp. ground ginger; 1/4 tsp. cayenne pepper. Combine all ingredients in a bowl and mix thoroughly. Transfer to an airtight jar and store in a cool place. Curry powder often accompanies fish, lamb, poultry, some salads, lentil soup, stews, and a number of other Far Eastern dishes.

Curries in Asia vary, but often contain onion, garlic, salt and usually a souring agent such as tamarind, lime, unripe mango or other sour fruit as well as other flavors derived from mustard, coconut, lemon grass and so forth. Using any of these with your curry powder will definitely accent the taste of any meal prepared.

U

UVA URSI
(ARCTOSTAPHYLOS UVA-URSI)

Brief Description

The leaves of bearberry or manzanita are leathery and plastic to the touch. The early Algonquian Indians enjoyed mixing the leaves with tobacco and having a good smoke. They called this interesting mixture "kinnikinnick." In Scandinavia the leaves have been used for tanning leather.

The flowers are either white, pink, or flesh-colored, each with five segments and formed like tiny narrow-mouthed urns, which eventually mature into small fruits with five seeds apiece.

The plant is a trailing vine and grows in thick carpets, depending on where it is. New growth in the spring can reach up to ten inches in height. The long trailing stems run just below ground level, usually in loose mulch.

Kidney Complaints Cured

Uva-ursi or manzanita is terrific for treating kidney problems. Nephritis (inflammation of the kidneys) and renal calculi (kidney stones) are overcome with a tea made from the berries and leaves of this plant. Cystitis (inflammation of the urinary bladder) and urethritis in women (inflammation of the urethra) have been successfully treated using the same tea. It is the astringency of the tannin acid on the berries and leaves that makes them work so well in such medical conditions.

It may be of interest to the reader to know that bearberry has been an official drug in the pharmacopoeias of Dublin, Ireland, Edinburgh,

Scotland, and London, England, as well as in the United States pharmacopoeia from 1820 to 1936, and the National Formulary from 1936 to 1950. Besides being recommended for the aforementioned kidney problems in some of these texts, it has also found favor in allaying the usual irritations that follow catheterization.

To make an all-purpose tea, bring a quart of water to a boil. Then add 3 tablespoons of dried, chopped berries and leaves. Reduce heat, cover, and simmer about 5 minutes. Turn off the stove and let the brew steep for a half hour. Strain one cup at a time and take when lukewarm on an empty stomach.

Bearberry Baths Useful for Female Problems

One of the most helpful recommendations I've given to many pregnant women over the years is for them to utilize a sitz bath made from bearberry tea immediately following childbirth. The tannins, including another compound called arbutin, act as mild vasoconstrictors to the endometrium of the uterus and reduce inflammation, infection, and further bleeding. This is only possible, though, if it is taken as a tea internally. However, a bearberry wash will eliminate inflammation on the perineum (the strip of tissue between the vagina and anus).

This is particularly useful if a woman has torn her perineum or had an episiotomy (surgical widening of the vagina).

Normally, a sitz bath is made by putting enough warm or hot herbal bath water in the tub so that it reaches your navel when you sit in it. The feet are propped up on a hassock set beside the tub. The body is wrapped from the neck down with large beach towels or blankets. About 4 inches of water are put into the bathtub, the knees are kept up and the water is splashed continually with the hand onto the abdomen. The person should remain in the tub for 30 minutes, then rinse with a short cold bath or shower.

However, a large oval-shaped enamel pan large enough for the average person to sit in will suffice in lieu of the tub. This space requires less liquid. The legs can hang over either side of the rim with the knees arched high. About three quarts of warm uva-ursi tea should suffice. An old cotton blanket or beach towel can be loosely draped over the person's midsection, while the individual washes the urogenital area with a cupped hand, while supporting the body upright with the other hand if necessary. Sitting with the back against a wall will help keep the upper torso erect while in this position.

Make the tea according to the instructions previously given. I should point out that this simple sitz bath arrangement will also go far in getting rid of hemorrhoids in the rectum. The buttock cheeks need to be firmly grasped by each hand and pulled apart in order for the tea to work this way. Hemorrhoids are quite common during pregnancy.

Cardiac Edema Helped

Cardiac edema means edema (fluid accumulation or swelling) of the limbs and other parts of the body due to congestive heart failure (CHF), not an accumulation of fluid around the heart per se. Pulmonary edema can occur, that is, excess water in the lungs, when CHF is bad. Decreased kidney function (actually a compensatory function due to the CHF) causes the edema but it does not cause the CHF. CHF results from a variety of health problems such as hypertension, mitral stenosis, and coronary artery disease. Dropsy is an old term formerly used to denote cardiac edema.

Rene Suscheaux lived in one of the parishes south of New Orleans. His diet was fairly typical of most native Louisianians: a lot of fatty meat, greasy foods, white bread, mashed potatoes and gravy, and pastries. Such meals he always consumed with gusto.

By the time he checked in with his physician to get a complete diagnosis of what was wrong, Rene was experiencing shortness of breath accompanied by an added sound every time he breathed. He had noticeable fluid accumulation in his hands and feet, engorged neck veins, and an enlarged liver that was very tender to surface skin touch.

Not happy with the drugs the doctor prescribed for his problems, Rene turned to a local Cajun folk healer who used herbs in her treatment program. She put him on a program of two cups of uva-ursi tea for the first two weeks and then two capsules of the powdered berries every day for the next six weeks. By that time his condition has improved enough to allow him to discontinue this natural medication.

Unfortunately, Rene didn't change his lifestyle habits and went back to his old ways of eating. He died several years later of congestive heart failure. But during the short time he took bearberry, he did feel a lot better.

Manzanita Cider for Allergies

"Manzanita" is the Spanish name given to bearberry. It means "little apple" and is quite apropos since the red berries do, indeed, look like miniature apples.

Here is an old recipe I got from an Hispanic curandera in Albuquerque some years ago. She washed approximately 4 cups of bearberries to remove accumulated debris. The berries were placed in a saucepan, covered with water, and gently simmered for about 20 minutes or until they were soft. She then drained them, reserving the liquid. The berries were mashed up a bit using a flat metal potato masher, but were not reduced to a pulp.

My friend then measured out the fruit and put it into a large mixing bowl. An equal amount of reserved liquid was added to the fruit. A cloth was put over the bowl and the mixture allowed to set for a day and a half until everything had properly settled. She then strained off the liquid and refrigerated it.

She mixed equal parts of this manzanita cider with orange or grape-fruit juice, added one tablespoon of apple cider vinegar, and gave it to those who came to her with allergy problems.

V

VALERIAN
(VALERIANA OFFICINALIS)

Brief Description

Common valerian is a perennial plant, about 2-4 feet high, which has escaped from cultivation to inhabit roadsides and thickets from New England south to New Jersey and west to Ohio. It is also very common all over Europe. The yellow-brown, tuberous rootstock produces a hollow, angular, furrowed stem with deeply dissected leaves each bearing 7-10 pairs of lance-shaped leaflets. The resulting smell of the dried, powdered rootstock is reminiscent of dirty socks or unwashed underwear.

Various constituents within the root account for the peculiar smell and the strong sedative properties. The butyl isovalerate present has been used in a synthetic, fermented egg product to attract coyotes and repel deer, while eremophilene has also been detected in ripe African mangoes. The valepotriates exert strong tranquilizing actions on the central nervous system.

Nature's Tranquilizer

Various Russian clinical journals indicate that valerian root has been successfully used throughout the Soviet Union for treating hysteria, high blood pressure, backache and occasional migraine headaches. Sometimes the tea, made by steeping 1-1/2 tbsps. of dried root in 1 pint of boiling water for 30 mins., was administered 1-2 cups daily. On other occasions, 2 tablets were prescribed twice or three times daily. The same amount also applies for taking capsules of this root.

458

How valerian root is able to do this is pretty amazing. A forty-year-old woman suffering from severe anxiety presented herself at the author's booth at the National Health Federation convention held in the Greater Pittsburgh ExpoMart in Monroeville, Pennsylvania in June, 1995. Eustace Mullens (a proponent of New World Order conspiracy theories) and I shared the exhibit. I was busily autographing copies of several of my health encyclopedias (*Healing Juices, Nuts, Berries and Seeds,* and *Fruits and Vegetables*) when she arrived.

She told me what she had been diagnosed with and then mentioned that she had been screened for below-normal levels of gamma-aminobutyric acid (GABA) in her blood serum. GABA is considered to be the major inhibitory neurotransmitter within the human central nervous system; it is found chiefly in the cerebral cortex, the thalamus gland, and many other regions of the brain. It is very necessary for glands controlled by the sympathetic nervous system (i.e., pancreas, duodenum and thymus). It also exerts a definite calming effect upon the nerves and, in greater concentrations, raises brain IQ.

I started her on 5 valerian root capsules daily—three in the morning on an empty stomach with a full glass of water and two in the evening around 7 pm. I told her to continue with this program for 3 weeks and then go back to her physician and have her blood tested again for GABA content. She did so and called me to report the results.

The doctor was surprised to see a marked increase in her blood GABA. He was even more surprised to see that she had gone off both the Valium and Antivan, which she had been taking faithfully prior to meeting me. She was remarkably calm and reported feeling more alert than before. The only side effect she noticed was some fatigue, probably brought on by an over-abundance of GABA production within her system.

I believe the valepotriates found in valerian root were directly responsible for the increase in her GABA output. (Consult *Planta Medica* 60:278-79, 1994 for more information on how valerian root influences the synthesis and transport of GABA in the brain and nervous system.)

VANILLA
(VANILLA PLANIFOLIA)

Brief Description

Liquid vanilla flavoring is obtained from the fully grown but unripe pods or beans found on large green-stemmed perennial herbaceous vines growing wild and extensively cultivated throughout the tropics (Mexico,

Malagasy Republic, Comoros Islands, Tahiti, Indonesia, Seychelles, Tanzania and Uganda, among others). Pollination is all done artificially, except in Mexico where it's performed partly artificially and partly by certain hummingbirds and butterflies not found anywhere else in the world. Because of the high price of vanilla and the low price of vanillin, vanilla extracts have been extensively adulterated. Vanillin is the major flavor component with over 150 other aroma chemicals present as well.

Sexual Stimulant

In various Central and South American countries such as Mexico, Argentina and Venezuela, an alcoholic extract of the dried pods is taken for increasing amorous desires. Generally 4-6 pods are steeped in 2 cups of tequila or imported cognac for 21 days in a well-stoppered flask or glass container of some kind. The bottle is shaken several times each day during this period of time. The tincture is then taken in doses of 10-20 drops 2-3 times a day, usually at night.

Calms Hysteria

Pure vanilla flavor fluid extract may be used to help calm hysteria and related emotional traumas. The best manner for successfully accomplishing this is to soak one or two cotton balls completely with the vanilla extract, lightly squeezing out any unnecessary excess fluid before placing them beneath the tongue, one on either side of that vertical fold which elevates the tongue as needed.

By so positioning each cotton ball, the vanilla can slowly penetrate the smallest of the salivary glands called the sublingual gland. The vanilla then travels through the tiny blood vessels which empty into the sublingual and submental arteries. These last two arteries, in turn, hook up directly with the much larger internal jugular vein and the external and internal carotid arteries.

Now the internal jugular vein and the internal carotid artery both supply blood directly to the brain, which suggests that this is the route by which vanilla travels in order to reach that part of the brain responsive to its calming effects in episodes of hysteria.

Tips on Using Whole Vanilla Beans

If you count yourself among the millions of people who love the sweet, richly fragrant aroma and comforting flavor of vanilla, you owe it to yourself to experience it straight from the bean.

Vanilla beans may be used over and over, and they're as easy to use as any spice. The essence of vanilla lies in thousands of tiny seeds found inside every bean. Actually the seeds look more like little specks, or superfine coffee grounds. They can be easily extracted from the whole bean.

To make your own intensely good vanilla extract (or a great gift), place six long beans, split open and cut into pieces into 1 quart of good quality vodka. Cap tightly and set in a cool, dark place. Leave for one month to six weeks, shaking the bottle occasionally. Before using, sieve through a strainer lined with cheesecloth (or use a coffee filter), rinse the bottle to remove residue, and pour the extract back into the bottle. Add one whole vanilla bean and cap tightly.

Here's how to slice a soft vanilla bean to extract the seeds: using a small, sharp paring knife or a one-sided razor blade, make a small cut down one side of the bean, about 3/4 inch from the tip. Place your index finger on the tip of the bean and slip the knife point into the small incision. Slowly slice the bean open lengthwise, cutting away from the direction of the finger holding the bean steady. Open the bean, laying the sides flat to the cutting surface and carefully scrape out the seeds with a teaspoon or knife blade.

Whole vanilla beans (left intact) are generally used for infusions. This means that when steeped in a liquid, such as warm milk or cream, the delicate flavor of the vanilla bean works a subtle magic as it permeates the liquid.

Try steeping a vanilla bean in your hot cocoa or coffee for four to five minutes for a light flavor. Or, leave it for about 20 minutes in egg custards to be used for pastry cream or ice cream. After steeping, the beans can be rinsed, well-dried, wrapped in plastic and refrigerated in an airtight container. This bean is good as long as the aroma is full and rich.

To make a delicately flavored, perfumed oil for cooking and to use as a salad oil, split a vanilla bean open and place it in a pint of good quality oil. Within a week, the oil will be flavored. Leave the bean in the oil and replenish your supply by adding oil to the container as needed. For more handy tips, consult *The Vanilla Cookbook* by Patricia Rain (Berkeley, CA: Celestial Arts, 1986).

W

WALNUT
(JUGLANS NIGRA, J. REGIA)

Brief Description

There are about fifteen different species of walnuts growing throughout the world. They are indigenous to eastern Asia, southeastern Europe, and North and South America. All walnuts are edible. However, the Persian or English walnut is probably the most delicious and certainly the most important.

Walnuts are oval-shaped, green, leathery, aromatic, and occur in groups of one to three. The hull encloses the familiar tan-colored fruit; the smooth, large nuts of the Persian walnut separate easily from the hulls at maturity. In the cultivated varieties, the shells are thin and easily broken. The kernel consists of two identical lobes, united at the apex; the ivory-colored nut meat is protected by a thin, light-brown testa. The hulls fall away from the shells more readily in the Persian or English walnut than in the black walnut. The kernel of the former is likewise easier to withdraw from the shell intact than that of the black walnut, which has a somewhat denser endocarp. The inner shell of the black walnut is more difficult to crack without damaging the kernels, so they are usually sold already shelled.

Effective Treatment for Diarrhea, Sore Throat, and Ringworm

In 1980 I had occasion to visit mainland China with the American Medical Students' Association (part of the larger A.M.A.). I had a chance to visit Hohhot (pronounced Hu-He-Hot), the capital of Inner Mongolia. There I learned from several local doctors some interesting applications for walnut.

462

Green walnut husks were routinely gathered and then boiled in enough water to cover them to a depth of about 2 inches for 1 1/4 hours or until half the liquid remained (no lid was put on the pot in which they were cooked). This bitter-tasting brew was strained and stored in corked jugs until ready to be used.

Some of the liquid would be heated to lukewarm and given to a patient in one-cup amounts twice daily on an empty stomach to stop diarrhea. One-half cup of the same lukewarm liquid was prescribed as an effective gargle for sore throats and tonsillitis with very good success. And poultices steeped in some of the cold juice and put on areas of the skin afflicted with ringworm would soon clear up that problem; powdered walnut bark was also liberally sprinkled over the area for the same purpose.

Runny Nose and Head Cold Cleared Up

A popular remedy in parts of Germany for many decades has been a tea made from walnut leaves to help dry up continual sinus discharges in young children and adults. Two tablespoons of walnut leaves are added to boiling water, stirred, covered, and removed from the heat and allowed to steep for 30 minutes. One-half cup of the lukewarm tea, strained, is given to young children every 4 hours to help stop a runny nose. One cup of the warm leaf tea every 3 hours is suitable for adults with head colds.

Acne, Eczema, and Psoriasis Benefitted

The same tea makes an excellent wash for a variety of skin afflictions. Some German teenagers suffering from bad cases of acne vulgaris who have been treated by their grandmothers or mothers with this remedy on a regular basis have regained clear complexions in time. They also drank the tea internally.

Older people who have been troubled with eczema and psoriasis reported considerable relief after washing their afflicted body parts with this same tea several times a day. The tea not only relieves the itching and inflammation, but actually helps to heal the skin, too. Sometimes, burdock root is added for greater effect; in such cases, one tablespoonful of coarsely chopped, dried root is simmered for 10 minutes before the walnut leaves are added and the mixture steeped for 40 minutes. The tea can also be taken internally.

Walnuts Head Off Heart Disease by Reducing Serum Cholesterol

In the summer of 1992 researchers at Loma Linda (California) University Medical School reported epidemiological data suggesting that Seventh Day

Adventists who rarely eat nuts suffer heart attacks and coronary deaths at roughly twice the rate of those who typically eat nuts five times a week. Then, in the spring of the following year, these same researchers came up with the reason for this. By comparing the results of two four-week-long dietary intervention trials in 18 men, they found that eating moderate amounts of walnuts, without increasing total dietary fat and calories, "decreases serum-cholesterol levels and favorably modifies the lipoprotein profile in healthy men."

Both experimental diets derived 30 percent of their calories from fat— a level recommended by the American Heart Association and 14 percent lower than the typical American diet, which contains a whopping 35 percent fat. Writing in the March 4, 1993 *New England Journal of Medicine*, Joan Sabate and her co-workers reported that substituting walnuts for two-thirds of the fat in such a relatively low-fat diet further lowers cholesterol concentrations in the blood by more than 10 percent.

Since the walnut diet contained roughly three times the ratio of polyunsaturated to saturated fat found in the other low-fat diet, some drop in cholesterol was expected anyway, said David Kritchevsky of the Wistar Institute in Philadelphia. But what no one anticipated, he noted, was the magnitude of the walnut's cholesterol-lowering and heart-saving effect.

WATERCRESS
(NASTURTIUM OFFICINALE)

Brief Description

Watercress is a perennial plant which thrives in clear, cold water and is found in ditches and streams everywhere. It's cultivated for its leaves, which are principally used as salad greens or garnishes. Connected to a creeping rootstock, the hollow, branching stem, 1-2 feet in length, generally extends with its leaves above the water. The smooth, somewhat fleshy, dark green leaves are odd-pinnate with 1-4 pairs of small, oblong or roundish leaflets.

Healing Mouth Sores

One of the most popular remedies among Chinese residing in Hong Kong and Canton, China is a special watercress soup used to treat canker sores on the tongue or lips, blisters in the mouth, swollen gums, bad teeth and foul breath. There are no specific amounts called for, but generally for one person, about 1/2 lb. each of cut watercress and chopped carrots are cooked in 2 qts. of water. The liquid is boiled down slowly to 1/3 or 1/4 of the original fluid volume and then the soup is consumed with the vegetables intact. It's also good for hot flashes when consumed cold.

Relieves Headaches

Watercress forms the basis of an excellent remedy for headaches brought on by some kind of sickness or general nervousness. A handful of watercress, having been first washed thoroughly, is put into a clean quart fruit jar and 2 cups of boiling apple cider vinegar added. After the solution becomes cold several hours later, it is strained and rebottled for use later on. When the headache occurs, a clean handkerchief or wash cloth should be dipped in the vinegar, wrung out and laid over the eyebrows and forehead.

Soothes Skin Ailments

An old and effective cure for eczema and dermatitis consisted of an infusion of watercress. A large panful should be thoroughly washed and put into a stainless steel saucepan that has just enough cold water added to cover the cress. Bring this to a boil, then reduce heat and simmer slowly until the watercress is quite tender. Strain through muslin cloth or several layers of gauze material and refrigerate.

The afflicted part should be bathed often with this infusion. It's better to use a piece of soft linen for this purpose. This infusion is excellent for roughness of the skin due to frequent exposure to the wind, sun and cold weather.

Diuretic and Expectorant

Watercress tea or juice is valuable for eliminating accumulated fluids in body tissue, such as in gout, and for clearing mucus congestion from the lungs. To make the tea steep 1 tbsp. chopped fresh cress in 1 cup boiling water for 20 minutes, then strain and drink. Fresh juice can be easily obtained from an electric juicer, but should be combined with some carrot or tomato juice before drinking.

WATERCRESS SOUP

Needed: 1 qt. chicken stock; 1 tbsp. honey; 1/2 tbsp. blackstrap molasses; pinch of kelp; 1 bunch watercress; water to cover stems; pinch of cardamom.

Heat stock and season with honey, molasses, kelp and cardamom. Before untying the bunch of purchased watercress, cut off stems. Wash stems and boil for about 10 minutes. Drain and add the cooking water to the stock. Cooked stems by themselves can be eaten when seasoned with a little tamari soy sauce.

Wash tops of watercress (flowers) and add to boiling stock just before serving. Boil soup 3 minutes, no longer, as you don't want to lose the emerald green color. Be sure to cook uncovered after you add the watercress or it will darken. Yields 4 cups.

WATERCRESS DIP

Needed: 3 cups watercress, stems removed; 1/2 cup small basil leaves; 1 tbsp. liquid Kyolic garlic (available from any health food store); 2 tbsps. extra-virgin olive oil; 1/2 cup parmesan cheese, grated; 3/4 cup Pet evaporated milk (or an equivalent brand); 1/4 cup walnuts, finely ground; 2 green onions, finely minced; and granulated kelp (a seaweed from any health food store) for flavor.

In a Vita-Mix whole food machine or similar blender, combine the watercress, basil, liquid Kyolic aged garlic extract, olive oil and parmesan cheese. Process until somewhat pasty. Then add the milk and pulse only until mixed; be careful to *not* overmix. Transfer the mixture to a bowl and stir in the walnuts and green onions. Add kelp for flavor. Dip will automatically thicken as it stands. Yield: Makes 1-1/2 cups.

NOTE: The fat content of this glorious dip is one-half that of standard commercial dips!

WAX MYRTLE
(see BAYBERRY)

WHEAT GRASS
(Triticum aestivum)

Brief Description

Wheat grass and barley grass look similar to the grass on your lawn or on a golf course, when they are young. They are leafy and of a deep green color. Starting at the University of Wisconsin in the mid 1930s and continuing on to the present time, considerable research has been done to prove the highly nutritive and healing properties of wheat and barley grass juices in tablet, powder, and water soluble extract forms.

There are essentially two types of wheat grass. The better one is the red winter wheat planted in the fall, grown for about 200 days through the winter in the Great Plains of North America, and finally harvested in the spring just prior to the "jointing" stage when the nutrients reach their fullest peak. The other kind is a grass-like plant sprouted at home from wheat grain. This plant is green and very sweet, but nutritionally inferior to the first. This indoor, tray-grown wheat grass only takes about five days to a week to get ready. The simple sugars produced in the shoots by photosynthesis are never converted to the complex nutrients found in the leaves of the young wheat plant grown in the soil in cold weather. As a result, this inferior wheat grass has a strong sweet taste; drinking even small amounts of this stuff straight can make first-time users sick to their stomachs. Tray-grown wheat grass may be all right for salads and sandwiches, but it definitely is no match for soil-grown winter wheat grass.

A Health Regeneration Food

Considerable space could be devoted to all of the wonderful things which wheat grass can do for the body. The list of diseases which respond very favorably to wheat grass would fill a couple of pages here. Basically, many problems ranging from acne to cancer, from dermatitis to lupus, from measles to ulcers, and from wounds to zits, can often be helped by including wheat or barley grass in the diet often.

My own experience with such cereal grasses has proven to me that they are of tremendous benefit in *regenerating* the system. A little common logic shows us how this can be possible. Frequent consumption of cooked and refined foods leaves the body feeling listless, tired, dull and dead. What it needs is some *live* nourishment that can refreshen and reinvigorate it. This is where wheat and barley grass come into play.

Because I spend an enormous amount of my time in my research center writing or studying, or in a classroom somewhere lecturing, I don't always get a chance to eat the way I'd like to. Instead I have to content myself with food that is, quite literally, cooked to death and not very nutritious. As a result, in time my body starts to feel sluggish.

So to give me some quick energy and "fire up" the system again, I will put some wheat and barley grass back into my system. I'm particularly fond of using Kyo-Green, a very nice powdered blend mix of different chlorophylls from Wakunauga of America (makers of Kyolic aged garlic extract). I add 1-1/2 heaping tablespoonfuls of this green powder to one full glass of water or tomato juice, stir and drink. Talk about a quick "pick-me-up." Is it ever good! It makes me feel as if new life has been breathed into my being again. And I'm *not* exaggerating when I say this either.

Now chlorophyll is to plants what blood is to us. It is the life-sustaining force for all things within the plant kingdom. Without it, trees, plants, flowers and grasses, as we know them, would turn an ugly brown and soon die. Imagine, though, if some of this life-giving "plant blood" is infused into the human system and comingles with some of our own blood. I mean, there is *no better* "transfusion from nature" than this stuff. It literally brings our near lifeless bodies back from the brink of oblivion to almost full activity again.

One word of caution, though, when using wheat grass powder on a regular basis. Some brands other than Kyo-Green are so heavily concentrated that they sometimes have a tendency to aggravate existing allergies. I know this for a fact! There was a brief period not too long ago when I was using another brand of chlorophyll powder and experienced a mixed reaction to it. On the one hand, I did have a lot more energy, but on the other, I started developing breathing problems almost symptomatic of asthma. So I quickly discontinued using this high-potency stuff and switched back to Kyo-Green; the symptoms quickly disappeared and my breathing returned to normal.

If there are two health food supplements that I recommend you take on a regular basis, they would have to be Kyo-Green (1 glass) and Kyolic garlic (3 capsules) every day. Along with this, add one level tablespoonful of Pines' organic beet root juice powder to your emerald green chlorophyll drink. With that take one tablespoon of Rex's Wheat Germ Oil every morning before breakfast.(See Product Appendix for more details.)

WHITE OAK
(QUERCUS ALBA)

Brief Description

The oaks as a genus (Quercus) consist of many species of deciduous and evergreen trees and shrubs and are the most important aggregation of hardwoods found on the North American continent, if not in the entire Northern Hemisphere.

The oaks are widely distributed and extend from Canada on the north southward to the mountains of Colombia in South America, and to the Indian Archipelago in the Eastern Hemisphere. There are 70 species native to the U.S. and about 58 of these reach tree size. There also are about 70 recognized hybrids.

The uses of oak include almost everything the human race has ever derived from trees: timber, food for people and animals, fuel, watershed protection, shade and beauty, tannin and extractive, and corks. Consequently, the oaks are widely planted for many purposes.

White oak can grow anywhere from 60 to 150 feet tall, and reach a trunk circumference of nearly 8-1/2 feet. White oak bark is pale gray, and the leaves have rounded or finger-shaped lobes. The fruit it bears is a kind of nut called an acorn and matures in one year.

Great Hemostatic

An infusion of white oak bark makes a wonderful hemostatic for hemorrhoids, excessive menstruation, blood urine, and internal hemorrhaging. In 1-1/2 pints boiling water, simmer 2 tbsps. white oak bark, covered, for 15 minutes on low heat. Set aside and steep for 30 minutes. Strain and drink 3 cups daily. Can also be used either as a douche or enema for any of the above problems.

A Cure for Stinky Feet

Many younger people suffer from sweaty feet, the smell of which is strong enough to knock the nostrils and brain for a loop! But early Native Americans had a sure cure for this and for smelly armpits and groins. They boiled handsful of crushed, green acorns in plenty of water until half of the original liquid remained. This they managed to strain off and preserve in crude containers. Smelly feet were routinely soaked in some of this green-acorn water each day until the problem cleared up. Other body parts were regularly washed with this same acorn water with good results.

Stops Diarrhea Quickly

An old Indian cure for diarrhea calls for 4 crushed acorns to be boiled in 1 quart of water on low heat for about 40 minutes, then strained. When cool, 1 cup of the tea is consumed. Within a matter of minutes even the worst case of diarrhea is known to stop, on account of the powerful astringency of the tannic acid present in the tea.

WHITE WILLOW

(see WILLOW)

WILD BLACK CHERRY
(PRUNUS SEROTINA)

Brief Description

Wild black cherry grows from Nova Scotia to Florida and as far west as the Dakotas, Utah and Arizona. It towers high at roughly 100 feet or so and has a trunk circumference somewhere between 4 and 5 feet. The trunk is covered with rough, black bark.

Cough Suppressant and Appetite Stimulant

Zeb Coltrin lives in the backwoods of Tennessee. Every so often we correspond with each other, albeit on a very elemental level due to his lack of education.

   In one of his occasional letters, he shared with me for the very first time his family's "secret remedy" for allaying the worst kind of hacking cough and also for stimulating the most depressed appetite. "Fill a likker jug [quart bottle] hav fool [1/2 full] 'o [wild black cherry] bark, and then pore [pour] sum gud [some good] moonshine [brandy or whiskey] inta thuh rist 'o et [into the rest of it]. Set in a dark plaz [place] for a weak [week], shakin' et evry day [shaking it every day]. Thin strane and put in 'nother likker jug, an' cork gud [then strain and put in another quart bottle and seal good]." For suppressing a hacking cough, he suggested putting 15-20 drops in one-half cup warm water and drinking slowly; for perking up the appetite, he mentioned taking 2 tablespoons before every meal.

   CAUTION: Wild black cherry contains a cyanonide compound called amygdalin (laetrile), which yields hydrocyanic acid on hydrolysis. Therefore, *never* use wilted leaves and *never boil* the bark (only steep it in hot water). And *do not* refrigerate the tea longer than 24 hours!

WILD MEXICAN YAM
(DIOSCOREA VILLOSA)

Brief Description

Wild yam is a climbing, stout-stemmed, non-hairy vine with white-fleshed branched tubers that are brown and corrugated on the outside. They resemble part of a skeleton and, because of this, once were called "devil's bones." These twisted roots grow up to 5 feet in length and can get 1-1/2 feet thick, sometimes reaching upwards of 12 lbs. The leaves are alternate, heart-shaped and somewhat leathery.

Wild yam is no relation to the delicious yams served at Thanksgiving or Christmas dinners. This perennial vine grows mainly in the central and southern parts of North America.

Proven Relief for Rheumatism

Wild yam was once widely used by slaves throughout the Deep South and the West Indies for rheumatism. An interesting historical note about how they came to discover its benefits was written up by W. Wright in a lengthy contribution entitled "An Account of the Medical Plants Growing in Jamaica" for the *London Medical Journal* (3(3):217-95) in 1787. He stated that "runaway negroes who absconded from the plantations" and found themselves having to make the best of things in the wild, often developed rheumatism as a result of having to sleep out a lot in damp conditions.

Out of necessity, "some of the early runaway Negroes started looking for relief for their body pains," and soon discovered that wild yam root was just the thing to help ease their terrible joint and muscle inflammations. Scientists now know that all species of wild yam carry varying amounts of a steroid-like material known as diosgenin, which has been shown experimentally to inhibit inflammation in laboratory animals. Up to 3 capsules or 25 drops of fluid extract twice daily can be taken for this problem.

Other Benefits

Penny Belding of Las Vegas, Nevada wrote me sometime ago that she had been taking wild yam supplements each day to help control her aging and weight, and as a prevention against cancer and heart attack. She noted that some of her wrinkles had disappeared after taking three capsules daily or 20 drops of the fluid extract for 2-1/2 months. Also she claimed her weight had stabilized: "I haven't lost any, but neither have I gained any more since I've been on this program of yam root."

Very few health stores or herb shops will carry this particular herbal product. But you can easily obtain it from one of two sources: call Enzymatic Therapy at (1-800) 783-2286 or Strength Systems USA at (1-800) 722-FIRM and ask them for information on their wild Mexican yam extracts.

WILD OREGON GRAPE
(BERBERIS VULGARIS OR MAHONIA AQUIFOLIUM)

Brief Description

This is an evergreen shrub found in mountain areas on wooded slopes below 7,000 feet from British Columbia to Utah, southward to Oregon and California. Although native to North America, it was introduced to Europe as a cultivated plant and has become naturalized. Its irregular, knotted rootstock has a brownish bark with yellow wood underneath. This yellow pigment is the antibiotic alkaloid, berberine—the same constituent found in goldenseal root. Its branched stems have 10 or more spiny, sessile leaflets adorning them. (NOTE: See GOLDENSEAL for more data on berberine.)

Inhibits Spinal Meningitis

One pharmaceutical study published a decade and a half ago demonstrated that berberine was even more potent against that species of bacteria (*Neisseria meningitidis*) which causes meningitis in the spine and brain than the antibiotic drug, chloramphenicol. Berberine also kills on contact a species of staph which infects stitches and other skin wounds, as well as *E.coli* and other infectious bacteria. Two to three capsules daily on an empty stomach is recommended. Or 1 cup of tea made by simmering 2 tbsps. of the rootstock in 1 pint of water for 7 minutes, then steeping for another 25 minutes, before straining and drinking. Infected wounds and herpes lesions can also be either dusted with the powder from some empty capsules or else frequently bathed with the tea.

Counteracts Scorpion Stings and Snakebites

The Ramah Navajo of northern Arizona use a strong solution of wild Oregon grape rootstock tea internally and compresses externally on the immediate site of injury to counteract the deadly effects of poisonous scorpion stings and deadly rattlesnake bites. The same tea has also been given immediately on an empty or evacuated stomach to those who've been bitten by a rabid animal or bat in 1-cup amounts 5-6 times daily until cured.

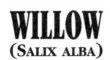

WILLOW
(Salix alba)

Brief Description

The willows consist of about 300 species of deciduous trees and shrubs widely distributed in both hemispheres from the Arctic region to South Africa and southern Chile. There are numerous hybrids. Of the some 70 North American species, some 30 attain tree size and form.

The tree grows up to 80 feet in height, but in some parts of the world may only reach 5 or 7 feet tall as a mere shrub! Its alternate, lanceolate, serrate leaves are ashy-gray in color and silky on both sides. Male and female flowers occur on separate trees, appearing in catkins on leafy stalks at the same time as the leaves do.

Tonsillitis, Sores, and Stinky Feet

Here's a simple method for making a decoction of white willow bark that will prove to be a very beneficial remedy for sore gums, tonsillitis, festering sores, open wounds, serious burns, and sweaty feet. Soak 5 tbsps. white willow bark in 5 cups cold water for 7 hours, or overnight. The next morning bring the contents to a slow, rolling boil. Cover, set aside, and steep until cool. Strain and refrigerate until needed.

> SORE GUMS: Soak 1 or 2 cotton balls in a little of the decoction, squeeze out excess liquid, and rub gums with them.
>
> TONSILLITIS: Gargle with 1/4 cup of cool tea every 1-1/2 hours.
>
> FESTERING SORES: Soak a few cotton balls in tea and then wash festering sores with them every few hours. Also a square strip of clean, white layered gauze can be soaked in the tea, the excess liquid squeezed out and then taped over the sores; change the dressing every few hours.
>
> WOUNDS: Same procedures as for sores.
>
> BURNS: Soak the burned area in a sufficient amount of the cool white willow bark tea; *loosely* apply layered gauze strips which have been previously soaked in the tea.
>
> SWEATY FEET: Soak the feet in cool tea every morning and evening for about 15 minutes. Be sure to wash in between the toes with some of the tea each time you do this.

First Aid for Medication Poisoning, Diarrhea, and Intestinal Distress

Activated charcoal powder, made from kiln-burned white willow logs, has long been recommended as an efficient antidote for prescription and over-the-counter drug poisonings, diarrhea, gas, heartburn and other general gastrointestinal distress. Stir one tablespoonful of charcoal powder, one teaspoonful of powdered ginger root, and 1/2 teaspoon white sugar in one large glass distilled water and drink. Repeat as necessary. To order this, write to:

> ACTIVATED CHARCOAL
> Reverend Tom Kopco
> P.O. Box 741551
> Orange City, FL 32774
> (904) 789-8198

WINTERGREEN
(GAULTHERIA PROCUMBENS)

Brief Description

The genus *Gaultheria* consists of about 100 species mostly native to Asia, Australia and South America, with 6 species found in North America. Salal has a distinctly woody stem, while creeping snowberry and wintergreen berry (also called checkerberry) are semi-shrubs. All three attain their best development in moist, acid soils. They provide cover and food for wildlife. The leaves of wintergreen contain an important oil (oil of wintergreen), which is extracted for pharmaceutical use. When the shiny, waxy, evergreen leaves are crushed and the winter-clinging little red berries are tasted, they give off a familiar wintergreen aroma.

The small trailing perennial creeps through and under the woodland humus, moss, and ground, thrusting up separate blooming and leafing clusters. The frosty flowers appear like chaste white miniature bells, with their unions of five petals, growing between stems and leaves about summertime, maturing into solid red fruits in fall and winter, each with a distinctive pucker on top. The leaves, which become leathery and ruddy with age, have tiny teeth, each with bristle-like tips.

Aspirin Alternative for Fever, Sore Throat, and Headache

Aspirin has been described as an "all-purpose" medicine, because tens of millions of people take it for a variety of general physical complaints. But aspirin is synthetic and not always good for the body, although its primary ingredient, acetylsalicylic acid, was originally synthesized from the true salicylic acid found in wintergreen berries and leaves. In fact, it was the Bayer Company in 1899 that first coined the term "aspirin" from the combination of "a" for "acetyl" and the original generic name *Spiraea* = spirin, from which salicylic acid was first isolated. [Salicylic acid was first observed in the flowerbuds of *Filipendula* (Spirae) *ulmaria* or Eurasian queen-of-the-meadow in 1839.]

A preferred alternative to this much overused medication would be wintergreen berries and leaves. Tea is the recommended form in which they are to be applied. A conservative way of making this tea is to immerse a tablespoonful of the chopped berries and a teaspoonful of the dried, cut leaves in one pint of boiling water. Stir, remove from heat, cover, and let steep for an hour.

Depending on what you're taking it for determines the temperature of the tea. For fevers, drink the tea *warm* on an empty stomach, in half-cup amounts every few hours. For a sore throat, gargle with some of the *cool* tea before swallowing every few hours. For any kind of headache, drink a cup twice daily when the tea is *cold*. But to apply compresses of the tea across the forehead to relieve throbbing pain and pressure, the tea should be somewhat *hot*.

WITCH HAZEL
(HAMAMELIS VIRGINIANA)

Brief Description

Witch hazel is a deciduous twisted shrub or small tree which prefers damp soil to grow in. It has gray-brown bark and grows to about 15 feet in height. The buds occur in clusters at the bases of the leaves. The flowers appear only from September to November and have petals resembling twisted yellow straps; they open after the leaves have fallen from the branches. The leaves are lopsided at the base, with shallow-toothed edges.

Witch hazel blooms in the fall, once its seeds have matured in capsules. At the same time that the flowers appear, the capsules split open, shooting the seeds as far as 20 feet from the plant. Its late flowering and explosive bursting of seed are commemorated in its other common names, winterbloom and snapping hazel.

Tincture of Witch Hazel

Witch hazel is a common drugstore item and is sold in the form of a liquid tincture. It is inexpensive, safe and reliable. Tincture of witch hazel may be used externally for relieving the following conditions: skin irritations, sunburn, insect bites and stings, bruises, abrasions, poison ivy/oak rash, diaper rash, eczema and bedsores. Either soak a cotton ball with some of the liquid and apply that way, or else put on the skin directly with a spray-on bottle applicator.

A tea can be made by adding 1/2 tablespoon each of the bark and leaves to one pint boiling water; cover, set aside and steep 45 minutes. Gargle with some of this tea for relieving a sore throat or drink 2 cups for stopping diarrhea. The tea can also be used as a vaginal douche for vaginitis.

WOOD BETONY
(STACHYS OFFICINALIS)

Brief Description

Wood betony is a perennial herb common to meadows, hilly slopes and forests. The plant's stem is hairy, unbranched or slightly branched, quadrangular, and reaches a height of 6 inches to two feet. The leaves of wood betony are somewhat hairy on both sides, opposite, with the top leaves lanceolate and the bottom ones more oblong-cordate in shape. The red-purple flowers are in bloom through the summer months of June, July and August.

Allergy, Headache, Hypertension

Wood betony was once a very popular remedy with many old-time herbalists, but now has been relegated to flavoring herb teas. A tea made of the stem, leaves and flowers was formerly used in the treatment of stomach problems, gout, intestinal worms, edema, kidney dysfunction, and bladder problems.

Currently it is included in the herbal formulas manufactured by some direct marketing companies that are intended for alleviating allergies and headaches and normalizing elevated blood pressure. About 3 capsules on an empty stomach with a glass of water is recommended for these problems.

A tea is even better for these disorders. Boil a pint of water; add 2 tablespoonfuls of dried leaves; stir, cover, and set aside to steep for 40 minutes. Strain and reheat enough for one cup until it is lukewarm. Drink two cups daily in between meals.

WORMWOOD
(ARTEMISIA ABSINTHIUM)

Brief Description

Wormwood is a shrubby perennial herb with grayish-white stems covered with fine silky hairs, and growing from 1-3 feet tall. The leaves are silky, hairy and glandular with small resinous particles and yellowish-green in color. The plant emits an aromatic odor and yields a spicy, somewhat bitter taste. It's native to Europe, northern Africa and western Asia, but now extensively cultivated.

Parts used are the leaves and flowering tops (fresh and dried), harvested just before or during flowering. Wormwood has been used in the manufacture of vermouth. Sweet wormwood, another species (*A. annua*), is often grown as an ornamental, but contains an essential oil that has strong antifungal and antibacterial activities.

Overpowering Relief for Pain

The team of Simon, Chadwick and Craker in their *Herbs—An Indexed Bibliography* (1971-1980) mentions that "wormwood has been used as a pain reliever for women during labor and against tumors and cancers." An alcoholic tincture of the same applied externally often has a profound effect in relieving the soreness of aching muscles, the hurt accompanying swollen, arthritic joints, and the terrific pain felt with a bad sprain, dislocated shoulder/knee or fractured bone.

The following episode was related by the eldest son of the Mormon prophet, Joseph Smith, Jr. The prophet's son was a teenager residing in Nauvoo, Illinois at the time he had this experience with wormwood.

> Our carriage had stopped by the roadside for lunch and to rest the horses. Upon getting back into my seat after the brief interval, I thought-

lessly put my hand around one of the carriage posts, and as the driver closed the door, two of my fingers were pretty badly crushed.

The wounds bled freely and Mother (Emma Smith) bound them up with some cloths from her bag, and we traveled on. My fingers became very painful, and after awhile we stopped at a farmhouse. Mother unwrapped them, soaking the temporary dressing off with warm water and rewrapped them with fresh cloths. Taking from her trunk a little bottle of whiskey and wormwood, she turned the tips of my fingers upward, and poured the liquid upon them, into the dressings —at which, for the first time in my life I promptly fainted! It seemed as if she had poured the strong medicine directly upon my heart, so sharply it stung and so quick was its circulatory effect.

When I returned to consciousness I was lying on a lounge against the wall and Mother was bathing my face most solicitously. I soon recovered and we proceeded on our journey, reaching home in good time and without further mishap.

To make an effective tincture for relieving excruciating pain, combine 1-1/2 cups of finely cut herb or else 8 tbsps. of the powdered herb in 2 cups of Jim Beam whiskey. Shake the jar daily, allowing the wormwood to extract for 11 days. Let the herbs settle and then pour off the tincture, straining out the powder through a fine cloth or paper coffee filter. Rebottle and seal with a tight lid until needed. Store in a cool, dry place. When using this tincture to relieve external pain, remember that because of its *strong potency* a little bit goes a long way! Wormwood oil used externally can relieve pain, too.

Destroys Intestinal Parasites

The wisdom of the ancients often holds up under modern scientific testing. A case in point has to do with a certain passage written in the *Zhou Hou Bei Ji Fang* (*A Handbook of Prescriptions for Emergencies*) by an herbalist named Ge Hong who lived to be 110 years old (231-341 A.D.): "Take a handful of sweet wormwood, soak it in a Sheng (about 1 liter) of water, squeeze out the juice and drink it all for malaria."

Now a researcher from the Institute of Chinese Materia Medica of the China Academy of Traditional Chinese Medicine, who has been perusing ancient medical texts in search of new antimalarial drugs, decided to find out if soaking this wormwood had been done to avoid the loss of antimalarial properties by boiling or brewing it instead. She and her colleagues not only proved this to be a fact, but also were able to actually test the herb on humans afflicted with the malaria parasites. The clinical results turned out to be very good.

Just recently chemists from the Division of Experimental Therapeutics, part of the Walter Reed Army Institute of Research in Washington DC, have begun to conduct their own lengthy investigations into sweet wormwood's ability to reduce fevers by killing intestinal parasites causing them.

The previously mentioned tincture may be used here for internal purposes. Using an eye-dropper, put 10 drops of tincture in with 1 tsp. of dark honey or blackstrap molasses. Mix well before eating. The honey or molasses helps to alleviate the bitter taste of the tincture.

Insect Repellant

Crush a handful of fresh wormwood leaves into a soggy pulp, then mix in with some apple cider vinegar. Next put a small amount of this wet mixture in a 6-inch square piece of gauze. Draw up the end corners together and tie at the top. Then rub the skin thoroughly with this to keep horse-flies, mosquitoes and gnats away from you while outdoors. The same mixture can also be rubbed directly onto household pets to keep flies, fleas and ticks away from them.

Remedy for Jaundice and Hepatitis

A study published in a recent issue of *Planta Medica* (37:81-85) points out that species of wormwood have been employed on a clinical basis for the treatment of hepatitis and to protect the liver from lesions produced by the ingestion of harmful chemicals. Another journal (*Chem. Pharm. Bulletin* 31:352) noted that wormwood is an important remedy for treatment of jaundice and inflammation of the gallbladder (cholecystitis). A tea might prove useful in these instances. Bring 2 cups of water to a boil. Remove from the heat and add 4 tsp. leaves or tops. Cover and steep until slightly lukewarm. Drink in 1/2-cup amounts morning, noon and night on an empty stomach. Sweeten with a little pure maple syrup to allay some of the bitterness. Or take 2 capsules of the powder twice daily for these problems, but on an intermittent basis. Remember that *wormwood is an herbal drug*, as are goldenseal root, chaparral and some of the other medicinal herbs cited in this text. And *they should be used with care only when needed*, and not taken indiscriminately.

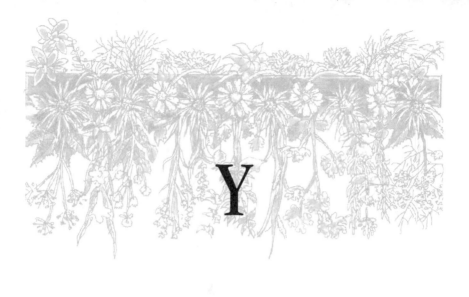

YARROW
(ACHILLEA MILLEFOLIUM)

Brief Description

Yarrow is a perennial herb found the world over in waste places, fields, pastures, meadows and along railroad embankments and highways where it should never be picked on account of the chemical spraying that's routinely done to keep the weeds down. The simple stem bears aromatic bipinnately parted and dissected leaves, giving a lacy appearance. The plant can grow up to a yard high, yielding pretty flower heads with white rays and yellow (turning to brown) disks in them. The light brown, creeping rootstock produces a round, smooth, pithy stem that branches near the top.

Extremely Useful for Inflammation

One of the most remarkable studies I've ever run across concerns yarrow's great ability to reduce tissue and joint inflammation in everything from wounds and edema to gout and arthritis.

The report which appeared in the August 1969 *Journal of Pharmaceutical Sciences* explained in clear detail that a number of closely-related protein-carbohydrate complexes, or glycoproteins, within the yarrow plant usually accumulate at the site of inflammation and remain there while injured tissue is being repaired. In one experiment a number of Swiss-Webster female mice were injected with a substance designed to induce swelling in their left foot pads. Later half of the group was injected with yarrow fractions, which reduced inflammation by 35% as compared with the untreated group.

Dennis Carman, who works for the Correlation Dept. of the LDS Church in Salt Lake City, related the following true incident to me sometime back:

About 12 years ago, myself and some other adults took a number of 'problem youth' from various Mormon wards on a weekend camping trip in a remote part of Yellowstone Park. One teenage boy happened to be scouring a nearby meadow for some dead firewood. In the process of pulling back on a dry limb jutting up from a fallen tree, he accidentally fell against another protruding piece of sharp wood, causing it to go into the side of his leg quite a ways.

We realized soon enough while attending to his injuries just how ill-prepared for this trip in terms of adequate first aid needs we really were. One adult picked a handful of yarrow and crushed it between two stones, then applied this poultice directly to the kid's wound. It was then bound up with adhesive tape. A couple of days later we were able to get the youngster to a hospital, where a doctor looked at his leg. In his opinion, nothing seemed wrong with the leg and so he released the boy immediately. We attributed this remarkable healing to yarrow.

Yarrow for Female Needs

Maria Treben, a renowned West German folk healer and popular herbalist, recounted for the benefit of a large audience her own experiences with yarrow some time ago:

I cannot recommend yarrow enough for women. They could be spared many troubles if they just took yarrow tea from time to time! Be it a young girl with irregular menstruation or an older woman during menopause or already past it, for everyone young and old, it is of importance to drink a cup of yarrow tea from time to time. It is very beneficial for the reproductive organs of women.

To make the tea, pour 4-1/2 cups of boiling water over 1-1/2 heaping tbsps. of yarrow, cover and steep for a while. The tea should be taken regularly. Or 100 grams (about 2 cups) of yarrow may be steeped in cold water overnight. The next day bring it to a boil, then add to just enough bath water in which the body can recline to soak the area of the kidneys.

Glaucoma Cured

Maria Treben insists that glaucoma is not an eye disorder, but rather a definite malfunction of the kidneys instead. A tea should be made, she observes, from equal parts of stinging nettle, yarrow, calendula, and horse-tail, and 2-3 cups consumed each day. Bring 1 qt. of water to a boil, add these herbs, cover and simmer for 7 minutes; then remove and steep anoth-er 45 minutes. Strain and sweeten with honey before drinking.

YELLOW DOCK
(RUMEX CRISPUS)

Brief Description

Yellow dock is a perennial plant considered by some to be a troublesome weed in many fields and waste places throughout Europe, the U.S. and southern Canada. Its spindle-shaped, yellow taproot sends up a smooth, rather slender stem, 1-3 feet high. Lanceolate to oblong-lanceolate in shape, the pointed light green leaves have predominantly wavy margins. The lower leaves are larger and longer-petioled than the upper. The numerous pale green, drooping flowers are loosely whorled in panicled racemes. The seed is a pointed, three-angled and heart-shaped kind of nut.

The Ultimate Purifier

What more can be said about this wonderful herb that hasn't been stated already with other cleansing herbs scattered throughout this book? Suffice it to say, this remarkable herb root is a dandy blood purifier for just about any kind of eruptive disease that may come to mind.

To make a useful decoction, just bring 1 qt. of water to a boil. Reduce the heat and add 1 cup of chopped, fresh or dried root, cover and simmer for 12 minutes. Remove and steep 1-1/2 more hours. Strain, sweeten with honey and drink up to 4 cups a day, especially during a *short*-weekend, *mild*-food fast in which much of your nourishment is derived only from liq-uids.

Many different kinds of skin afflictions may also be judiciously bathed with this same tea, when it's cool, to relieve some of the itching and inflam-mation. Equal parts of this root and sage make a great tea to drink while using a sauna or sitting in a jacuzzi (those with hypertension, however, should avoid excess heat like this).

A cup of warm tea improves digestion when consuming a particular-ly heavy meal or rich foods. Yellow dock tea also stimulates the liver and colon as well.

Comforts Emphysema

Yellow dock syrup is a good remedy for relieving upper respiratory problems such as emphysema. A half-pound of the root is boiled in a pint of *distilled* water until the liquid is reduced to a mere cupful. Strain and discard the spent root, and to the liquid add 1/2 cup dark honey, 1/2 cup blackstrap molasses and 1 tbsp. pure maple syrup, then a dash of genuine vanilla flavor. Mix everything together by hand until you have an even syrup. Take 1 tsp. at a time for bronchitis, asthma and the like to stop tickling sensations in the throat or lungs.

Strengthens Eyes in Night Blindness

The late plant forager, Euell Gibbons, asserted that " yellow dock greens are richer in vitamin A than carrots are." He believed that by eating many helpings of these greens, one could definitely improve his or her night vision, particularly if it had become somewhat dim with age.

Gibbons' Greens

Gibbons stated that the best time for collecting dock greens was either in the early spring or the late winter just after the first or second frost. A real treat for him was to combine equal parts of fresh dock greens and watercress in a little water and cook for about 15 minutes. Then the greens were drained, chopped and seasoned with kelp, butter, minced raw Bermuda onion, some crumbled crisp bacon, thin slices of a hard-cooked egg and a dash of lime juice (something I've added for good measure).

"This will make a hearty supper dish that I would enjoy for taste alone," he once confessed, "even if it weren't fairly bulging with all those healthful vitamins and minerals. A little apple cider vinegar, he believed, also adds zest to dock greens.

Because dock is a large plant and grows in great patches, one gathering can furnish many meals. Cook dock alone or mix it with other spring greens. It doesn't cook down much, so it's particularly good for canning—just follow standard directions for canning greens. It also freezes well. Enclose it, after blanching in boiling water for a couple of minutes, in plastic bags, then wrap it again in freezer paper to keep it from turning dark in your freezer later on.

YOHIMBINE
(CORYNANTHE YOHIMBE)

Brief Description

Yohimbine is the popularized name of a real tongue-twisting chemical known officially as 17 alpha-hydroxyyohimban-16 alpha-carboxylic acid methylester. Yet it has clinically verified aphrodisiac effects and is obtained from the bark of an African evergreen by the same name and growing in Cameroon, West Africa.

Ultimate Sexual Rejuvenators

During a 1984 stopover visit I made in Singapore on my way to Indonesia, I had the good fortune to be introduced to an old Chinese herb doctor by the name of Hsu Ching-tso. Through an acquaintance who spoke both languages fairly well, I was able to obtain a very old sexual rejuvenating formula which had been in this man's family for at least 17 generations.

What had attracted me to this old gentleman was the wide number of claims I had heard from many others (especially men) concerning the amazing effectiveness of his simple formula. I learned that his only three ingredients were yohimbine bark, dried schizandra berries, and ginkgo leaves and seeds.

Now I already knew about the medical success of yohimbine as reported in the August, 1984 issue of *Science.* Therein scientists from Stanford University discovered to their astonishment that when impotent male rats were given yohimbine, they went absolutely wild and mounted female rodents up to 45 times in less than 15 minutes—about twice as often as they normally would. Even when castrated rats were given a shot of the stuff, they climbed longingly on females.

And I also was aware of the in-depth study on yohimbine published in Volume 35 of *Pharmacological Reviews* concerning its fantastic erection-promoting ability when sexual desires were present in men, but when their penile veins weren't up to much contracting.

So the old fellow's inclusion of one-third yohimbine bark in his powerful sexual stimulant obviously made sense. I also knew about the warm, sexual energies attributed to schizandra berries by ancient Chinese herbalists. But I couldn't for the life of me figure out why he included one-third ginkgo leaves and seeds along with his other one-third schizandra fruit. He explained to me that gingo helped to increase the vital "life energies" passing through the brain. He said it wasn't enough to lift a man's copulating organ —holding up a drooping, bony finger that quickly became firm and elevated as he spoke—but it was also necessary to raise his *mental* powers of sex as well. This, he believed, is what ginkgo essentially accomplished with the mind, while the other two ingredients worked on the reproductive organs themselves.

He made and sold this concoction in tablet form, instructing those who purchased it to take 6-8 tablets at a time at least 30 minutes before sexual activities commenced. In recommending this same formula to different men here in the States who were unable to buy it directly from him, I soon found that an alcoholic tincture of the yohimbine worked better than when taken in capsule form with the other two ingredients.

Mix 1-1/2 tablespoons of powdered yohimbine bark with one pint brandy. Shake daily and let set for about two weeks. Strain through layered gauze and pour into bottle with eye-dropper cap. Put 14 drops beneath the tongue every day. Follow this by taking two capsules each of schizandra fruit and ginkgo biloba with a glass of water. All of these herbs are readily available at most health food stores or herb shops, or can be obtained through the mail (see Product Appendix).

Obesity Modified

One study a few years ago demonstrated that yohimbine may be of some value in treating overweight. Obese subjects were put on a low-calorie diet (1,000 calories per day) and also given a supplement of yohimbine (5 milligram capsules taken 4 times a day). The test patients were instructed to take the herb capsules 1-1/2 hours before eating. Yohimbine worked better in reducing overall weight than did a placebo. The herb did this by increasing the process of thermogenesis, which helps to chemically "burn up" accumulated fat.

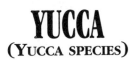

YUCCA
(YUCCA SPECIES)

Brief Description

This acclaimed "Guardian of the Desert" stands silently silhouetted against an azure-blue sky, its many sharp, lance-like leaves assuming a defensive position of sorts against all manner of unwanted intruders. And as in the imagination of the naturalist's mind, so too does this ubiquitous plant perform similar service when it comes to protecting our health. Yuccas can be either tall trees ranging in heights from 15 to 60 feet as it were (Mojave yucca and the Joshua tree), or much humbler-looking specimens averaging no more than a couple of yards in height.

Potential Cancer Remedy

A team of scientists working at the AMC Cancer Research Center and Hospital in Lakewood, Colorado several years ago isolated a strong anti-tumor factor from *fresh* yucca flowers, which disappears when the flower wilts or dries. In mice with B16 melanoma, a crude extract of yucca flowers caused a 50-100% increase in their lifespan, as mentioned in *Growth* (42:213-23) for 1978.

Similar findings were also confirmed by Dr. Kanematsu Sugiura of the prestigious Sloan-Kettering Cancer Research Institute in New York City. There the partially purified extract of yucca flowers inhibited almost completely both sarcoma 180 and Ehrlich carcinoma. Also Dr. Jonathan l. Hartwell, formerly with the Cancer Chemotherapy National Service Center, reported in the scientific press that extracts of certain yucca flowers *strongly* inhibited Lewis lung mouse tumor and the Friend virus leukemia in mice by some 70%. This data appeared in a back issue (1968) of Oncology (22:57), a well-respected cancer research journal.

What all of this means then to those of us interested in finding natural solutions to the problems of cancer is that the fresh blossoms or flowers of different yucca species may be picked and *immediately* be included in a carrot-mixed greens juice concoction whipped up in a food blender. Not that yucca alone will do the job, but it's merely another good weapon in the natural arsenal to be used in combating this dreaded disease.

Arthritis Under Attack

During the mid-1970s Drs. Bernard A. Bellew and Robert Bingham conducted studies with 101 arthritic patients, giving half yucca tablets and the other half lookalike placebos. Of the 50 receiving an average of 4 yucca tablets daily, 61% reported feeling less pain, stiffness and swelling in their arthritis than did those on the placebo. These tests were conducted at the National Arthritis Medical Clinic in Desert Hot Springs, California, and later published in *Journal of Applied Nutrition* (Fall 1975). Four capsules of yucca from any local health food store twice daily on an empty stomach is suggested.

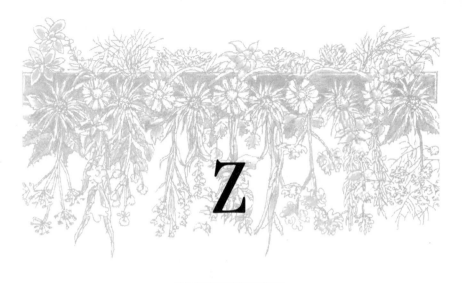

ZEDOARY
(Curcuma zedoaria)

Brief Description

Zedoary is common to the wet forests and humid jungles of the Eastern Himalayas and may be found in northeastern India, Sri Lanka, and China. The plant is propagated by tubers, which are cut into small pieces bearing buds and then planted in raked soil at the beginning of the monsoon season. Zedoary looks a lot like turmeric plant in appearance; the roots of both are valuable in food as well as in medicine.

Zedoary grows to a height of about 1-1/2 feet and bears green leaves with brownish-purple veins somewhat resembling the bulging varicose veins on the legs of older, heavy-set women. The rhizomes are large and fleshy. They are cut into thin transverse sections and dried. I've been through some of the Indian bazaars in the cities of Bombay and Calcutta in times past and have immediately detected the very agreeable musky odor with a hint of camphor that is emitted by these dried slices of buff gray zedoary root. Once or twice I've nibbled some of the root out of curiosity and discovered that the flavor is quite pungent and a tad on the bitter side.

Gets Rid of Sticky Taste in the Mouth

Ever eat something so sweet that it left a sticky taste in your mouth for a while? Occasionally, an illness of some type may also produce the same effect. Chewing a tiny piece of zedoary root and thoroughly mixing it with some saliva will quickly get rid of any unpleasant sticky taste.

Amish "Bitters" for Liver and Digestive Problems

Amos Yoder is an old Amish folk healer I've known for years. He is recognized by many of the old-order Amish and Mennonite groups (those who don't use electricity or drive cars or trucks) as a first-rate "herb doctor." He formulated an interesting "bitters tonic" of his own based on the famous "Swedish bitters" of Europe. One of the principal ingredients is zedoary root, of course, along with aloes, rhubarb, gentian, anise, camphor, manna, angelica, senna, carline thistle, myrrh, ginger, galangal, goldenseal and saffron. All of these herbs are in an alcohol and sorbitol base.

Old Amish Herbs of St. Petersburg, Florida (see Product Appendix) markets this fine product for him. He routinely recommends it for sluggish liver, mild constipation, stomach problems of all kinds, and gall bladder attacks. He claims it's also useful for treating cuts, sprains and varicose veins. He suggests taking one tablespoonful first thing in the morning upon getting up and the same amount again at night last thing before going to bed. Some of the liquid can be applied for external purposes using cotton balls, gauze pad, or put directly on the skin if you wish.

"It's good for what ails ya'!" he bragged one time, while stroking his foot-long white beard. After I had cocked my head to one side and rolled my eyes around in my head in mock disbelief, he reassured me: "Johnny Boy! I'm not yanking your beard on this one." Fine thing for him to say, since I've *never* had a beard to begin with!

> And so you've reached the end at last
> With all your reading in the past;
> The time we've spent, both you and I,
> Somehow wonderfully did fly
> In the pursuit of fact and lore
> To guard your health forevermore!
>> John Heinerman
>> July 12, 1995
>> Salt Lake City, UT

To Contact the Author of this Book:

John Heinerman, Ph.D.
Director
Anthropological Research Center
P.O. Box 11471
Salt Lake City, UT 84147
(801)-521-8824 before 8am MST

PRODUCT APPENDIX

There are obviously a number of companies which carry herbs and spices for medicinal and culinary uses. However, in my many years of working with plants I've found just a few that I consider to be reputable enough to place my confidence in. Therefore, the following companies come highly recommended by me, and will be able to supply you with any of the herbs, spices, or flowers (in dried and prepared forms) mentioned in this book. You can trust the integrity of their products for sure!

Great American Natural Products, Inc.
4121 - 16th Street North
St. Petersburg, FL 33703
(813) -521-4372

Old Amish Herbs
4141 Iris St. North
St. Petersburg, FL 33703

(Old-order Amish *don't* have telephones or fax machines; it's against their religious beliefs!)

Pines International, Inc.
P.O. Box 1107
Lawrence, KS 66044
(913)-841-6016

You would just order organic beet root juice and rhubarb juice powder from them.

Vita-Mix Corporation
8615 Usher Road
Cleveland, OH 44138
(1-800) -848-2649

It makes the best whole food/ herb machine in America. Its unit in indispensable when using *fresh* herbs or spices for medicinal or culinary purposes.

Southern Utah Herb Co.
P.O.Box 160
Tropic, UT 84776

Wakunauga of America Co., Ltd.
23501 Madero
Mission Viejo, CA 92691
(714) - 855-2776

This company manufactures and distributes the world's premier selling and best researched garlic—Kyolic Garlic. It also makes a superior ginkgo biloba product called Ginkolic. In addition, this company also markets one of the finest wheat grass/ barley grass powdered juice drinks in America; it is called Kyo-Green. All of these fine products are readily available at most health food stores, nutrition centers and herb shops. Of the many different forms of Kyolic available, I personally like Kyolic EPA and liquid Kyolic Aged Garlic Extract the best. I alternate between the two on a regular basis to keep my serum cholesterol and triglycerides down and my heart in good shape. I use Ginkolic to keep my blood circulation in good shape and regularly drink Kyo-Green to carry me through a busy day with lots of energy and stamina!

INDEX

490